The Clinician's Guide to Ethical Non-Monogamous Relationships

This book is a comprehensive guide designed to help mental health professionals understand and meet the unique needs of individuals in ethical non-monogamous relationships.

Drawing on a wealth of research, case studies, and expert insights, Dr. Stephanie Sigler offers invaluable guidance on fostering healthy communication, managing jealousy and insecurities, and addressing the emotional dynamics that arise in non-monogamous relationships. With a compassionate and inclusive approach, this book helps mental health practitioners develop a deep understanding of diverse relationship structures. This book covers topics such as polyamory, open relationships, and swinging, addressing the specific needs and concerns of clients engaged in these relationships. It also encourages discussions of self-care for practitioners, ethical considerations, and addressing stigma within the therapeutic process. Sigler provides clinicians with step-by-step strategies and interventions mental health practitioners can implement in their sessions.

An invaluable resource for practitioners new to ethical non-monogamy, this book is equally essential for therapists looking to expand their knowledge and skills and can help practitioners provide meaningful support to clients in this often misunderstood and underrepresented community.

Stephanie Sigler, PhD, is a licensed professional counselor, certified sex therapist, and clinical sexologist with expertise in alternative relationships and sexual health. She is a professional member of ASSECT and an affiliate of the National Coalition for Sexual Freedom.

The Clinician's Guide to Ethical Non-Monogamous Relationships

Working with Clients with Alternative Lifestyles

Stephanie Sigler

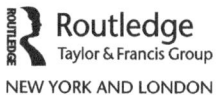
Routledge
Taylor & Francis Group

NEW YORK AND LONDON

Designed cover image: ©Getty

First published 2025
by Routledge
605 Third Avenue, New York, NY 10158

and by Routledge
4 Park Square, Milton Park, Abingdon, Oxon, OX14 4RN

Routledge is an imprint of the Taylor & Francis Group, an informa business

© 2025 Stephanie Sigler

ISBN: 978-1-032-72981-7 (hbk)
ISBN: 978-1-032-72978-7 (pbk)
ISBN: 978-1-003-46489-1 (ebk)

DOI: 10.4324/9781003464891

Typeset in Times New Roman
by MPS Limited, Dehradun

This project is dedicated to those who aspire to be better humans, treating others with the respect they deserve, regardless of their love interests or preferences. It is also dedicated to those who wholeheartedly love and accept me as I am, embracing my dramatic and passionate nature.

~ Dramatically Yours!

Contents

Acknowledgments

I am incredibly grateful to the individuals who have helped me bring this volume to life. I would like to express my sincere appreciation to Joe Kort for agreeing to be my committee chair and for his enthusiasm about my project which helped me to realize its potential. I am also grateful to Dr. Laurie Betito, whose inspiration and encouragement helped me to keep going, even when the going got tough. Dr. Stacy Friedman offered me invaluable wisdom and guidance, which gave me the confidence to complete this project.

To my daughter Kadence, your unwavering support and presence throughout this project bolstered me during many long nights of research. I want you to always remember that you are enough, even when you feel that you're not doing enough. To Adrianna, I cannot express how thankful I am for your arrival in my life, and for being there for me when I needed you most. Liz, your unwavering encouragement, support, and positive attitude helped me through uncertain times. Boots, your no-nonsense attitude and kind words of support pushed me toward the finish line. I am blessed to have each of you in my life.

To my fellow Lifestyle community members, this volume is a product of our collective experiences and love. We have all sought help with our intimate relationships, but too often have been dismissed or told that monogamy is the only solution. Your stories and support are why I have invested in educating therapists, counselors, and coaches about working with our community. You are seen, loved, and appreciated.

Preface

I believe everything in my past has led me to create this project. I have always wanted to explore various subjects and experiences throughout my educational journey. This curiosity is reflected in my academic choices. After completing my Associate degree in Business Administration, I took a leap of faith and moved to New York City to pursue film school. While at film school, I had a transformative experience with one of my instructors, who helped me discover my passion for teaching. This revelation prompted me to return to Texas and earn my Bachelor's degree in Education Theater.

After graduation, I embarked on a fulfilling career as a theater teacher in public schools, dedicating eight years of my life to nurturing young minds through the power of performance. However, toward the end of my teaching career, I felt a strong therapeutic call-to-action. This desire stemmed from my own traumatic childhood experiences and the burning need to understand and help others who have gone through similar challenges. This led me to become a Licensed Professional Counselor (LPC).

While becoming an LPC, I encountered a partner who introduced me to alternative love dynamics. As someone who grew up in a conservative environment in East Texas, I carried a great deal of religious guilt and shame surrounding sex. These beliefs severely limited my understanding and experience in this domain. However, upon discovering the lifestyle community, I immediately found an immense sense of belonging and acceptance. The beauty of this new world fascinated me and opened up a new path for growth and exploration.

The idea for this book was sparked when I began exploring the world of ethical non-monogamy (ENM). As word got out that I was an LPC specializing in couples, people started sharing their troubling therapeutic experiences with me. These individuals opened up about counselors who shamed their choices, pressured them to return to monogamy, or attempted to impose their religious ideologies upon them. These stories left me appalled and ignited a passion for sex therapy within me. In response to these revelations, I began my journey to become a Clinical Sexologist.

My education to become an LPC provided minimal attention to sex therapy, with only one course dedicated to human sexuality. Realizing that I was ill-prepared to work with individuals and couples seeking sex therapy, I delved into researching sex therapy certification programs. I embarked on the path to becoming a clinical sexologist. As I expanded my knowledge and comfort in sex therapy, I gradually opened my practice to couples in alternative relationships, evolving into the practical and talented certified sex therapist I am today.

The outline for this book emerged over time through extensive work with clients in alternative relationships, extensive research into limited literature on best practices for these couples, interviews with pioneers in the ENM field, and my journey in ENM with my partner at the time. Entering the world of alternative relationships can be complex and challenging. It defies societal norms and pushes boundaries you may have never known existed. However, it also opens up incredible opportunities for self-exploration, new desires, and mind-blowing experiences. Through trial and error, the steps for helping couples navigate the ENM lifestyle gradually took shape, forming a program that has allowed me to educate and support more individuals and couples than I ever imagined possible.

One aspect of this book that I am particularly proud of is the inclusion of treatment plans. Currently, no pre-written treatment plans are available specifically tailored to supporting individuals and couples in ENM relationships. By providing readers with this resource, I hope to offer a template for their therapeutic notes, removing the guesswork and empowering them to support their clients effectively. By including handouts, worksheets, and treatment plans, readers can effortlessly incorporate this book into their practices, ultimately ensuring that more couples receive the support they need.

Drawing from my journey in ENM, I use my experiences to guide and empower others in discovering their own paths. This book is a valuable resource for anyone seeking to work with individuals and couples in ENM or for current practitioners looking to enhance their knowledge and improve their therapeutic skills. Let us embrace the beauty and complexity of the ENM world, making it a safe and transformative space for all.

Introduction

Welcome to the world of Ethical Non-Monogamy (ENM)! This book is here to help you expand your therapeutic skills, practice, and appreciation of ENM. Ethical non-monogamy (ENM) is growing in popularity, and it is becoming more common to come across individuals or couples who may seek therapeutic services to address their ENM relationship dynamics.

The initial part of this book aims to provide therapists new to ENM with essential knowledge. It will explore into the origins of ENM, explore the motives behind people choosing ENM relationships, discuss different relationship dynamics, and address potential biases that may impact the therapeutic relationship. This section aims to equip therapists with the necessary tools to effectively work with the ENM population and ensure successful outcomes.

The second part of this book is designed to serve as a comprehensive and detailed guide for therapists who are supporting couples at the beginning of their ENM journey. It is structured in a step-by-step manner, providing therapists with a clear progression of activities, treatment plans, and homework assignments that are specifically tailored to ensure successful outcomes for their clients.

This part of the book offers critical insights into the complexities that arise when navigating multiple relationships as both an ENM community member and a therapist specializing in ENM. It strives to provide therapists with the necessary tools and knowledge to effectively address the unique challenges and dynamics associated with ENM. With a lesson plan format, the second part of the book offers detailed explanations on how to utilize each resource effectively. However, it is crucial for clinicians to recognize that the usage and implementation of these tools may vary depending on the specific circumstances of their clients. Therefore, it is essential for therapists to adapt and customize these resources as needed, tailoring them to suit the preferences and unique needs of their individual clients.

This flexibility allows therapists to modify the format and style of the resources according to their own preferences and the specific requirements

DOI: 10.4324/9781003464891-1

of their clients. By doing so, therapists can effectively support couples as they navigate the complexities of ENM and work towards building healthy and fulfilling relationships.

When utilizing these resources in therapy, it is essential to follow up with clients to gather feedback on the impact of the assignment on their emotional, mental, and physical well-being. This will help identify which tools are practical and which need further modification.

In conclusion, this book is an essential resource for therapists new to ENM as it helps them understand the benefits, challenges, and uniqueness of ENM relationships. We hope this book will provide invaluable insights and a comprehensive view of assisting individuals and couples navigate the complex and beautiful world of ENM.

Part 1

Understanding ENM

Chapter 1

Foundational Knowledge

Foundational Knowledge

Congratulations on taking the first step toward expanding your therapeutic skills, practice, and appreciation of ethical non-monogamy (ENM). According to a recent study in *Frontiers in Psychology*, ENM is a reality for one in nine Americans, with one in six Americans expressing a desire to explore ENM (Moors et al., 2021). Even prominent figures like Liliana Bakhtiari, a Georgia lawmaker, have openly identified as non-monogamous, underscoring the growing recognition and acceptance of ENM (Mayer, 2022).

In the first part of this book, we will lay the foundation of knowledge for therapists new to ENM. By reading and completing the exercises, you will gain a deeper understanding of ENM, its origins, why individuals choose to engage in ENM relationships, the various relationship dynamics involved, and how to address potential biases that could impact therapeutic relationships. While this book cannot cover every aspect of ENM, it aims to equip therapists with the tools they need to succeed when working with the ENM population.

Part 2 of this book is a detailed, step-by-step guide on how to assist couples as they embark on their ENM journey. This part offers practical activities to be conducted in therapy sessions, suggestions for documenting treatment plans, and homework assignments to ensure the best possible outcomes. As a member of the ENM community and a therapist specializing in ENM, this book offers a comprehensive view of the beautiful world of loving multiple partners.

Welcome to a new chapter in your therapeutic practice—prepare to embrace the wonders of ENM!

What Is ENM?

Moors et al. (2021) defined ethical non-monogamous relationships as "the consenting agreements to engage in varying degrees of romance and sex with more than one partner."

DOI: 10.4324/9781003464891-3

According to the Merriam-Webster dictionary, "ethical" is defined as (*Ethic Definition & Meaning*, n.d.):

1 Of or relating to ethics
2 Involving or expressing moral approval or disapproval
3 Conforming to accepted standards of conduct

According to the Merriam-Webster dictionary, "consensual" is defined as (*Consensual Definition & Meaning*, n.d.):

• Existing or made by mutual consent without an act of writing
• Involving or based on mutual consent

Based on these definitions, all parties involved agree to participate (or not participate) in simultaneous romantic and/or sexual relationships. The keyword for this relationship dynamic is "consent," which sets ENM apart from infidelity or cheating.

Designer relationships are built on equality and mutual respect rather than possessiveness. In this context, having multiple partners is not considered cheating. In traditional monogamous relationships, one person is seen as the property of the other, which is a more outdated viewpoint. In designer relationships, both parties willingly uphold values such as open communication, emotional support, and honoring agreements (Michaels & Johnson, 2015).

Because relationship dynamics vary, practitioners must avoid biases and preconceived notions when working with ENM individuals. It is crucial to ask ENM individuals what their relationship dynamics look like. Some common forms of ENM are open relationships, swinging relationships, and polyamorous relationships. We will take an in-depth look at each dynamic of ENM in Chapter 2.

ENM Requires Honesty

Honesty is a foundational aspect that is crucial in fostering successful ENM relationships. It is vital to ensure that all willing participants are heard, understood, and respected, regardless of the specific dynamics within the relationship.

It is important to note that honesty does not imply perfection. In the context of ENM, it refers to a commitment toward open and transparent communication, where individuals involved are aware of one another, and there is no deliberate withholding of information or keeping secrets.

By embracing honesty, individuals in ENM relationships create an environment of trust and authenticity. Openness allows for open dialogue, sharing desires and boundaries, and fostering a deep sense of mutual understanding. Honesty cultivates an atmosphere where partners can speak their truth without fear of judgment or rejection, laying the foundation for healthy and fulfilling connections.

Furthermore, honesty plays a vital role in managing expectations and ensuring that all individuals clearly understand the respective boundaries and agreements within the relationship. It allows for ongoing negotiation and consent.

ENM Exists on a Spectrum

ENM is a broad term that encompasses various forms of consensual non-monogamous relationships, including polyamory, open relationships, swinging, and other related practices. ENM exists on a spectrum, with different individuals and couples placing themselves at various points along this spectrum.

The concept of sexual orientation complexity clarifies the spectrum of ENM. The Kinsey Scale, developed by Dr. Alfred Kinsey, Wardell Pomeroy, and Clyde Martin in 1948, illustrates this concept. Their research uncovered that sexual behavior, thoughts, and feelings toward the same or opposite sex could vary over time and that bisexuality encompasses various attraction patterns.

The Kinsey Scale allows individuals to self-report their sexual orientation on a continuum ranging from 0 (exclusively heterosexual) to 6 (exclusively homosexual), reflecting their lifestyle preferences and attitudes toward sexuality. While the Kinsey Scale has limitations in capturing the full complexities of contemporary sexual and gender orientations, it remains a valuable tool in understanding and portraying the diversity of sexual expression and desire.

Similarly, ENM relationships exist on a continuum, with some individuals and couples practicing strict monogamy while others engage in more fluid, open structures. For instance, individuals who describe themselves as "monogamish" may engage in occasional sexual encounters outside their primary relationships while still maintaining strong emotional bonds with their partners. Polyamorous relationships, in contrast, involve multiple committed partners with equal emotional investments and some degree of interconnectivity.

While labels may not be necessary for everyone, to many marginalized individuals, there is comfort in finding a community of like-minded individuals who are knowledgeable and sympathetic to their trials and tribulations. Each couple, throuple, or pod that a therapist works with will have its terminology and may have developed its definitions of its own. It is vital for the success of the therapeutic relationship that the therapist fully understands what labels and language mean specifically to the clients they

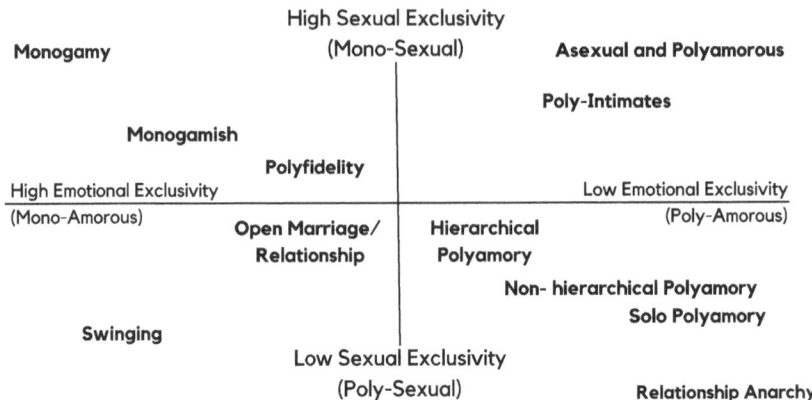

Fern, J. (2020). Polysecure: Attachment, Trauma and Consensual Nonmonogamy. Thorntree Press, LLC.

Figure 1.1 The Different Types of Non-Monogamy.

Source: Adapted from *Polysecure* by Jessica Fern (2020).

are working with when establishing the framework for each member's expectations and roles within the dynamic.

The author of *Polysecure* (2020), Jessica Fern, explains that each style of ENM and/or relationship dynamic "will have different degrees of openness to sexual and/or emotional engagement with others" (Fern, 2020, p. 109) as indicated in the double spectrum later.

Where Did ENM Begin?

Managing multiple ethical sexual and loving relationships is not new; however, it is not widely accepted. While the exact origins are not fully understood due to the secrecy of those in ethically non-monogamous relationships, we do know that the consensus agrees that in the United States, swinging has roots beginning during the Roaring Twenties with "petting parties" (Blakemore, 2017).

Terry Gould, the author of *The Lifestyle: A Look at the Erotic Rites of Swingers*, reported that modern swinging or "wife-swapping" stems from U.S. Air Force fighter pilots during World War II (2010). The pilots formed close bonds by sexually sharing their spouses to feel more relative to each other. Gould posited that this practice took place before deployment to ensure that widows would be emotionally and sexually cared for if their husbands did not return from their missions (Gould, 2010). Toward the Korean War's end, media reports that swinging had spread from the military and extended into the American suburbs.

According to Dr. Elisabeth Sheff, a certified sex educator and expert on polyamorous families, ENM and polyamory in the United States can be categorized into different "waves" spanning the nineteenth to the twenty-first centuries (Sheff, 2022). Sheff identified the first wave as Nineteenth-Century Transcendentalism and cited the example of John Humphrey Noyes, who founded the Oneida community in 1848. Noyes introduced a "complex marriage" system in which every male and female community member was considered married, viewing everyone else as a brother or sister (Muncy, 1973, p. 160).

The rejection of monogamous marriage aimed to provide an alternative to the exclusive and selfish nature of such relationships, which went against the ideals of communism (Muncy, 1973, p. 168). Likewise, children lived together in a communal children's house. Parents were not allowed to favor their children but were required to treat all children in the community equally.

In Dr. Elisabeth Sheff's classification, the second wave of ENM and polyamory in the United States is called Twentieth-Century Countercultures (Sheff, 2012). This period, specifically the 1960s and 1970s, witnessed the emergence and evolution of polyamory as a direct outcome of the sexual revolution. It became intertwined with other alternative forms of sexuality previously discussed, particularly the bisexual and free love movements. However, the history of the polyamorous movement does have points of contention.

During this second wave, communes experienced a revival and became a focal point. These communes aimed to forge chosen families, emphasizing intimate relationships. They emphasized spiritual growth cooperation over competition and actively rebelled against societal norms. The era also saw an interest in group marriage and partner swapping. Researchers such as Constantine and Constantine (1974, p. 49) delved into the exploration of "sexual alternatives in marriage," including the concept of "multilateral marriages," where three or more partners were considered married or committed to one another similarly.

In the third wave, Dr. Elisabeth Sheff's classification, known as the Impact of the Internet, the polyamorous community experienced a transformative shift due to the advent of the World Wide Web (Sheff, 2022). The Internet served as a super highway for sexual non-conformists, providing a platform for individuals to connect and form personal and sexual relationships online (Bargh & McKenna, 2004). The impact of the Internet on the polyamorous community cannot be overstated.

The online realm became a crucial hub for the polyamorous community, enabling various activities such as online dating, discussions on managing jealousy, and seeking advice on navigating the intricacies of polyamorous relationships. It became a space where individuals could connect, share experiences, and receive support. This virtual landscape facilitated the formation of virtual communities, paving the way for polyamorous individuals to find like-minded individuals, regardless of geographical constraints.

The Internet provided a new level of accessibility, enhancing communication avenues and creating a sense of community for those embracing ENM. It allowed individuals to explore and express their non-conventional relationships in a safe and supportive environment. Furthermore, the Internet became a valuable resource for education, research, and the dissemination of information on polyamory, contributing to the understanding and acceptance of this relationship style.

Reasons for Opening a Relationship

If couples are coming to your office requesting guidance on opening up their relationship, it is likely they have already researched the lifestyle and may need assistance and encouragement with a deeper dive. As with any couple coming to therapy, a thorough intake is required, including their sexual history and a clear understanding of why they want to open their relationship.

Open relationships allow curious couples to experience erotic encounters or romantic relationships with those outside their initial primary relationship. Initial primary relationships are relationships that began the ENM journey for a couple, but that does not mean they stay the primary relationship for the couple. The couple can design their relationship(s) any way they feel is best for them. Wanting to open a relationship does not mean that one or both partners reject the other to be with someone else. Instead, it should be seen as an opportunity for self-discovery and growth with their initial primary partner.

Dossie Easton and Janet Hardy, the authors of *The Ethical Slut: A practical guide to polyamory, open relationships, and other freedoms in sex and love*, provide that open relationships are a version of ethical sexual exploration where partners have permission to have erotic and emotional rendezvous with individuals outside of their initial primary relationship without the fear of betrayal.

Liz Powell, the author of *Building Open Relationships: Your Hands on Guide to Swinging, Polyamory, & Beyond*, explains that the three main reasons for opening a relationship are having an abundance of love to give, exploring yourself, and being turned on when watching your partner having an intimate moment with someone else. Further, the author provides examples of behaviors that indicate you have a lot of love to give, including tending to fall in love with more than one person at a time, having a history of "emotional affairs," or cultivating several deep, meaningful relationships at one time.

Everyone should have their reason for wanting to open the relationship and a common goal as a couple. Esther Perel said it best in her book, *The State of Affairs*, "contained within the small circle of the wedding band are vastly contradictory ideals. We want to choose one to offer stability, safety, predictability, and dependability, and we want that person to supply awe, mystery, adventure, and risk."

Believing one person can supply your needs and desires for the rest of your life is unrealistic. That is a tremendous expectation to put on one individual and a recipe for failure. Research has shown that those in ethically non-monogamous relationships have more vital communication skills, feel less jealousy over time, put more trust in their partners, and are more sexually and emotionally fulfilled than their contemporaries in monogamous relationships (Sheff, 2015).

Identifying Sexual Coercion

Sexual coercion in intimate relationships occurs when one partner uses nonviolent behaviors, such as manipulation and intimidation, to press another partner to comply with sexual requests (Fontes, 2023). According to the research study, *Intimate Partner Sexual Violence: A Review of Terms, Definitions, and Prevalence*, intimate partner sexual violence (IPSV) is often overlooked by those who study intimate partner violence because of the "difficulties with identifying, defining and measuring IPSV, and research lacks consistency in terminology and measurement" (Bagwell-Gray et al., 2015, p. 1).

The CDC released a new report, *The National Intimate Partner and Sexual Violence Survey: 2016/2017 Report on Intimate Partner Violence*, highlighting the following key findings:

- Approximately one in two individuals identifying as women and more than two in five individuals identifying as male reported sustaining "contact sexual violence, physical violence, and/or stalking victimization by an intimate partner at some point in their lifetime".
- About one in five women reported contact with sexual violence from an intimate partner.
  - 13.7% experienced sexual coercion.
- Almost one in five men reported contact with sexual violence from an intimate partner.
  - 5% experienced sexual coercion.

Acquaintances can sexually coerce individuals, for example, someone they met at a bar, coworkers, friends, play partners, etc., or by their romantic partners/spouses. In ENM, there is no place for sexual coercion; however, it is prevalent. Participants of ENM preach consent and equality, but unfortunately, as with any romantic relationship, coercion exists.

According to Bagwell-Gray et al. (2015), there are eight general ways partners use coercion for unwanted sex:

- Exploitation
- Bullying
- Pressure
- Relational Threats or Manipulation
- Humiliation/Intimidation
- Learned Helplessness
- Physical Harm/Threats of Physical Violence

Exploitation

Coercion through exploitation is indeed prevalent in many romantic relationships, and this issue extends to non-monogamous relationships as well. However, the dynamics of coercion can vary when multiple partners are involved. It is essential to acknowledge and actively address the presence of exploitation in non-monogamous relationships in order to promote the well-being and personal growth of all individuals involved.

Exploitation can take various forms in non-monogamous relationships. For example, one partner may exert undue influence or pressure on others to engage in activities or relationships against their will or comfort levels. This could manifest as emotional manipulation, gaslighting, or even threats of abandonment or exclusion. Additionally, power imbalances within the relationship, such as a hierarchical structure where one partner has more decision-making authority or control, can contribute to exploitation.

Recognizing and addressing exploitation in non-monogamous relationships requires a commitment to open, honest, and transparent communication among all partners involved. It involves actively seeking and obtaining enthusiastic consent from all parties and ensuring that each individual's boundaries, needs, and desires are respected and considered. By fostering an environment of trust, respect, and consent, individuals can work toward building healthier and more egalitarian, non-monogamous relationships.

Unfortunately, societal norms and expectations regarding monogamy often perpetuate harmful behaviors and attitudes, including the normalization of coercion and exploitation. Many people are unaware of the potential harm they can cause in their relationships due to a lack of awareness or understanding. It is crucial, therefore, to engage in ongoing education and discussions surrounding healthy relationship dynamics, consent, and ENM to challenge these harmful norms and promote more inclusive and respectful relationship practices.

By raising awareness about the presence of coercion through exploitation in non-monogamous relationships and promoting a culture of consent and respect, we can work toward creating a safer and more supportive environment for all individuals involved in non-monogamous dynamics. This consists of taking responsibility for our actions, actively dismantling harmful beliefs and behaviors, and continuously striving for healthier, more equitable relationships.

Key Behaviors of Exploitation
- Claiming to be in love or using their partner's love against them

  - "If you loved me, then you would do this … ."
  - "If you truly loved me as much as you say you do, then … ."

- Encouraging their partner to drink more alcohol as a means of lowering inhibitions so there is less resistance to sexual requests.
- One partner is pushing to move faster than the other is comfortable with regarding ENM.
- Evidence of a power imbalance between the couple.
- Weaponizing guilt.
- Gaslighting
- Being dishonest about

Bullying

Bullying within relationships can take on various forms and may be disguised as harmless jokes or playful banter. Fang's research in 2017 suggests that people with low self-esteem are more likely to accept bullying behaviors in romantic relationships (Choi & Park, 2021). The partner engaging in bullying may use insults, name-calling, and demeaning behavior and dismiss it as playful banter. This behavior can create a toxic and unhealthy dynamic within the relationship.

In a recent interview, Backer explains that relationship bullying is a deliberate act of one partner bullying the other within the context of the relationship. Backer suggests that the bullying partner brings personal traits or an exclusive attitude toward the partnership, assuming a dominating role and making the other person feel vulnerable, undermined, and disrespected (Chatterjee, 2022).

The effects of relationship bullying can be damaging and long-lasting, leading to decreased self-esteem, increased anxiety, and a sense of worthlessness. It can also erode trust and intimacy, leading to emotional disconnection between partners.

To foster healthier relationships, it is vital to recognize and address bullying behaviors. Open and honest communication is essential in addressing this issue by initiating conversations about boundaries and respect to create a space where both partners feel safe expressing their needs and concerns.

Seeking professional help, such as couples therapy or counseling, can benefit people in navigating the impact of relationship bullying. Therapists can provide guidance and support in developing healthy communication skills, building self-esteem, and identifying and addressing power imbalances in the relationship.

Education and awareness of healthy relationship dynamics are also valuable for combatting bullying behaviors. Creating a culture of kindness, respect, and empathy is essential in promoting healthy and fulfilling partnerships where individuals feel valued and respected. It is crucial for both partners to actively work toward fostering a supportive and nurturing environment free from bullying and harmful behaviors.

Key Behaviors of Bullying
- Invalidated opinions
- Constant judgment
- Depreciation of accomplishments
- Dictating or controlling everything
- Physical abuse

Pressure

The decision for a couple to pursue an open relationship can sometimes lack autonomy, which can have negative implications for the individuals involved. Research has shown that when one partner feels pressured to engage in ENM, it can harm their mental well-being. The anxiety and fear of losing their primary partner can intensify the sense of being coerced into moving at a pace they are not ready for, leading to feelings of resentment (McNichols, 2022).

In my experience working with couples, I have observed cases where, initially, both partners may express openness to ENM. Still, as one partner becomes hesitant or resistant, the other exerts pressure to engage in activities or relationships they are uncomfortable with. As therapists, it is crucial to be aware of the presence of coerced consent and its impact in these situations.

Coerced consent is when someone is pressured or manipulated into consenting to something against their will. It can occur through overt threats or more subtle forms of manipulation, such as withholding affection, giving silent treatment, criticizing, pressuring, or even threatening to end the relationship if the other person does not comply with their terms. In these instances, there is a lack of negotiation, recognition of individual wants and needs, and agency within the relationship. The dynamic becomes one-sided, with the person exerting control and expecting compliance without considering the autonomy and desires of the other person involved (Stray, 2019a).

To address coerced consent and promote healthier dynamics within non-monogamous relationships, therapists should prioritize open communication, consent, and negotiation. Creating a safe and non-judgmental space where individuals can express their concerns, boundaries, and desires without fear of retribution or coercion is essential. Therapists can help couples explore the underlying reasons behind the pressure for non-monogamy and work toward finding mutually satisfying solutions that respect the autonomy and well-being of all parties involved.

Key Behaviors of Pressure
- Frequent arguments
- Constant nagging
- Relentless begging

Relational Threats or Manipulation

When a partner resorts to threats of ending the relationship to coerce the other into agreeing to ENM, it is crucial to recognize this behavior as emotional manipulation. Emotional manipulation occurs when one partner tries to manipulate and control the thoughts and feelings of the other to satisfy their desires (Stray, 2019b).

The threat of ending the relationship creates a power dynamic where the manipulated partner may feel pressured, frightened, or guilty if they do not comply with the manipulator's wishes. This can lead to significant emotional distress, as the individual may be forced to act against their genuine thoughts and feelings to avoid losing the relationship. The manipulated partner may experience a sense of internal conflict, as they have to suppress their needs and desires to please their partner and maintain the relationship.

It is crucial for therapists to be aware of these signs of emotional manipulation within non-monogamous relationships and to address them appropriately. This may involve exploring the underlying motivations behind the manipulator's actions and helping the manipulated partner regain a sense of agency, autonomy, and self-worth. Setting boundaries and promoting open communication can be crucial in addressing emotional manipulation and creating a healthier dynamic within the relationship.

Key Behaviors of Relational Threats or Manipulation
- Crossing boundaries
- Unable to take no for an answer
- Dramatic statements that cause guilt and shame
- Ability to cry on cue
- The requirement to prove your love for them
- Expected to react in a specific way
- Love bombing
- Playing the role of the victim
- Frequently, they are "just joking" when the victim stands up for themselves.

Humiliation/Intimidation

Humiliation and intimidation in romantic relationships can have severe and long-lasting effects, similar to physical abuse. Both behaviors can undermine an individual's confidence, create self-doubt, and result in a loss of self-esteem. It is essential to recognize that these forms of abuse can be just as damaging as physical abuse, as they can significantly impact a person's emotional well-being and overall quality of life.

Humiliation is characterized by deliberately demeaning or degrading someone, causing a loss of status and standing in their eyes or the eyes of others. This can include disparaging comments, public embarrassment, or any action intended to belittle and erode an individual's sense of honor and dignity (Burton, 2014). Humiliation can have a profound psychological impact, leading to feelings of shame, powerlessness, and a distorted self-image.

Intimidation in romantic relationships involves using fear, manipulation, or threats to control and overpower the other person. It can manifest through a variety of behaviors, such as verbal aggression, constant criticism, gaslighting, stalking, or physical intimidation (Niolon et al., 2017). Intimidation can instill fear and create a toxic atmosphere, making it difficult for the victim to assert their wants and needs or to leave the relationship.

Humiliation and intimidation undermine an individual's ability to defend themselves against their aggressor. The power dynamics in these abusive relationships leave the victim feeling trapped, helpless, and unable to assert their autonomy. Over time, this can lead to emotional trauma, anxiety, depression, and a diminished sense of self-worth (Duhigg, 2016).

Recognizing the signs of humiliation and intimidation is crucial for both individuals experiencing these behaviors and for therapists working with clients in such situations. Therapy can provide a safe space for victims to explore their experiences, develop coping strategies, and work toward regaining their self-esteem and independence. It is vital to provide support and validate the experiences of those who have endured humiliation and intimidation in romantic relationships, as they deserve to be free from these harmful dynamics.

Key Behaviors of Humiliation/Intimidation
- Dominates conversations
- Screaming
- Shouting
- Creating a scene
- Unnegotiated degradation
- Punching structures to cause fear
- Breaking things to induce fear

Learned Helplessness

Learned helplessness is a psychological concept that occurs when individuals feel they have no control over a situation, leading them to believe that their actions will not make a difference. In the context of a romantic relationship, this can manifest when a partner lacks sexual autonomy and feels powerless to advocate for their needs and desires. As a result, they may stop supporting themselves, believing their efforts will be futile (Nickerson, 2022).

Abusive relationships often perpetuate learned helplessness by subjecting victims to repeated acts of abuse, creating an environment where the victim is acclimatized to the mistreatment and loses their sense of control over the situation. This can be particularly evident regarding sexual dynamics within the relationship (Nickerson, 2022).

When individuals feel helpless in their relationship, especially regarding sexual autonomy, they may experience a range of negative consequences. These can include decreased self-esteem, a diminished sense of agency, and an overall loss of empowerment (Bempechat, 2021). By feeling that their actions would not make a difference, individuals may refrain from expressing their desires, setting boundaries, or seeking help, perpetuating a cycle of powerlessness.

It is crucial to recognize and address learned helplessness in the context of abusive relationships. This can be done through therapy, support groups, and education that promote empowerment, self-advocacy, and the development of healthy boundaries. By fostering an environment of safety and support, individuals can regain control over their lives and work toward creating healthier relationship dynamics.

Key Behaviors of Learned Helplessness
- Passive behavior
- Low self-esteem
- Avoiding decisions
- Quick to give up
- Lack of solid effort

Physical Harm/Threats of Physical Violence

In abusive relationships, victims may engage in behaviors that make them uncomfortable or go against their personal preferences to avoid potential violence or physical harm from their abuser. The fear of what may happen if they do not comply with their abuser's requests can be significant, creating a sense of threat and intimidation that can be difficult to escape. Over time, this can lead to psychological trauma, diminished self-worth, and a pervasive sense of powerlessness in the victim (Campbell & Raja, 2005).

The phenomenon of engaging in unwanted behaviors to avoid abuse has been studied in the context of intimate partner violence, where victims may endure sexual, emotional, or physical violations out of fear for their safety (Arriaga et al., 2017). Research has shown that when individuals feel trapped in an abusive relationship, they may engage in what is known as "survival sex," where they trade sex for necessities such as food, shelter, or access to money (Williamson et al., 2010).

In these situations, it is essential to recognize that the victim is not freely consenting to the behavior but is instead acting out of fear and necessity. It is crucial to provide support and resources to help victims regain their agency and work toward ending the cycle of abuse. This can be done through counseling, safety planning, and interventions that focus on empowering the victim breaking the cycle of control established by the abuser (Dichter et al., 2015).

In summary, when abuse is present in a relationship, victims may engage in behaviors that they are uncomfortable with to avoid violence or physical harm from their abuser. The fear of what may happen if they stand up for themselves can be overwhelming, creating a sense of threat and intimidation that can be challenging to escape. Recognizing and addressing this behavior is crucial to helping victims regain their agency and work toward a healthier relationship dynamic.

Key Behaviors of Physical Harm/Threats of Physical Violence

- Extreme jealousy
- Isolation from friends and family
- Accusations without evidence
- Intense anger
- One partner is "allowed" to do things the other is not permitted to do
- Emotional dysregulation

When perpetrators of sexual coercion employ various abusive tactics, it can have a detrimental impact on their partner's mental health. It is common for abusers to use a combination of tactics, such as emotional manipulation, threats, physical violence, and control, to maintain power and control over their partner's sexual autonomy (Bonomi et al., 2012).

These tactics can create an environment that causes significant harm to the victim's mental well-being.

Therapists play a crucial role in addressing situations where one partner is stifling the other's sexual autonomy. They need to be attuned to signs of sexual coercion and advocate for the victim's well-being. Therapists should provide a safe and non-judgmental space for clients to express their concerns and experiences. By openly discussing issues related to power dynamics and consent, therapists can help victims recognize the coercive tactics being used against them and work toward reclaiming their sexual autonomy (Fontes, 2023).

Unwanted sexual experiences within dating or marital relationships can be challenging to label accurately due to the complexities of intimacy involved. Coercion tactics may not always apply direct pressure or physical force, leaving individuals confused and uncertain about their experiences. Victims may engage in sexual activity without fully consenting, feeling frozen, or offering sex as a means to avoid negative consequences (Fontes, 2023).

It is important to note that victims of sexual coercion may struggle to identify their experiences as assault because they may have engaged in some form of compliance or attempted to exert limited control over the encounter. Victims may perceive themselves as "willing victims" and internalize a sense of responsibility for the sexual encounter, further complicating their understanding of the situation (Fontes, 2023).

By providing support, validation, and education, therapists can assist victims in recognizing the coercive tactics used against them, challenging victim-blaming narratives, and helping them restore their sense of agency and autonomy in their sexual relationships.

Instructions for Using a Brain Dump Chart on Sexual Coercion

- Prepare the brain dump chart: Create a visual chart or use a digital tool to organize your thoughts. Divide the diagram into sections for different aspects of your ideas on sexual coercion, such as client education, information presentation, and identifying coercion in couples.

List Thoughts on Client Education

- Brainstorm all the ideas you have for ensuring your clients are adequately educated on sexual coercion. This could include providing resources, sharing educational materials, conducting workshops or group therapy sessions, or discussing consent and healthy boundaries in individual sessions.
- Once you have brainstormed all your ideas, choose and list your top three approaches or strategies for educating clients about sexual coercion on the chart.

List Thoughts on Presenting the Information to the Client

- Brainstorm different ways to present information on sexual coercion to your clients. This may involve explaining the dynamics of coercion, discussing consent, identifying warning signs, and offering strategies for assertiveness and self-protection.
- Freely jot down all your ideas and suggestions related to presenting this information.
- Select the three ideas or approaches from your list that will be most effective in conveying the information to your clients.

List Thoughts on Identifying Sexual Coercion in Couples

- Consider various methods for recognizing signs of sexual coercion in couples. This may include assessing power dynamics, communication patterns, levels of control, and instances of consent violation.
- Generate all your thoughts and ideas on how to catch sexual coercion in couples.
- Choose the following three ideas that you find most promising or feasible for recognizing and addressing sexual coercion within couples.

Reflect and Review: Once you have completed the brain dump chart, take a moment to review your ideas in each category. Consider each approach or strategy's potential strengths, limitations, and possible challenges.

Develop an Action Plan: Based on your brainstormed ideas and the top priorities you identified in each category, create an action plan to implement these strategies in your therapy practice. Consider timelines, resources, and any necessary adaptations to your therapeutic approach.

Table 1.1 Brain Dump

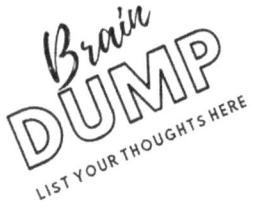	**List Thoughts on Client Education:** 1. 2. 3. **List Thoughts on Presenting the Information to the Client:** 1. 2. 3. **List Thoughts on Identifying Sexual Coercion in Couples:** 1. 2. 3.

Source: Created by author.

Chapter Highlights

- ENM refers to the consensual agreement to engage in romantic and sexual relationships with multiple partners.
- Common forms of ENM include open relationships and polyamorous relationships.
- Honesty is a fundamental principle of ENM.
- ENM exists on a spectrum, with each style of ENM varying in the level of openness and boundaries.
- If a couple seeks guidance in opening up about their relationship, it is likely they have already conducted some research. However, it is advised and encouraged for therapists to conduct a more in-depth exploration of the topic.
- When working with any couple, therapists should conduct a thorough intake process that includes assessing the couple's sexual history and gaining a clear understanding of their motivations for pursuing an open relationship.

References

Arriaga, X., Capezza, N. M., Daly, C. A., & Johnson, K. (2017). Influence of intimate partner violence survivor-centered behavior and global rating on survivors' medical and legal system satisfaction. *Journal of interpersonal violence, 32*(24), 3728–3757.

Bagwell-Gray, M. E., Messing, J. T., & Baldwin-White, A. (2015). Intimate partner sexual violence. *Trauma, Violence, & Abuse, 16*(3), 316–335. 10.1177/152483 8014557290

Bargh, J. A., & McKenna, K. Y. (2004). The Internet and social life. *Annual Review of Psychology, 55*(1), 573–590. 10.1146/annurev.psych.55.090902.141922

Bempechat, T. (2021). Sexual coercion, consent, and demands in adolescent romantic relationships. *Journal of Adolescent Health, 69*(6), 794–797.

Blakemore, E. (2017, October 20). *The scandalous sex parties that made Americans hate flappers*. History.com. Retrieved January 9, 2023, from https://www.history. com/news/the-scandalous-sex-parties-that-made-americans-hate-flappers

Bonomi, A. E., Anderson, M. L., Nemeth, J., Bartle-Haring, S., & Buettner, C. (2012). Dating violence victimization across the teen years: Abuse frequency, number of abusive partners, and age at first occurrence. *BMC Public Health, 12*(1), 637.

Burton, J. W. (2014). Human dignity and humiliation studies. In M. Lutz-Bachmann & A. Føllesdal (Eds.), *Human rights and the impact of religion* (pp. 415–438). Nomos Verlagsgesellschaft mbH & Co. KG.

Campbell, J. C., & Raja, S. (2005). Secondhand and community effects of partner violence. In J. C. Campbell (Ed.), *Handbook of family violence* (pp. 389–406). Springer.

Centers for Disease Control and Prevention. (2021, July 19). *The national intimate partner and sexual violence survey*. Centers for Disease Control and Prevention. Retrieved January 9, 2023, from https://www.cdc.gov/violenceprevention/ datasources/nisvs/index.html

Chatterjee, P. (2022, November 20). *Relationship bullying: What is it and 5 signs you are a victim.* Bonobology.com. Retrieved January 9, 2023, from https://www.bonobology.com/relationship-bullying/

Choi, B., & Park, S. (2021). Bullying perpetration, victimization, and low self-esteem: Examining longitudinal reciprocal relationships in Korean adolescents. *Journal of Youth and Adolescence, 50*(6), 1114–1128. 10.1007/s10964-020-01379-8

Constantine, L. L., & Constantine, J. M. (1974). *Group marriage: A study of contemporary multilateral marriage.* Collier Books.

Dichter, M. E., Cerulli, C., & Bossarte, R. M. (2015). Intimate partner violence victimization among women veterans and associated heart health risks. *Women's Health Issues, 25*(6), 658–665.

Duhigg, C. (2016). *The power of habit: Why we do what we do in life and business.* Random House.

Easton, D., & Hardy, J. W. (2017). *The ethical slut: A practical guide to polyamory, open relationships, and other freedoms in sex and love.* Random House Inc.

Fang, Q. (2017). *Attachment, bullying, and romantic relationships in college students* (dissertation).

Fern, J. (2020). *Polysecure: Attachment, trauma and consensual nonmonogamy.* Thorntree Press, LLC.

Fontes, L. A. (2023, January 9). *Sexual coercion in intimate relationships: Eight tactics.* DomesticShelters.org. Retrieved January 9, 2023, from https://www.domesticshelters.org/articles/identifying-abuse/sexual-coercion-in-intimate-relationships-eight-tactics

Gould, T. (2010). *The lifestyle a look at the erotic rites of Swingers.* Random House of Canada.

Kinsey, A. C., Pomeroy, W. B., & Martin, C. E. (1948). *Sexual behavior in the human male.* Ishi Press Int.

Mayer, E. (2022, September 30). What is ethical non-monogamy?: U.S. politician comes out as polyamorous. Newsweek. Retrieved January 8, 2023, from https://www.newsweek.com/what-ethical-non-monogamy-us-politician-comes-out-polyamorous-1747639

McNichols, T. (2022). Pressured to be polyamorous? Study shows negative mental health effects. PsyPost. Retrieved from https://www.psypost.org/2022/05/pressured-to-be-polyamorous-study-shows-negative-mental-health-effects-65790

Merriam-Webster. (n.d.). *Consensual definition & meaning.* Merriam-Webster. Retrieved January 8, 2023, from https://www.merriam-webster.com/dictionary/consensual

Merriam-Webster. (n.d.). *Ethical definition & meaning.* Merriam-Webster. Retrieved January 8, 2023, from https://www.merriam-webster.com/dictionary/ethical

Michaels, M. A., & Johnson, P. (2015). *Designer relationships: A guide to happy monogamy, positive polyamory, and optimistic open relationships.* Cleis Press.

Moors, A. C., Gesselman, A. N., & Garcia, J. R. (2021, March 23). *Desire, familiarity, and engagement in polyamory: Results from a national sample of single adults in the United States.* NCBI. Retrieved October 12, 2022, from https://www.ncbi.nlm.nih.gov/pmc/articles/PMC8023325/

Muncy, R. L. (1973). *Sex and marriage in Utopian communities: 19th century America.* Indiana University Press.

Nickerson, A. K. (2022). Intimate partner violence: Incidence, prevention, and intervention. In H. S. Friedman (Ed.), *Encyclopedia of mental health* (2nd ed., pp. 520–526). Elsevier.

Niolon, P. H., Vivolo-Kantor, A. M., Latzman, N. E., Valle, L. A., Kuoh, H., Burton, T., … & Taylor, B. G. (2017). Prevalence of intimate partner violence and associated risk factors among adolescents in seven Caribbean countries. *Journal of Interpersonal Violence, 32*(23), 3603–3629.

Perel, E. (2019). *The state of affairs: Rethinking infidelity*. Yellow Kite.

Powell, D. L. (2018). *Building open relationships: Your hands on guide to swinging, polyamory, and beyond!* Dr. Liz Powell.

Sheff, D. E. (2012, October 23). *Three waves of non-monogamy: A select history of polyamory in the United States*. Dr. Elisabeth "Eli" Sheff. Retrieved September 25, 2022, from https://elisabethsheff.com/2012/09/09/three-waves-of-polyamory-a-select-history-of-non-monogamy/

Sheff, E. (2015). *The polyamorists next door: Inside multiple-partner relationships and families*. Rowman & Littlefield.

Sheff, E. A. (2022, April 12). *A select history of consensual nonmonogamies in the U.S. Psychology Today*. Retrieved September 25, 2022, from https://www.psychologytoday.com/us/blog/the-polyamorists-next-door/202204/select-history-consensual-nonmonogamies-in-the-us#:~:text=Nineteenth%2Dcentury%20consensual%20nonmonogamy%20was,together%20in%20experimental%20utopian%20communities

Stray, A. (2019a). Negotiating coercion in non-monogamy: Ethical frameworks and personal strategies. *Sexualities, 22*(5–6), 924–942.

Stray, S. M. (2019b, August 17). *Power, privilege and coerced consent in polyamory*. Medium. Retrieved January 9, 2023, from https://medium.com/@loveinthesuburbs/power-privilege-and-coerced-consent-in-polyamory-9244ae314105

The Kinsey Scale and the Klein Grid. (n.d.). Bi.org. Retrieved October 12, 2022, from https://bi.org/en/101/Kinsey-Klein

Williamson, E., Dutch, N., & Clawson, H. (2010). The nature and extent of known cases of trafficking in persons: Identifying victims of international trafficking and their exploitation in the United States. Research Report. US Department of Justice.

Chapter 2

Relationship Structures

Relationship Dynamics in Ethical Non-Monogamy

Ethical non-monogamy (ENM) is an umbrella term that includes various consensual relationship models that are non-exclusive and allow for multiple romantic or sexual partners (Barker, 2019). ENM practices challenge traditional social norms and expectations regarding romantic relationships, including the belief in monogamy as the only acceptable relationship model. This concept includes various non-monogamous relationships, such as polyamory, open relationships, swinging, and relationship anarchy, among others (Barker, 2019).

Polyamory is a type of ENM where individuals can form multiple romantic, emotional, or sexual relationships with the knowledge and consent of everyone involved (Sheff, 2019). Open relationships include partners having sexual relationships with other people with the knowledge and consent of their primary partner (Moors & Conley, 2020). Swinging is an ENM model where partners engage in sexual activities with other couples or individuals as a couple (Moors & Conley, 2020). Relationship anarchy is a style of ENM where individuals prioritize individual autonomy and create relationships that suit their needs and desires rather than conforming to social norms or hierarchical frameworks (Andie & Green, 2020).

These different models of ENM can be confusing to navigate since they challenge entrenched norms about what relationships should look like and how people should behave within them. However, ENM allows individuals to explore relationship models that fit their needs and desires. Non-monogamous relationships, when conducted ethically, can involve clear communication, informed consent, and consideration of everyone's emotional and physical boundaries (Barker, 2019).

Furthermore, ENM can positively impact individuals and society by challenging heteronormative monogamous ideals and providing alternatives that reduce the constraints of those expectations. ENM can promote sexual education, communication skills, self-awareness, and openness,

DOI: 10.4324/9781003464891-4

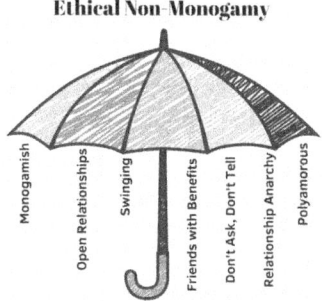

Figure 2.1 Ethical Non-Monogamy Umbrella.

Source: Created by the author.

potentially leading to personal, relational, and societal growth (Horne & Sweeney, 2015).

ENM is an umbrella term for various relationship models prioritizing respect, autonomy, and consent. While it can be confusing to navigate, exploring honest, non-monogamous relationships challenges traditional social norms, promotes personal growth, and offers alternative relationship models that fit individual needs and desires.

Monogamish

The term "monogamish" was coined by Dan Savage, a well-known sex advice columnist and author of the column, Savage Love. It refers to a type of relationship where a couple, who would typically identify as monogamous, occasionally invites other individuals into their sexual experiences (Savage, 2011). Unlike traditional monogamy, where sexual engagement is exclusive between the two partners, monogamish couples have negotiated boundaries that allow for some level of sexual exploration with others.

These boundaries can vary widely among monogamish couples and are typically established through open communication and mutual consent. Some couples may choose to engage in occasional threesomes, where all sexual activities involve all parties present. On the other hand, some couples may only allow certain types of sexual activities (e.g., kissing, but no penetrative intercourse) or establish limitations on the times and locations permitted for outside sexual encounters (Savage, 2011).

It is crucial to note that the boundaries and rules within monogamish relationships are unique to each couple, and no standard template applies universally. Each couple must have open and ongoing discussions to establish clear boundaries, ensure consent, and address any concerns or insecurities that may arise. Building trust and maintaining strong communication are essential components for the success of monogamish relationships.

Counselors must understand their dynamics and boundaries when working with a monogamish couple. Here are some questions that can help you better understand their boundaries:

1   What do you consider to be cheating in your relationship?
2   Are your boundaries universal for the relationship, or do you have specific boundaries for each other? If so, can you tell me more about those boundaries?
3   Do you have specific boundaries for times and locations with a play partner?
4   Do you have time limits for play partners? For example, partners can only play with a specific play partner for one week (specific timeframe) before ending the agreement and becoming monogamous again.

Polyamorous

Polyamory is a type of ENM, and it involves engaging in multiple romantic and often sexual relationships with the consent of all parties involved (Polyamory Definition & Meaning, 2022). However, polyamory is not a one-size-fits-all relationship style. Instead, polyamorous relationships can take on various forms, each with its unique dynamics and expectations.

One of the most common types of polyamorous relationships is a V-shaped relationship, where one person is involved with two people who are not romantically involved with each other (Veaux & Rickert, 2014). Similarly, a triad relationship is a polyamorous relationship where three people are romantically and sexually involved. Another type of polyamorous relationship is a quad relationship, where four people are interested in a romantic and sexual relationship.

It is crucial to understand each dynamic because each relationship type has different expectations and boundaries. For example, all three people have an equal say in a triad relationship, and the communication dynamic differs from a V-shaped relationship. In contrast, physical and emotional intimacy boundaries may vary from a triad or V-shaped dynamic in a quad relationship.

Therefore, counselors need to understand the nuances of each polyamorous dynamic and assist clients in navigating the complexities of these relationships. Counselors can support clients through open communication, boundary-setting, and developing healthy and fulfilling relationships with multiple partners.

Mono-Poly

This type of relationship occurs when one partner identifies as polyamorous, meaning they have the desire and capacity for multiple romantic and sexual relationships. In contrast, the other partner identifies as

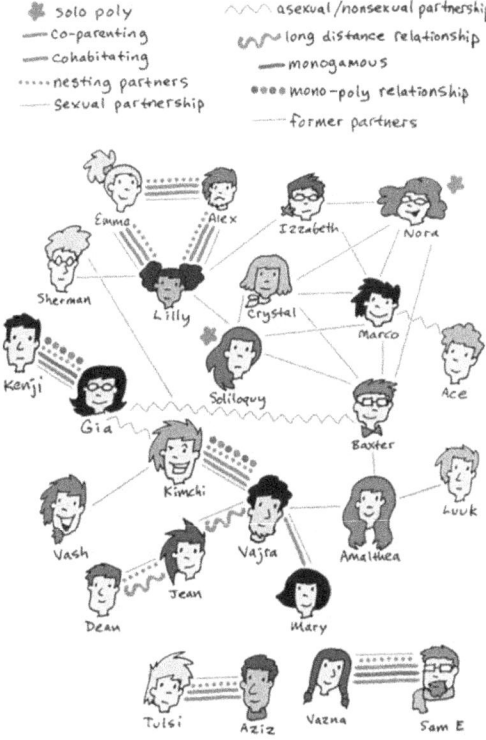

Figure 2.2 Polyamorous Dynamics.

Source: Created by Tikva Wolf: TikvaWolf.com

monogamous, preferring and being fulfilled by exclusive romantic and sexual involvement with one person (Pallotta-Chiarolli, 2020).

Mono-poly relationships can present significant challenges due to the inherent differences in relationship orientation. The monogamous partner may struggle with feelings of jealousy, insecurity, and fear of abandonment when their polyamorous partner explores multiple connections. The poly-amorous partner, on the other hand, may struggle with feelings of restriction and unfulfilled desires for multiple partners (Pallotta-Chiarolli, 2020).

Navigating a mono-poly relationship requires open and honest com-munication, empathy, and compromise from both partners. It is crucial for therapists to actively engage with the couple to understand their specific dynamics, boundaries, and needs. This understanding allows therapists to tailor their therapeutic approach and provide the best care possible to support the couple's unique challenges and navigate the complexities of their relationship (Pallotta-Chiarolli, 2020).

Therapeutic interventions for mono-poly relationships may focus on addressing jealousy and insecurity concerns, fostering trust, exploring individual needs and boundaries, and developing effective communication strategies between partners. Additionally, therapists can help partners develop strategies for finding balance and meeting the needs of both the monogamous and polyamorous partner to maintain a fulfilling and sustainable relationship dynamic (Pallotta-Chiarolli, 2020).

Solo Polyamory

Solo polyamory, also known as solo poly, is a relationship style in which individuals prioritize their autonomy and independence while engaging in ethical, non-monogamous relationships. In solo polyamory, individuals do not seek a traditional primary partnership and do not subscribe to conventional relationship timelines or commitments (Freedman, 2017).

Individuals in solo polyamorous relationships have a strong focus on personal growth, self-awareness, and boundary-setting. Firm emotional and physical boundaries can aid in maintaining independence while still engaging in meaningful relationships. Solo polyamory allows individuals to explore and nurture connections without sacrificing their independent lifestyle or personal identity (Freedman, 2017).

Individuals who practice solo polyamory do not equate their value or self-worth to their relationships, and they take accountability for navigating their own emotional and physical needs. In contrast to traditional relationship models prioritizing stability and long-term commitment, solo polyamory prioritizes growth and self-awareness.

It's important to note that while individuals who practice solo polyamory may not desire or prioritize a primary long-term partner, that does not mean they are detached or uncaring about their relationships. Instead, individuals in solo polyamorous relationships strive to form meaningful and fulfilling connections while maintaining autonomy (García & García, 2021).

Therapeutic interventions for individuals in solo polyamorous relationships may focus on developing healthy and practical communication skills, exploring boundaries and expectations, and building self-awareness around personal needs and relationship goals. In addition, counselors can assist individuals in navigating the difficulties of ENM and maintaining fulfilling relationships while prioritizing independence and personal growth.

Closed V

The closed V relationship dynamic is a form of polyamorous relationship structure where two partners are involved in a romantic and sexual relationship with a third person but not with each other. In this dynamic, the person who is romantically and sexually involved with both partners is often referred to as the "hinge partner," as they act as the bridge or connection between the two "leg partners" (Conley et al., 2013).

The hinge partner, who is romantically and sexually involved with both leg partners, maintains separate and distinct relationships. The leg partners typically do not engage in sexual activities with each other but can have varying levels of closeness, emotional connection, and involvement with the hinge partner. The dynamics of the relationships can differ depending on the desires, boundaries, and agreements made by all parties involved (Conley et al., 2013).

Unlike a traditional triad relationship where all three partners are romantically and sexually involved with each other, the closed V relationship does not necessarily affect all three individuals being sexually involved with one another. Instead, the focus is on the interactions and connections between the hinge partner and each leg partner (Conley et al., 2013).

Living arrangements in a closed V relationship can vary, but it is common for all three individuals to live together. This living arrangement allows for shared spaces and a sense of family or household while maintaining the unique dynamics of the closed V relationship (Conley et al., 2013).

It is crucial to recognize that relationships within the closed V dynamic can have different complexities and considerations compared to other types of polyamorous relationship structures. Open communication, negotiation of boundaries, and ongoing consent among all parties involved are essential for building and maintaining healthy and fulfilling relationships (Conley et al., 2013).

Counselors working with individuals in closed V relationships can support them in navigating the unique challenges and dynamics of this relationship structure. This can involve exploring communication strategies, managing jealousy and insecurities, and establishing clear boundaries and agreements to ensure the emotional well-being of all individuals involved (Sheff, 2019).

Triad

A triad relationship, also known as a throuple, is a polyamorous relationship structure in which all three individuals involved have a sexual and emotional relationship with each other. Unlike the closed V relationship dynamic where two "leg partners" are not sexually involved with each other, in a triad relationship all three individuals are romantically and sexually involved with each other equally (Conley et al., 2013).

In a triad relationship, the connections between the individuals involve four distinct relationships: the relationships between person 1 and person 2, person 1 and person 3, person 2 and person 3, and all three people together. Each of these relationships can have unique dynamics, boundaries, and levels of emotional and sexual intimacy based on the individuals involved (Conley et al., 2013).

Establishing healthy communication and boundaries is essential for a successful triad relationship. All individuals must be open and transparent about their needs, desires, and expectations. Negotiating boundaries around physical intimacy, time spent together, and decision-making processes can help ensure that all individuals feel respected and fulfilled in the relationship (Sheff, 2019).

Triad relationships can also face challenges in navigating societal stigma and discrimination against non-traditional relationship structures. In addition, jealousy and feelings of exclusion can arise if one individual feels left out or less connected to the group dynamic. Counseling can help address these issues and support positive outcomes for all individuals involved (Conley et al., 2013).

Overall, triad relationships allow individuals to create a unique and fulfilling dynamic of polyamorous connection. By prioritizing open communication, clear boundaries, and mutual respect, all individuals can experience meaningful and positive relationships.

Hierarchical Polyamory

Hierarchical polyamory is a relationship structure within polyamory where a primary couple forms the foundation of the relationship and invites other individuals to join and form secondary relationships. In this dynamic, the primary relationship is prioritized over the secondary relationships, and the couple maintains a higher level of commitment and decision-making power within the structure (Sheff, 2019).

In hierarchical polyamory, the primary couple may have established rules or agreements prioritizing their relationship, such as having veto power over the relationships or limiting emotional involvement or commitment with the other partners (Veaux & Rickert, 2014). The secondary partners know their position and understand that the primary couple's relationship takes precedence.

Jealousy can be a common challenge in hierarchical polyamory. The primary couple may experience jealousy or fear of losing their connection or intimacy when their partners form connections with others. It is crucial for all individuals involved to engage in open and honest communication to address and manage jealousy effectively. Failure to do so can lead to toxicity and damage the relationships (Sheff, 2019).

It is noteworthy that hierarchical polyamory is not as widely practiced within the broader polyamorous community as other relationship structures. Many individuals prefer non-hierarchical arrangements where all relationships are given equal weight and importance. However, hierarchical polyamory can still come up in client conversations when dealing with presenting issues, and therapists should be prepared to navigate the unique challenges and dynamics that may arise within this relationship structure.

When working with clients who are engaged in hierarchical polyamory, therapists need to create a supportive and non-judgmental environment to explore the dynamics and emotions involved. They can help clients in developing skills in effective communication, managing jealousy, and establishing boundaries within the structure. Encouraging ongoing consent and mutual respect among all individuals involved is essential for maintaining healthy relationships within a hierarchical polyamory framework (Sheff, 2019).

Non-Hierarchical Polyamory

Non-hierarchical polyamory is a relationship structure where individuals have multiple partners and loved ones are equally important. In this dynamic, there is no ranking or hierarchy among the relationships; each connection holds equal significance to the individual involved. Unlike hierarchical polyamory, where there is a primary couple with priority over secondary relationships, non-hierarchical polyamory emphasizes the value and equality of all relationships (Duck-Chong, 2017).

According to Aggie, the author of solopoly.net, non-hierarchical polyamory typically does not involve intimate relationships heading toward merging life infrastructure in a primary-style manner. This means that individuals practicing non-hierarchical polyamory may not have the goal of creating a primary partnership with shared living arrangements, shared finances, or other markers of traditional relationships (Duck-Chong, 2017).

Non-hierarchical polyamory allows individuals to maintain their autonomy and personal freedom while still forming deep and meaningful connections with multiple partners. This relationship structure often values independence and individuality, allowing everyone involved to prioritize their needs, goals, and relationships without imposing hierarchy or ranking (Sheff, 2019).

It is important to note that non-hierarchical polyamory is just one approach within the broader polyamory spectrum. Many individuals find fulfillment and happiness in non-hierarchical arrangements, allowing for more flexibility, freedom, and diverse connections. However, it is crucial for all individuals involved to engage in open and honest communication, negotiate boundaries, and address any potential feelings of jealousy or insecurity that may arise (Duck-Chong, 2017).

Polyandry

Polyandry is a rare form of polyamorous relationship where one woman is married to multiple men. This relationship structure is distinct from polygamy, where an individual can have multiple spouses regardless of gender. Polyandry's distinguishing feature is that it specifically features women marrying multiple male partners (Leone, 2019).

Polyandry is a relatively rare form of non-monogamy around the world and more often occurs in isolated and rural areas in Asian countries such as Tibet, Nepal, and India (Hirschberger & Oman-Reagan, 2018). In these cultures, where polyandrous relationships occur, it is often necessary based on practical and cultural considerations, such as land ownership, inheritance rights, and population control (Kiriushcheva, 2021).

In polyandrous relationships, all the male partners share in the marriage to one woman, and the woman has equal status and commitment to each of them. While jealousy can still arise, its expression is often drastically different than in other forms of polyamory. The men involved may be relatives or titled dissents who wish to keep assets within a group or family. Therefore, allocating one woman as the incubator or household organizer will ensure that any offspring can be traced back to reliable members of the family lines (Hirschberger & Oman-Reagan, 2018).

Polyandrous relationships can be challenging to navigate, especially in cultures where they are not shared or accepted. However, many who practice polyandrous forms of relationships have found it to be rewarding in terms of commitment, support, and economic stability. The woman involved does not need to bear sole responsibility for household and child-rearing duties but rather shares it with multiple male partners (Kiriushcheva, 2021).

Polyandry remains a controversial and relatively understudied relationship form and requires further exploration to gain insight into its dynamics, benefits, and challenges.

Polygyny

Polygyny is indeed a common form of multiple-partner relationships, where one man is married to multiple wives. In this dynamic, the man has various exclusive and sexual relationships with his wives. Unlike polyandry, which involves one woman having multiple husbands, polygyny emphasizes a male-centric structure (Hooks, 2000).

Historically, polygyny has been practiced in various cultures around the world, including some African, Middle Eastern, and South Asian societies. It often reflects these communities' social, cultural, and religious norms (Altman, 2003). In some cases, polygyny may be seen as a symbol of wealth, power, or social status, with men taking on multiple wives as a means of demonstrating their success or fulfilling cultural expectations (Hamzeh, 2017).

While polygyny may vary across different cultures, it typically involves a hierarchical structure, where each wife has a different status level and influence within the family. The husband usually holds a higher position and has authority over his wives, making important household decisions (Shankar, 2016).

It is important to note that the practice of polygyny is not without its challenges and complexities. Jealousy, competition, and unequal power dynamics can arise within polygynous relationships. Moreover, the husband's unequal access to resources, time, and attention can create tensions and conflicts among the wives (Elder & Greene, 2020).

In modern times, polygynous relationships are not legally recognized in many countries, primarily due to concerns around gender equality, women's rights, and consent. The emphasis on male privilege and potential exploitation within such relationships has led to legal restrictions and social opposition in several jurisdictions (Tremayne, 2012).

Overall, polygyny as a form of multiple-partner relationships remains a complex and culturally diverse phenomenon, with variations in practice and perception around the world.

Polyfidelity

Polyfidelity is a form of consensual non-monogamy where three or more individuals are involved in a closed relationship. In this dynamic, all individuals have equal status within the relationship and are sexually and emotionally exclusive to the group (Easton & Liszt, 2018). Polyfidelity is characterized by a sense of commitment, fidelity, and exclusivity, similar to monogamy but with multiple partners.

In a polyfidelitous relationship, the group members have agreed upon specific boundaries and agreements regarding their involvement with other partners outside the group. This can vary depending on the particular dynamics and preferences of the individuals involved. The goal is to maintain emotional and sexual exclusivity within the group while allowing for a larger sense of connection and support (Easton & Liszt, 2018).

Polyfidelity can provide a sense of security and stability for those who prefer committed relationships but also desire multiple partners. The focus is on building deep emotional connections and maintaining high trust and communication within the group (Mackenzie & Scott, 2018).

It is important to note that polyfidelity is not the same as polyamory, as polyamory involves the potential for having multiple romantic and sexual relationships with individuals outside the primary group (Weitzman, 2011). In polyfidelity, the commitment and exclusivity are limited to the group members only.

Maintaining a successful polyfidelitous relationship requires open communication, negotiation of boundaries, and ongoing reassessment of the dynamics within the group. Jealousy and conflict can still arise, but the emphasis is on addressing these issues within the group and finding resolutions that maintain the stability and well-being of all involved (Easton & Liszt, 2018).

While polyfidelity may not be as well-known or practiced as other forms of non-monogamy, it is a valid and consensual relationship style chosen by some individuals who seek a committed and exclusive connection with multiple partners.

Polyaffective

Polyaffective relationships are a type of non-monogamous relationship where individuals form emotionally intimate partnerships linked through polyamorous relationships. This type of relationship involves multiple individuals who may have different romantic and sexual relationships with each other. Still, a deep emotional connection exists between all members of the polyaffective network (Klesse, 2020).

In a polyaffective relationship, the connection between individuals is not necessarily sexual but rather emotional and intimate. The focus is on building meaningful relationships and prioritizing emotional bonding and support between all network members. For example, two individuals who are partners may have close friendships with each other's partners, creating a web of emotional connectivity within the group (Klesse, 2020).

Co-spousal relationships are another type of polyaffective relationship where two or more individuals are partnered with the same person and form a close connection with each other. Sometimes, co-spouses may live together and function as a family unit despite not being legally recognized. These relationships prioritize emotional intimacy and support between all members rather than specific sexual or gender-based dynamics (Klesse, 2020).

Polyaffective relationships can be challenging to navigate, as they require a high level of trust, communication, and emotional intelligence between all members. Some members may feel jealousy or insecurity, and ongoing work is needed to maintain the emotional connection and support within the group (Meyer, 2015).

Despite the complex nature of polyaffective relationships, many individuals find fulfillment and support within them. They can provide a sense of community and emotional bonding that may be less present in traditional monogamous relationships (Klesse, 2020).

Overall, polyaffective relationships are a unique and valid form of non-monogamy that prioritizes emotional intimacy and support between all members of the network.

Open Relationships

Open relationships are a broad term that encompasses a range of non-monogamous dynamics, including swinging, polyamory, monogamish, and others. In these relationships, individuals or couples choose to pursue sexual or romantic connections with other partners outside of their primary relationship while maintaining clear boundaries and communication.

Swinging involves couples engaging in sexual activities with other couples or individuals with the explicit consent and participation of both partners. It may include attending events or parties designed explicitly for swinging or arranging meetings with other couples or individuals on a case-by-case basis (Barker & Langdridge, 2010).

Polyamory involves individuals or couples who have romantic and sexual relationships with more than one partner, with an emphasis on building ongoing connections and emotional intimacy with all partners involved. Polyamory often involves a high level of communication and negotiation of boundaries between all partners (Easton & Liszt, 2018).

Monogamish relationships are those where the primary couple has agreed to some level of non-monogamy, such as engaging in sexual activities with other individuals on occasion, but with clear boundaries and rules to ensure that the primary relationship remains the focus (Finn, 2017).

While open relationships can provide opportunities for individual growth and exploration, they are not without challenges. They require an exceptional level of trust and communication between all parties involved. Open relationships may not work for everyone, and individuals should take the time to explore their needs, desires, and boundaries before engaging in any non-monogamous relationship (Weitzman, 2011).

In summary, open relationships are an umbrella term that covers a range of non-monogamous relationship dynamics. These relationships involve clear boundaries and communication, with the primary focus being to ensure that the primary relationship remains solid and stable.

Swinging

Swinging, also known as wife swapping or partner swapping, is a type of open relationship in which committed couples engage in sexual activities with other couples or individuals with the explicit consent and participation of all partners involved. Swinging can take many forms, from brief interactions with other couples to long-term arrangements with a significant couple (Barker & Langdridge, 2010).

One common form of swinging is full-swap, where couples engage in sex with another couple, including penetrative sex. Another form is soft-swap, where couples engage in sexual activities with another couple but without penetration. Group sex can also be a part of swinging, where multiple couples engage in sexual activities with one another. These activities are usually conducted at events or parties designed for swingers or through arranged meetings with other couples or individuals (Maticka-Tyndale et al., 2011).

A significant couple is a long-term relationship with a deeper emotional or romantic bond. In a significant couple arrangement, two couples may engage in sexual activities with one another exclusively, with each couple having a presence in the other's life that goes beyond sex. This kind of relationship can provide a sense of emotional intimacy and support beyond that found in casual swinging arrangements (Easton & Liszt, 2018).

Swinging can be a way for couples to explore their sexuality, expand their sexual experiences, and strengthen their connection through the trust and communication required in the arrangement. However, swinging also has inherent risks, such as the possibility of jealousy, emotional attachment, and the spread of sexually transmitted infections. It requires high communication, trust, and mutual respect between all parties involved (Maticka-Tyndale et al., 2011).

In conclusion, swinging is a form of ENM in which committed couples engage in sexual activities with other couples or individuals with full consent and participation from all. It can take various forms, including full-swap, soft-swap, and group sex, and may involve long-term arrangements with significant couples.

Casual Sex/Friends with Benefits

The relationship model of friends with benefits (FWB) involves two people who engage in non-committed, casual sex while maintaining a friendship-based relationship. Unlike other types of open relationships, such as swinging or polyamory, FWB relationships involve sexual encounters with only one partner at a time. In these relationships, fidelity is not part of the dynamic; all involved partners understand and accept this (Owen et al., 2011).

While FWB is often used interchangeably with "casual hook-up," the two concepts differ. A casual hook-up generally refers to a one-time sexual encounter without any expectation of future involvement. In contrast, FWB implies a longer-term arrangement based on a foundation of friendship, with a mutually agreed-upon emphasis on sex (Mongeau et al., 2013).

FWB relationships can offer several benefits, including physical pleasure and emotional support, without the pressure or commitment of a typical romantic relationship. However, they can also have negative consequences, such as jealousy, miscommunication, or unrequited feelings. Establishing clear boundaries and maintaining open communication is essential to avoid misunderstandings and potential hurt (Owen et al., 2011).

In summary, the FWB relationship model involves two people engaging in casual, non-committed sex while maintaining a friendship-based relationship. While similar to a casual hook-up, it is based on a mutual, agreed-upon emphasis on sex and often involves a longer-term arrangement.

Relationship Anarchy

Relationship anarchy is a relationship approach that rejects hierarchical structures and prioritizes certain forms of intimacy over others. According to this approach, all forms of intimacy, whether romantic or platonic, are equally valid and should be valued and respected. Relationship anarchists prioritize individual autonomy and the freedom to create relationships based on mutual consent rather than conforming to societal norms or expectations (Barker, 2017).

Relationship anarchists view each relationship as unique and constantly evolving, with each individual having complete agency to decide what intimacy they want to share with others. This allows for a wide range of possibilities in terms of relationship dynamics, from deep emotional connections to casual sexual encounters. The approach emphasizes communication and ensuring that everyone is aware of their own boundaries and those of others (Barker & Langdridge, 2010).

Relationship anarchists often reject labels such as "polyamorous" or "monogamous," as these labels imply a commitment to a specific form of relationship structure. Instead, they see themselves as free to explore and create relationships that fit their desires and needs without being tied down by conventional expectations (Barker, 2017).

While relationship anarchy can offer benefits, such as increased freedom and the potential for meaningful connections with various people, it can also present challenges for individuals used to more traditional relationship structures. Building and maintaining healthy relationships requires a significant amount of self-awareness, introspection, and communication without the guidance of societal norms (Barker & Langdridge, 2010).

In summary, relationship anarchy is an approach to relationships that prioritizes individual autonomy, rejects hierarchical structures, and values all forms of intimacy equally. It emphasizes open communication and encourages individuals to create relationships that fit their desires and needs.

Don't Ask, Don't Tell

The "Don't Ask, Don't Tell" (DADT) relationship dynamic is a relatively common arrangement where there is an understanding between primary partners that one partner will engage in clandestine affairs or sexual encounters with others, but the other partner does not want to know any details about those encounters (Conley et al., 2018). This model often resembles an extramarital affair but with the element of deceit removed, as both partners are aware of the arrangement (Conley et al., 2018).

In DADT relationships, one partner typically desires to open the primary relationship, while the other partner may be resistant to or uninterested in engaging in non-monogamous activities (Conley et al., 2018). One common scenario is when one partner's sexual interests or desires don't align with the other partner's, resulting in a desire to seek those experiences outside of the primary relationship. This dynamic allows the partner who wants more sexual variety or exploration to do so discreetly while not sharing the details with the other partner (Conley et al., 2018).

DADT relationships can offer a way for couples to address sexual needs and desires while maintaining the stability and primary bond of their relationship. It can also be a solution when one partner wants to explore non-monogamy, but the other is uncomfortable knowing or discussing those experiences (Conley et al., 2018).

However, DADT relationships also come with potential challenges and risks. Lack of communication about outside encounters can lead to difficulties in addressing emotions such as jealousy or insecurity. It can also create a disconnect between partners when one partner has meaningful experiences that the other is unaware of, potentially impacting overall intimacy and trust (Conley et al., 2018).

To navigate a DADT arrangement successfully, couples need to establish clear boundaries and rules, including safe sex practices and expectations of discretion. Communication, trust, and frequent check-ins ensure that both partners feel heard, respected, and supported within the arrangement (Conley et al., 2018).

In conclusion, the DADT relationship dynamic is a model where primary partners agree that one partner can engage in clandestine affairs while not sharing any details with the other partner. It can be a way to address sexual needs and desires when one partner wants to explore non-monogamy while the other partner prefers not to be involved. Effective communication and clear boundaries are essential to navigating DADT arrangements' challenges and potential risks.

Deconstruction of "Relationship Escalator"

Aggie Sez, a relationship blogger and activist, introduced the concept of the "relationship escalator," a linear model of a typical romantic relationship that begins with dating, moves on to commitment, cohabitation, marriage, and eventually having children (Sez, 2012). The traditional relationship escalator model can be constraining for couples who do not fit into the mold of a "typical" relationship. Deconstructing the relationship escalator can allow couples to find alternative routes to building meaningful connections and commitments, which can involve creating unique models that focus on mutual growth and appreciation of individuality (Barker, 2019).

Prioritizing individual growth and autonomy is essential to establish a significant relationship outside of the traditional relationship escalator. Couples who communicate openly and have shared values while respecting each other's individuality can build a healthy and fulfilling partnership (Reis & Holmes, 2019). Promoting autonomy in a relationship can lead to higher satisfaction and commitment levels by allowing each partner to express themselves and grow alongside each other. This can also increase intimacy as both partners are respected as independent individuals (Reis & Holmes, 2019).

Building shared experiences fostering individual interests is essential to preserving a sense of self within a relationship. For couples, seeking out

Table 2.1 Creative Space

Use this space to write things you want to
remember from this chapter for future use:

shared experiences and communities outside of the relationship can be a powerful way of enhancing their relationship as it allows them to bond over meaningful things while promoting individual interests (Oya, 2017). Participation in activities that give the couple a sense of adventure and connectedness helps to redefine the boundaries of the relationship and influence the level of vulnerability between couples. Encouraging each partner to pursue their passions and identity-building fosters intimacy, vulnerability, and emotional intelligence, leading to a stronger bond between the two partners (Oya, 2017).

In conclusion, deconstructing the conventional relationship escalator model can alleviate feelings of entrapment for couples and empower individuals to create meaningful connections and commitments outside of traditional norms. Prioritizing individual growth and autonomy, building shared experiences, and fostering personal interests are essential to promoting successful romantic relationships.

Chapter Highlights

- Many labels fit underneath the umbrella of ENM.
- These labels include but are not limited to Cheating, Monogamish, Polyamorous, Triad, Swinging, Casual Sex, and DADT.
- Cheating occurs when a couple has agreed to be sexually exclusive. Still, one or both have had a secret sexual engagement outside the relationship while lying to their partner and pretending to be monogamous.
- Monogamish is when a monogamous couple occasionally invites other people into their sex life. Counselors must understand their dynamics and boundaries when working with a monogamish couple.
- Polyamorous is engaging in multiple romantic (and typically sexual) relationships with the consent of all the people involved. However, there are many polyamorous dynamics that your clients might practice, and it is essential to understand each of these dynamics.
- In a triad relationship, commonly referred to as a throuple, all three participants have a sexual and emotional relationship.
- Swinging is a relationship model where committed couples have ethical sex with others outside their primary relationship.
- Casual sex involves one person engaging in casual sex with multiple partners. Commitment and fidelity are not a part of the dynamic.
- DADT is a dynamic relationship with an agreement between primary partners where they understand that their primary partner will engage in clandestine affairs but do not want to know any details. This model often resembles an extramarital affair; however, the element of deceit has been removed.

References

Altman, D. (2003). Polygyny, secondary-infidelity, and the structure of Nagovisi families in southern Bougainville, Papua New Guinea. *Ethnology, 42*(1), 55–69. 10.2307/3774042

Andie, C., & Green, E. D. (2020). What is relationship anarchy? Here's what it means and why it's important. Healthline. Retrieved from https://www.healthline.com/health/non-monogamy-relationship-anarchy

Barker, M. (2017). What is relationship anarchy? *Psychology Today*. Retrieved from https://www.psychologytoday.com/us/blog/the-polyamorists-next-door/201707/what-is-relationship-anarchy

Barker, M., & Langdridge, D. (2010). *Understanding non-monogamies*. Routledge.

Barker, M. J. (2019). *Rewriting the rules: An integrative guide to love, sex, and relationships*. Routledge.

Conley, T. D., Matsick, J. L., Moors, A. C., & Ziegler, A. (2013). Investigation of consensually non-monogamous relationships: Theories, methods, and new directions. *Perspectives on Psychological Science, 8*(2), 685–688. 10.1177/1745691613489837

Conley, T. D., Piemonte, J. L., Gusakova, S., & Rubin, J. D. (2018). Sexual satisfaction among individuals in monogamous and consensually non-monogamous relationships. *Journal of Social and Personal Relationships*. 10.1177/0265407517743078

Duck-Chong, L. I. (2017, June 20). *Non-hierarchical polyamory: Stepping off the relationship escalator*. Archer Magazine. Retrieved January 10, 2023, from https://archermagazine.com.au/2017/06/non-hierarchical-polyamory/

Easton, D., & Liszt, C. A. (2018). *The ethical slut: A practical guide to polyamory, open relationships & other adventures* (2nd ed.). Ten Speed Press.

Elder, C., & Greene, S. M. (2020). *Introduction to ethnology: A reader for the introduction to ethnology*. University of Toronto Press.

Finn, M. (2017). Monogamish? Non-monogamous? Ethical slut? What open relationships mean in 2017. *Independent*. Retrieved from https://www.independent.co.uk/life-style/love-sex/open-relationships-ethical-sluts-monogamish-meaning-definition-a7909331.html

Freedman, L. (2017). What is solo polyamory? *Psychology Today*. Retrieved from https://www.psychologytoday.com/us/blog/the-polyamorists-next-door/201710/what-is-solo-polyamory

García, M. J., & García, A. L. (2021). Attachment, autonomy, and self-compassion in solo polyamory. *Journal of Sex & Marital Therapy, 47*(2), 151–165. 10.1080/0092623X.2020.1840349

Hamzeh, M. (2017). Polygamy is not polygyny: On the relationship between the stages of Sufism and the rightful practice of polygamy. *Journal of Islamic Studies, 28*(3), 259–281. 10.1093/jis/etx010

Hirschberger, L., & Oman-Reagan, M. P. (2018). Analysis of polyandry: When one woman has multiple husbands. *Sexual and Relationship Therapy, 33*(1), 109–123. 10.1080/14681994.2017.1417618

Hooks, B. (2000). *Feminism is for everybody: Passionate politics*. Routledge.

Horne, S. G. & Sweeney, R. B. (2015). Ethical non-monogamy and social justice: A case for relationship anarchy. *Journal of Feminist Family Therapy, 27*, 66–82. 10.1080/08952833.2015.1007858

Kiriushcheva, E. (2021). Polyandry. *Encyclopedia Britannica*. Retrieved July 12, 2021, from https://www.britannica.com/topic/polyandry

Klesse, C. (2020). Polyamory and queer anarchism: Contemporary debates and challenges. *Sexualities*, *23*(1–2), 127–144. 10.1177/1363460718824494

Leone, R. (2019, January 17). The truth about polygamy and polyamory. *Psychology Today*. Retrieved July 12, 2021, from https://www.psychologytoday.com/ca/blog/talking-about-men/201901/the-truth-about-polygamy-and-polyamory

Mackenzie, D. A., & Scott, R. T. (2018). Polyamory and the ethical slut: The importance of sexual freedom and relationship choice. *Journal of Contemporary Ethnography*, *47*(3), 349–376. 10.1177/0891241617699184

Maticka-Tyndale, E., Herold, E. S., & Mewhinney, D. (2011). Casual sex among swingers. *Journal of Sex Research*, *48*(4), 346–361. 10.1080/00224499.2010.481421

Meyer, M. (2015). *Beyond monogamy: Polyamory and the future of polyqueer sexualities*. NYU Press.

Mongeau, P. A., Knight, K., Williams, J., Eden, J., & Shaw, C. (2013). Scripts, sexual identity, and disclosure in Friends with Benefits relationships. *Western Journal of Communication*, *77*(4), 377–397. 10.1080/10570314.2012.756055

Moors, A. C., & Conley, T. D. (2020). Polyamory and relationship diversity. *Annual Review of Psychology*, *71*, 671–690. 10.1146/annurev-psych-010419-050912

Owen, J., Fincham, F. D., & Moore, J. (2011). Short-term prospective study of hooking up among college students. *Archives of Sexual Behavior*, *40*(2), 331–341. 10.1007/s10508-010-9690-2

Oya, A. (2017). Cultivating relationships with yourself, your partner and your community. *Flourish Counseling and Coaching*. Retrieved from https://www. flourishcounseling.co/blog/cultivating-relationships-with-yourself-your-partner-and-your-community

Pallotta-Chiarolli, M. D. (2020). Mental health for sexual and gender minority polyamorous and consensually non-monogamous individuals. In E. D. Rothblum (Ed.), *The Oxford handbook of sexual and gender minority mental health* (pp. 369–379). Essay, Oxford University Press.

Polyamory Definition & Meaning. (2022). Merriam-Webster. Retrieved from https://www.merriam-webster.com/dictionary/polyamory

Reis, H. T., & Holmes, J. G. (2019). Perceived partner responsiveness as an organizing theme for the study of relationships and well-being. In L. Campbell & T. J. Loving (Eds.), *Interdisciplinary research on close relationships: The case for integration* (pp. 27–52). American Psychological Association. 10.1037/13486-002

Savage, D. (2011). Monogamish. *Savage Love*. Retrieved from https://www. thestranger.com/seattle/SavageLove?oid=10195681

Sez, A. (2012). On the subject of the "relationship escalator." *Solo Poly*. Retrieved from https://solopoly.net/2012/11/29/on-the-subject-of-the-relationship-escalator/

Shankar, S. (2016). *Harems, hijabs, and hijras: Muslims and media in the global era*. Indiana University Press.

Sheff, E. (2019). *The polyamorists next door: Inside multiple-partner relationships and families* (2nd ed.). Rowman & Littlefield Publishers.

Tremayne, S. (2012). *More than one: Plural marriage, polygamy, and polyamory* (1st ed.). Paradigm Publishers.

Veaux, F., & Rickert, E. (2014). *More than two: A practical guide to ethical polyamory*. Thorntree Press.

Weitzman, G. (2011). Negotiating non-monogamy: Exclusive monogamy agreements in gay male couples. *Symbolic Interaction*, *34*(2), 186–208. 10.1525/si.2011.34.2.186

Chapter 3

Examining Clinician's Bias

Be Respectful and Considerate

Participation and public interest in ethical non-monogamy (ENM) or relationship dynamics where all involved partners agree to extradyadic sexual/romantic relationships have increased. According to Schechinger et al. (2018), the increased interest is evidenced by positive and negative media coverage, expanded scientific research exploration, mainstream books, and increased Internet search rates (Moors et al., 2017). Even the increased interest in ENM, mononormativity, or society's standard of monogamy as the only acceptable practice for engaging in romantic relationships impacts the success of those who participate in ENM relationships by inadvertently prioritizing monogamous relationships above other relationship dynamics (Cassidy & Wong, 2018b).

A research study where individuals in ENM relationships responded to survey questions regarding their past and current therapeutic experiences indicated that among therapists seen by those practicing ENM, approximately 29% lacked the basic knowledge of ENM needed to be effective, with only 27% considered knowledgeable about ENM (Schechinger, 2015). Furthermore, the research revealed that 15% viewed their therapist as unhelpful, 11% felt their therapist was "destructive," and one in ten ENM clients terminated sessions before achieving their therapeutic goals due to negative therapist bias.

A therapist who can explore the client's subjective experience without inserting assumptions is more likely to help them achieve their goals. In addition to the fundamental considerations for cultural sensitivity, there are unique challenges that those in ENM relationships encounter.

Weitzman (2017) constructed a list of common themes while working with ENM clients:

1 A primary partner having feelings of or being neglected
2 Acquiring more lovers than they have time for

DOI: 10.4324/9781003464891-5

3 Rushing into new relationships
4 Believe that jealousy should not be experienced or felt
5 Relationships comparisons
6 Dishonesty

Moors and Schechinger (2014) recommend five essential elements for practitioners to consider "to avoid reinforcing mononormative assumptions within the therapy context":

1 Become well-versed in sexual practices and dynamics outside normative expectations.
2 Understand that sexual exclusivity is not a requirement for a healthy relationship.
3 Attend therapeutic training for alternative relationship styles.
4 Provide various opportunities for clients to disclose their specific relationship structure during intake.
5 Disconnect deceit and desire when discussing infidelity.

Clients and couples who actively engage in ENM relationships might approach therapeutic services seeking support for a range of concerns that may not directly relate to their relationship dynamics. These diverse issues can include financial matters, general communication challenges, or past trauma. Amidst providing assistance on these matters, therapists must remain mindful of the cultural significance and unique experiences of individuals involved in ENM relationships.

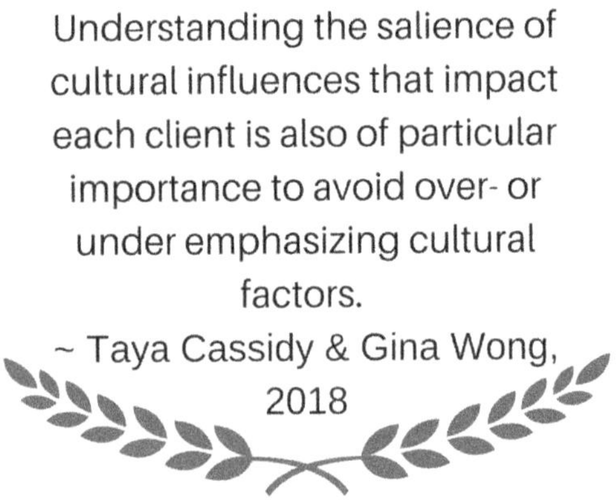

Understanding the salience of cultural influences that impact each client is also of particular importance to avoid over- or under emphasizing cultural factors.
~ Taya Cassidy & Gina Wong, 2018

Figure 3.1 Quote by Cassidy and Wong.
Source: Created by the author.

To ensure ethical therapeutic practice, it becomes essential for therapists to examine and assess their attitudes and values concerning minority populations, specifically those identifying as ENM (Cassidy & Wong, 2018b). Acknowledging the cultural salience of ENM-identified individuals allows therapists to approach their clients with sensitivity, respect, and a genuine understanding of their lived experiences.

By fostering such awareness and cultural competence, therapists can create a therapeutic environment that promotes trust, empathy, and inclusivity. This approach enables therapists to effectively address not only the immediate concerns clients bring to therapy but also to navigate the complexities and nuances of their ENM lifestyles with sensitivity and understanding.

The Aftereffect of Microaggressions

Microaggressions can have a significant impact on marginalized individuals, and it can be challenging for the offender to hear and recognize when they occur. Microaggressions are defined by Merriam-Webster (n.d.) as "a comment or action subtly and often unconsciously or unintentionally expresses a prejudiced attitude toward a marginalized group member" (2021). It is important to understand that individuals in alternative relationships may experience microaggressions and bias from therapists and healthcare providers and may not feel safe or understood in the therapeutic environment.

Holding a negative bias toward alternative relationships can manifest in the clinician's perception of presenting issues. It is essential to acknowledge that a client's ENM relationship status may not be the primary reason for seeking therapy. For instance, a client who is engaging in an alternative relationship may seek treatment for a financial stressor. Still, if the therapist holds a negative bias toward their client's relationship structure, it may impede their clinical judgment and lead to projection and microaggressions within the therapeutic relationship (APA, 2002).

In a research dissertation by Shelton (2009), eight themes emerged from a focus group composed of LGBTQIA+ individuals receiving therapeutic services from licensed professionals. This research is valuable because the Society for the Psychology of Sexual Orientation and Gender Diversity expressed that the LGBTQIA+ community is twice as likely to participate in ENM. The themes that emerged include "invisible minority prejudice and discrimination," "expectation of heterosexuality," "negative media images," "identity confusion," "self-doubt," "internalized oppression," "isolation," and "hopelessness" (Shelton, 2009). These themes highlight the need for healthcare providers and therapists to engage in self-reflection and awareness of potential biases toward marginalized communities and create a safe therapeutic environment for all clients.

The eight sexual orientation microaggression themes are as follows (Sprott et al., 2020):

1   The assumption that sexual orientation *[and/or ENM] is the cause of all presenting issues.
2   Avoidance and minimizing of sexual orientation *[and/or ENM].
3   Attempts to overidentify with LGBTQIA+ *[and/or ENM] clients.
4   Making stereotypical speculations about LGBTQIA+ *[and/or ENM] clients.
5   Assumed dominancy of heterosexuality *[and/or monosexuality].
6   The assumption that LGBTQIA+ *[and/or ENM] individuals need psychotherapeutic services.
7   Practitioners have a "Duty to Warn" LGBTQIA+ individuals about the dangers of identifying with a non-exclusively heterosexual orientation.
8   Underdeveloped themes.

> *This information was added by the author (and was not part of the original research study) to indicate that sexual and relationship orientation can be interchangeable.

Cassidy and Wong (2018a) emphasize that therapists need to explore ways to address the pervasiveness of mononormativity and how it can influence the counseling process. They suggest adopting a culturally aware perspective that involves considering the impact of attitudes from the client and therapist toward ENM in the therapeutic relationship; utilizing theoretical orientations that do not reflect a monocentric bias; and being aware of mononormativity throughout the counseling process, including assessments, intervention strategies, and outcome evaluations (Cassidy & Wong, 2018b).

In situations where therapists unintentionally commit a microaggression toward a client, it is essential to take responsibility and discuss the problem with the client. Miller (2020) emphasizes that avoiding uncomfortable conversations due to discomfort or ignorance is not a valid reason and could be another microaggression. It is more detrimental to the therapeutic relationship to deny or invalidate the client's experience, as this can cause further harm. Instead, therapists should take responsibility for their words or actions and genuinely apologize to the offended client (Miller, 2020).

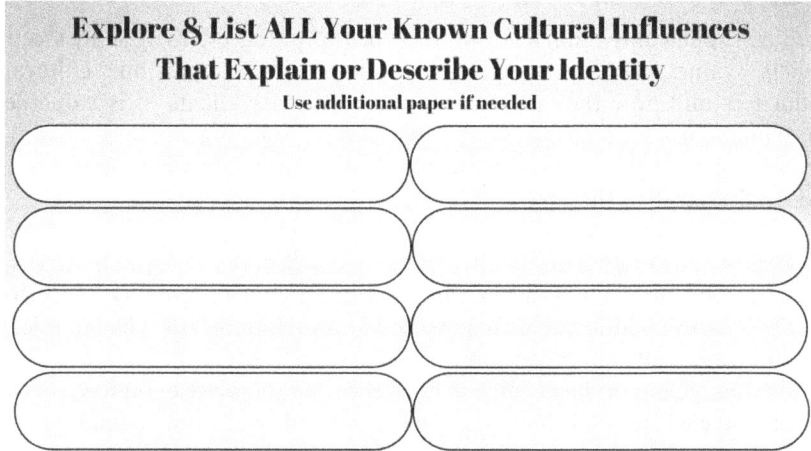

Figure 3.2 Addressing Microaggressions.

Source: Created by the author.

Clinicians' Examination of Own Bias

According to the American Psychological Association (APA), therapists must understand themselves as cultural and racial beings (2002). This means creating a safe therapeutic environment for those seeking therapy for alternative relationships. Therapists should evaluate their biases and acknowledge that monogamous relationships may not be the only healthy and successful relationship structures. Thus, clinicians serving those in alternative relationships need to understand what polyamory, swinging, and other forms of ENM are and what they are not to adequately hold space for the couple (APA, 2002).

To be an effective therapist for this population, one must accept and recognize that ENM is ethical, understand the specific terminology used by clients, and avoid judgment. As with any other population group, all individuals need to feel safe and accepted when seeking therapy, even if the therapist is still learning about alternative models for relationships and families.

A systematic review conducted by FitzGerald and Hurst (2017) found that healthcare providers' preferences may predict their behavior more than initially realized. This review highlights that it is crucial for healthcare providers, including therapists, to check their biases regularly. Failure to check biases can impact interpersonal interactions, leading to biased decision-making or invalidating clients' experiences (FitzGerald & Hurst, 2017).

Suggestions for Exploring Your Bias About ENM

Culture significantly impacts our therapeutic practices, as it shapes our beliefs, values, and perspectives. To better understand our cultural influences and how they may affect our work with clients, it is valuable to explore our past and present experiences. Engaging in the following activities can deepen our self-awareness and enhance our ability to provide culturally sensitive therapy:

1 Reflect on Your Family of Origin: Consider the cultural patterns, traditions, and values instilled in you during your upbringing. How do these aspects influence your perspective on relationships, gender roles, and other cultural dimensions?
2 Examine Geographical Influences: Reflect on the places you have lived or traveled to and how they have shaped your understanding of diversity and cultural differences. How have these experiences expanded your worldview and informed your account of clients from diverse backgrounds?
3 Evaluate Religious and Spiritual Beliefs: Assess how your religious or spiritual beliefs impact your therapeutic approach. Consider how these beliefs may intersect or clash with the values and practices of clients from different religious or spiritual backgrounds.
4 Reflect on Gender and Sexuality: Explore how your own gender identity and sexual orientation inform your understanding of these aspects in therapy. Reflect on any biases or assumptions that may arise and the potential impact on working with clients who have different gender identities or sexual orientations.

Consider Educational Influences: Reflect on the educational institutions you have attended and how they have contributed to your cultural perspectives. How have your educational experiences influenced your understanding of diversity, privilege, and power dynamics in therapy?

Therapists can gain valuable insights into their cultural influences and biases by engaging in these activities, allowing for a more informed and sensitive therapeutic practice.

The influences above have shaped you into the clinician you are today and could permeate your practice if not adequately addressed. To become aware of cultural biases toward ENM, one should evaluate their therapeutic blind spots. The following activities can help you identify and process some of your therapeutic blind spots.

For each cultural influence listed, create an action plan for addressing them when they appear in a therapeutic setting.

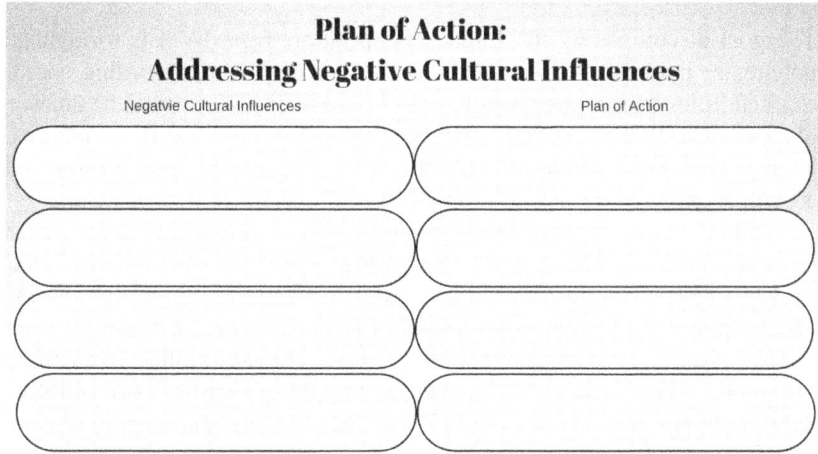

Figure 3.3 Cultural Influences.

Source: Created by the author.

CULTURAGRAM

Time in Community	Legal Status	Language Spoken

Values: Family, Power Myths & Rules

FAMILY MEMBERS

Additional Partners

Impact of Crisis Events	Holidays & Events	Health Beliefs

MULTIPLE PARTNERS

Figure 3.4 Plan of Action.

Source: Created by the author.

Activity 1: Take the Implicit Association Test

The goal of completing the Implicit Association Test (IAT) is to highlight potentially harmful attitudes and beliefs you may have regarding specific characteristics such as age, skin tone, and/or sexuality. You could be unaware of a bias or feel embarrassed or ashamed for having it, leading to avoidance of learning and more stifling self-growth. The departure of learning and self-growth is expected when one is unaware of or ashamed of their biases.

While there are several variations of the IAT, I suggest Project Implicit because of their scope of tests (*Harvard Implicit Association Test*, 2011). Project Implicit is a 501(c)(3) non-profit organization and an international collaboration of researchers interested in implicit social cognition (*Harvard Implicit Association Test*, 2011). The mission of Project Implicit is to educate the public about bias and to provide a "virtual laboratory" for collecting data on the Internet. Project Implicit scientists produce high-impact research that forms the basis of our scientific knowledge about bias and disparities.

*To find Project Implicit, visit https://implicit.harvard.edu/implicit/takeatest.html.

Activity 2: Find Poly and Kink Support Groups in Your Area

When working with creative couples and individuals in alternative relationships, it is crucial for therapists to continue learning and expanding their understanding of these populations. Cultural differences play a significant role in communication styles, problem-solving approaches, and family dynamics, all of which can influence how clients perceive the therapist's assistance (Cassidy & Wong, 2018b).

In order to navigate these complexities, therapists can benefit from attending support groups or establishing relationships with other therapists who specialize in working with alternative relationship dynamics. These connections can provide valuable guidance and support when facing uncomfortable situations or encountering unfamiliar territory (Miller, 2012). Engaging in these professional networks can also contribute to ongoing education and awareness of the diverse experiences and needs of clients in alternative relationships.

While it is essential for therapists to be knowledgeable and informed, it is also important to recognize the expertise that clients possess in their own lives. Each client brings their unique terminology, definitions, and mannerisms that may require clarification. It is acceptable and encouraged for therapists to ask questions and seek clarification from clients to enhance their understanding of their dynamics. However, therapists should be mindful of maintaining the therapeutic role and ensuring that clients do not feel burdened with the responsibility of educating their therapist instead of receiving therapy (Savage & Cruikshank, 2020).

Activity 3: Create a Culturagram

Culturagrams can be a useful tool for clinicians to gain a better understanding of their clients' cultural and familial backgrounds (Furnham & Bochner, 1986). Through the visual representation of a culturagram, clinicians can explore different aspects of their clients' lives, such as language spoken at home, the impact of trauma and crisis events, and family, occupational, and educational influences that have shaped their values. Culturagrams can provide a comprehensive picture of their clients' experiences, which can be particularly helpful when working with clients from diverse backgrounds (D'Andrade, 1995).

When working with clients in open or polyamorous relationships, culturagrams can be modified to help understand the relationship

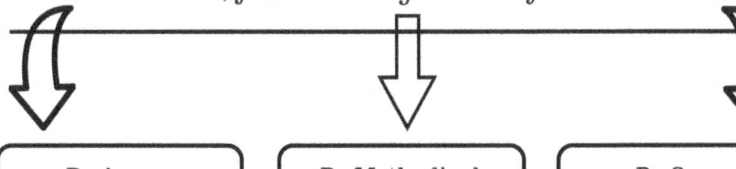

Addressing Microaggressions (Before They Occur)

We all have bias and while you cannot dictate someone else's actions, you can be cognizant of your own actions.

Be Aware	Be Methodical	Be Open
Explore you own biases and how they could present in a therapeutic environment	Utilize guidelines and checklists as a means of transparency when making decisions.	Put yourself in uncomfortable situations that foster learning about various identities

Addressing Microaggressions (After They Occur)

What if you unintentionally commit a microaggression?

INTENT VS IMPACT
~ Your intent does not invalidate the impact
~ Take into consideration the receiver's past experiences

OWN YOUR ACTIONS
~ Own your actions & acknowledge they were biased
~ Accept the consequences

REINFORCE & REPAIR
~ Make contact & begin to rebuild trust in the therapeutic relationship
~ Review your plan of action for addressing the bias

Figure 3.5 Culturagram.

Source: Created by the author.

dynamics between multiple partners with various cultural differences. Relationship dynamics in ENM relationships can be complex, and clients may find it challenging to explain these nuances to their therapists repeatedly. By creating a culturagram that visualizes these complexities, clinicians can better understand their clients' experiences and provide more effective support (Savage & Cruikshank, 2020).

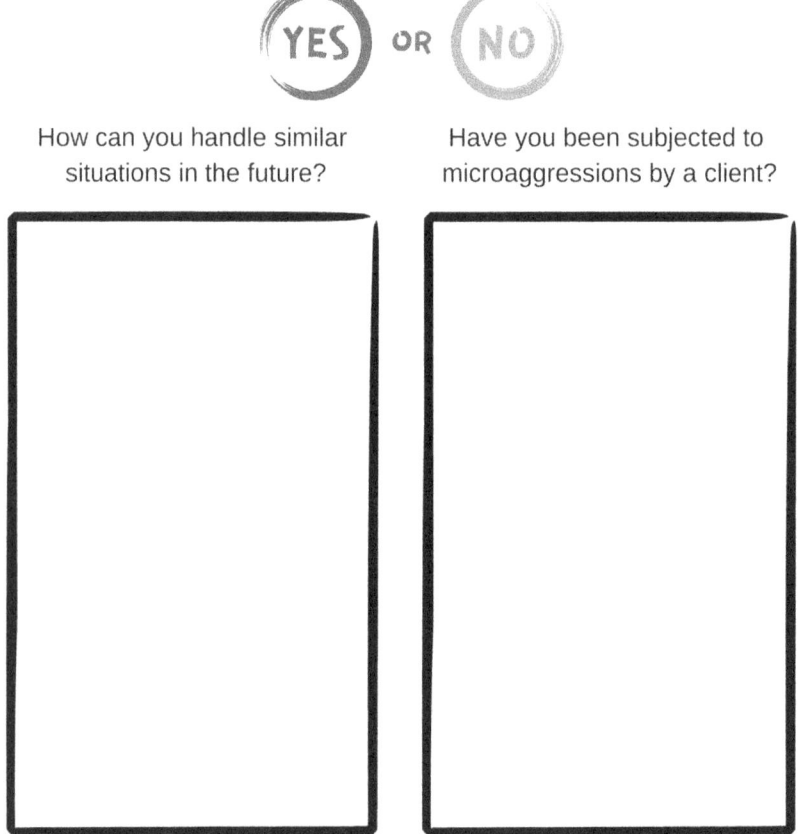

Figure 3.6 Reflection Time.

Source: Created by the author.

As clinicians working with complicated relationship dynamics, it is essential to recognize that mistakes can be made. It is crucial to be honest and open about processing discomfort when mistakes occur. Practitioners who are receptive to their biases and demonstrate a willingness to acknowledge uncertainty and unintentional microaggressions can create a supportive therapeutic environment that enhances the client's experience (Miller, 2020). Addressing errors with honesty and an open mind can lead to a more significant therapeutic relationship, preventing clients from reaching a stressful crisis point.

Chapter Highlights

- Interest in ENM has increased. Therapists who can explore their clients' subjective experiences are more helpful than those who cannot do so. A significant part of the ethical therapeutic practice involves the evaluation of the therapist's attitude, values, and biases toward the ENM lifestyle. As with any clientele, the therapeutic environment must be safe and judgment-free.
- Activity 1: Take the IAT. The objective of completing the IAT is to highlight potentially harmful attitudes and beliefs you may have regarding specific characteristics such as age, skin tone, and/or sexuality.
- Activity 2: Find Poly and Kink support groups in your area. You might have been a therapist for many years and feel nothing can shock you any longer, but nothing is taboo regarding creative sexual couples. If this is a new population you are adding to your practice, there could be some cultural differences that should be considered.
- Activity 3: Create a culturagram. Creating a visual tool like a culturagram can help a clinician understand the client's familial and cultural background.

References

American Psychological Association. (2002). Guidelines on multicultural education, training, research, practice, and organizational change for psychologists. *American Psychological Association*.

Cassidy, C., & Wong, S. (2018a). Multicultural and social justice counseling competencies in the 21st century. In S. D. Brown & R. W. Lent (Eds.), *Handbook of counseling psychology* (5th ed., pp. 119–135). Wiley. 10.1002/97811193 74333.ch5

Cassidy, T., & Wong, G. (2018b, March 25). Consensually non-monogamous clients and the impact of mononormativity in therapy. *Canadian Journal of Counselling and Psychotherapy*. Retrieved October 12, 2022, from https://cjc-rcc. ucalgary.ca/article/view/61124

D'Andrade, R. G. (1995). *The development of cognitive anthropology*. Cambridge University Press.

FitzGerald, C., & Hurst, S. (2017). Implicit bias in healthcare professionals: A systematic review. *BMC Medical Ethics, 18*(1). 10.1186/s12910-017-0179-8

Furnham, A., & Bochner, S. (1986). *Culture shock: Psychological reactions to unfamiliar environments* (Vol. *13*). Methuen.

Harvard Implicit Association Test. (2011). *About us*. Project Implicit. Retrieved January 12, 2023, from https://implicit.harvard.edu/implicit/aboutus.html

Merriam-Webster. (n.d.). *Microaggression definition & meaning*. Merriam-Webster. Retrieved January 12, 2023, from https://www.merriam-webster.com/dictionary/microaggression

Miller, A. (2020, December 5). *Fellow white therapists—We need to talk about our microaggressions toward clients immediately*. Medium. Retrieved January 12, 2023, from https://medium.com/amalgam/fellow-white-therapists-we-need-to-talk-about-our-microaggressions-toward-clients-c632ed452fb3#:~:text=Discomfort%20is%20not%20a%20valid,with%20clients%20of%20many%20cultures

Miller, E. (2020, June 11). How to handle accidentally committing microaggressions. Verywell Mind. https://www.verywellmind.com/how-to-handle-accidentally-committing-microaggressions-5085779

Miller, K. (2012). A therapist's primary questions when the unexplored happens in therapy. *Journal of Family Psychotherapy, 23*(3), 235–246. 10.1080/08975353.2012.704434

Moors, A. C., Matsick, J. L., & Schechinger, H. A. (2017). Unique and shared relationship benefits of consensually non-monogamous and monogamous relationships: A review and insights for moving forward. *European Psychologist, 22*(1), 55–71. 10.1027/1016-9040/a000278

Moors, A. C., & Schechinger, H. (2014). Understanding sexuality: Implications of Rubin for relationship research and clinical practice. *Sexual and Relationship Therapy, 29*(4), 476–482. 10.1080/14681994.2014.941347

Savage, S., & Cruikshank, M. L. (2020). Therapy with polyamorous and consensually non-monogamous clients: Guidelines for practice. *Family Process, 59*(2), 488–503. 10.1111/famp.12464

Schechinger, H. (2015, May 15). *Toward guidelines for psychological practice with consensually non-monogamous clients: Results from a mixed-method analysis of therapy practices and outcomes*. KU ScholarWorks. Retrieved April 30, 2022, from https://kuscholarworks.ku.edu/handle/1808/22028

Schechinger, H. A., Sakaluk, J. K., & Moors, A. C. (2018). Harmful and helpful therapy practices with consensually non-monogamous clients: Toward an inclusive framework. *Journal of Consulting and Clinical Psychology, 86*(11), 879–891. 10.1037/ccp0000349

Shelton, K. L. (2009). *Sexual orientation microaggressions: The experience of lesbian, gay, bisexual and queer clients in psychotherapy* (dissertation). The University of Georgia, Athens, GA.

Sprott, R. A., Vivid, J., Vilkin, E., Swallow, L., Lev, E. M., Orejudos, J., & Schnittman, D. (2020). A queer boundary: How sex and BDSM interact for people who identify as kinky. *Sexualities, 24*(5–6), 708–732. 10.1177/1363460720944594

Weitzman, G. D. (2017). Counseling clients in polyamorous relationships. *Foundations for Couples' Therapy*, 310–319. 10.4324/9781315678610-31

Clinical Misconceptions about Alternative Relationships

Clinical Misconceptions About Alternative Relationships

Most therapists who received their training in the United States were taught a monocentric point of view, essentially stating that any other relationship dynamic is wrong. Clients in alternative relationships seek therapeutic services for the same reasons monogamous clients do and for the controversy surrounding having multiple partners. However, when clinicians automatically assume that all of the difficulties and issues within their relationship stem from being ethically non-monogamous, they are left unassisted on their journey to cultivating their version of a healthy relationship.

According to research conducted by Haupert et al. (2016), "people engaged in ethical non-monogamy (ENM) experience unjustified stigma, as empirical evidence does not support the belief that these individuals are fundamentally flawed citizens, poor relationship partners, or inadequate parents." Furthermore, clinicians who lack adequate training are at a higher risk of causing more harm to the clients, perpetuating their mental distress.

To fully understand the complexities of ENM, one must explore common misconceptions made by those not living an alternative lifestyle. Unfortunately, a large portion of misinformation is aimed at polyamory, relationships consisting of multiple partners living together as a family raising children or in different locations but still considered family. As previously mentioned, other alternative relationships are swinging, open relationships, and various other dynamics discussed in Chapter 2.

Common misconceptions include the following:

- ENM violates all religious tenets
- ENM is against the law
- ENM perpetuates child abuse and neglect
- ENM promotes sex addiction
- ENM indicates attachment disorders

DOI: 10.4324/9781003464891-6

- ENM is cheating
- ENM as a means to repair a marriage
- ENM means never experiencing jealousy
- ENM promotes sexually transmitted infections (STIs).

Does ENM Violate All Religious Tenets?

Religious attitudes toward ENM vary widely. For conservative or fundamentalist sects of Christianity, Islam, and Judaism, extramarital sex is strongly condemned, and the family structure is based on sexual exclusivity for women. These religions prioritize sexual fidelity within a monogamous marriage, and polyamorous relationships are not accepted (Sheff, 2015).

Christianity, Islam, and Judaism all place importance on sexual relationships within the confines of a recognized marriage and discourage sexual relationships outside of that union. These religions value a woman's purity on her wedding day and expect continued fidelity throughout the marriage to her husband (Sheff, 2014a,b).

Within Christianity, beliefs about sexuality are derived from the Bible, which emphasizes the importance of physical intimacy within marriage for procreation and as a symbol of the union between Christ and His Church. While there are examples of polygynous marriages in the Bible, modern branches of Christianity generally reject polyamory because it allows women to have multiple partners (Focus on the Family, 2023).

In Islam, polygyny is accepted, with men being allowed to have up to four wives as long as they can financially support them. However, women are held to strict standards and are only permitted to have sexual experiences with their husbands. Adultery is severely punished, and a woman's virginity and fidelity to her husband are emphasized (Sheff, 2014a,b).

It is important to note that these are generalizations, and each religious community may interpret and apply their beliefs differently. Some individuals within these religions may have more open and accepting attitudes toward ENM, while others may strongly oppose it. The level of acceptance will largely depend on the specific denomination or interpretation of the religion.

Is ENM Against the Law?

While ENM itself is not illegal, the legal consequences of adultery can impact those practicing non-monogamy. According to Edward Stein, Professor of Law and Director of the Gertrud Mainzer Program in Family Law, Policy, and Bioethics at Cardozo School of Law, 38 states have laws related explicitly to adultery but are rarely enforced (2019).

Adultery is grounds for divorce in the majority of states, and some states have family laws that punish adultery. Adultery can also have indirect legal consequences, such as losing a job or being denied housing. Additionally, the courts may award smaller percentages of shared assets to the adulterer in a divorce settlement (Stein, 2019).

Professor Stein notes that both adultery and ENM are often treated similarly in the judicial system, which can be problematic for those practicing consensual non-monogamy. For example, some states have "heart balm" tort suits that allow emotionally damaged spouses to recover damages from the offending spouse's paramour for wrongful behavior (Stein, 2019).

Overall, while not illegal, the legal landscape of ENM is complex and can have significant consequences for those who practice it. Individuals need to be aware of the laws in their state and take steps to protect themselves legally and emotionally in consensual non-monogamous relationships.

Does ENM Perpetuate Child Abuse and Neglect?

Research suggests that ENM does not perpetuate child abuse or neglect more than monogamous relationships (The Conversation, 2023). Though child abuse is universal, the author of "The Polyamorists Next Door," Dr. Elisabeth Sheff, expressed that children in poly families may receive better care and attention from their parents than those in monogamous homes. Sheff explains that polyamorous relationships provide three or more participating parents with the time to practice healthy self-care, which gives them more energy and resources to invest in the children within the household. In comparison, monogamous two-parent homes are often sleep-deprived, do not take care of their personal needs, and may require working longer hours to support the family (The Conversation, 2023).

Furthermore, according to Sheff, the assumption that individuals who engage in unconventional relationships have no sexual boundaries is erroneous (The Conversation, 2023). This assertion holds for all non-monogamous relationships, including polyamorous ones, as research indicates individuals in these relationships are not more likely to molest children than individuals in conventional relationships (Sheff, 2015).

Does ENM Promote Sex Addiction?

The notion of "sex addiction" as a clinical diagnosis has been rejected by the American Psychiatric Association (APA) in the fifth edition of the Diagnostic and Statistical Manual (DSM-V) published in 2013. Within the field of clinical sexology, the concept of addiction concerning sex is not widely accepted (APA, 2013). The American Association of Sex Educators, Counselors, and Therapists (AASECT), founded in 1967, released a statement in 2016 stating that it does not endorse or recognize the diagnosis of sex addiction (2016). AASECT does acknowledge that individuals may experience significant physical, psychological, spiritual, and sexual health consequences due to their sexual urges, thoughts, or behaviors. Still, it recommends using models that do not pathologize ethical sexual behaviors (2016).

AASECT explicitly states that it does not find sufficient empirical evidence to support the classification of sex addiction or porn addiction as mental health disorders, and it does not see the training and treatment methods related to sexual addiction to be adequately informed by accurate knowledge of human sexuality (2016). Therefore, AASECT does not advocate for the use of sex addiction as a standard of practice for sexuality education, counseling, or therapy (2016).

Instead, the term "out-of-control sexual behavior" (OCSB) is often used by sexologists to describe unhealthy and compulsive sexual behaviors (Vigorito et al., 2016). It is important to note that no universally determined or recommended amount of sex is considered "normal" or "too much." Sexuality researcher Rhea Orion, the author of "A Therapist's Guide to Consensual Nonmonogamy: Polyamory, Swinging, and Open Marriage," highlights that ENM, with its emphasis on honesty, safe practices, and open communication, is not conducive to fostering compulsive sexual desires (Orion, 2018).

Does ENM Indicate Attachment Disorders?

The study of attachment theory is exceedingly mononormative; therefore, the research and resources regarding ENM are limited. Jessica Fern, the author of *Polysecure: Attachment, Trauma, and Consensual Non-Monogamy*, provided that a large portion of the study conducted to understand romantic attachment further is with monogamous couples, and the available information regarding how to establish secure attachment in relationships indicates that monogamy is necessary for creating safety and security.

The limited research conducted at the time of this book has found that there is little to no difference in attachment anxiety levels among monogamous and non-monogamous. A study by Moors et al., *Multiple Loves: The Effects of Attachment with Multiple Concurrent Romantic Partners on Relational Functioning* (2019), explored the attachment styles of over 350 individuals who identify as polyamorous and are currently in two or more different relationships. The research indicated that those practicing polyamory demonstrated secure attachment styles with all involved partners, and "having more of an insecure style with one specific partner did not affect the attachment functioning of their other relationships" (Fern, 2020).

Does ENM Constitute Cheating?

Cheating can be defined as when two individuals in a relationship have agreed to be sexually exclusive. Still, one or more partners engage in emotional and/or sexual activities outside of the relationship without the knowledge or consent of their partner(s) while implying that they are monogamous (Mark et al., 2011).

In contrast, ENM involves creating agreements and boundaries between partners that outline expectations for the relationship (Fern, 2020). In ENM relationships, all participants are aware of and consent to the non-monogamous nature of the relationship, and any changes in the relationship dynamic are carefully and thoughtfully negotiated and communicated among all involved parties (Fern, 2020). Jessica Fern, the author of *Polysecure: Attachment, Trauma, and Consensual Non-Monogamy*, explains that ENM means that all parties involved have agreed to the arrangement (Fern, 2020).

By openly discussing and defining the terms of their relationship, individuals in ENM relationships can maintain trust, transparency, and honesty among all partners. This allows for a consensual exploration of multiple relationships or sexual experiences outside of the primary partnership.

Does ENM Indicate Marriage Issues?

While some couples may consider ENM as a solution to their marital problems, it is essential to note that most couples who practice ENM did not enter this lifestyle to save their marriages. Research suggests that couples who engage in ENM have healthy communication patterns and experience increases in sexual satisfaction, suggesting that ENM does not necessarily indicate marital issues.

A study conducted by Murphy, Joel, and Muise titled "A Prospective Investigation of the Decision to Open Up a Romantic Relationship" in 2021 explored the motivations and experiences of individuals who chose to open up their romantic relationships to non-monogamy. The findings of this study indicated that couples who practiced ENM reported higher levels of relationship satisfaction, sexual satisfaction, and overall communication compared to monogamous couples. It also found that those who opened up their relationship to ENM did so as a mutual choice and intending to explore and expand their sexual and emotional connections rather than as a desperate attempt to fix underlying marital issues (Murphy et al., 2021).

Therefore, it is crucial to challenge the misconception that ENM is solely pursued to save troubled marriages. Many couples who engage in ENM do so to nurture and enhance their existing relationships by embracing the principles of open communication, consent, and exploration of multiple connections.

Does ENM Mean That There Is No Jealousy Experienced?

Jealousy is a common experience within ENM relationships. However, research suggests that individuals who practice ENM can process and manage feelings of jealousy by engaging in open communication with their partner(s) and negotiating agreements regarding acceptable extradyadic sexual or romantic behaviors (Mogilski et al., 2019). By having open and honest conversations about boundaries, participants in ENM relationships can effectively navigate and manage jealousy.

A study conducted by Mogilski et al. (2019) examined the experiences of individuals in consensually non-monogamous relationships, including how they handle jealousy. The study's findings indicated that when individuals in ENM relationships experienced jealousy, they were more likely to communicate openly with their partner(s) about these feelings. Through these conversations and negotiations, the participants established mutual understanding and agreements regarding behaviors and boundaries within the relationship. This process helped them manage feelings of jealousy and prevent consent violations when negotiated agreements are transgressed, leading to interpersonal distress (Mogilski et al., 2019).

By engaging in open and honest communication, individuals in ENM relationships can address and navigate their jealous feelings healthily and constructively. This approach allows for establishing clear boundaries and agreements, promoting trust, understanding, and overall relationship satisfaction.

Does ENM Promote the Spread of STIs?

Research studies indicate that individuals who make monogamous agreements are not immune to cheating and that such behavior often occurs with less attention to safe sex practices and health risks. In contrast, people practicing ENM show more significant concern and care for their sexual health and that of their partners.

A study conducted by Lehmiller (2015) explored the sexual behavior of individuals who engage in consensual non-monogamy versus monogamy, specifically concerning safe sex practices and health risks (Lehmiller, 2015). The findings indicated that individuals who practice consensual non-monogamy tend to report more responsible sexual behavior, including greater condom use, more frequent STI testing, and a lower likelihood of transmitting infections to their partners compared to individuals in monogamous relationships (Lehmiller, 2015).

Moreover, the study revealed that individuals in monogamous relationships who engage in extramarital affairs are likely to take fewer precautions to protect their sexual health and the health of their partners during such encounters. This pattern has heightened the potential for STI transmission and other health risks (Lehmiller, 2015).

These findings highlight the importance of prioritizing safe sex practices and taking proactive measures for maintaining sexual health, especially in the context of non-monogamous relationships. By engaging in open and honest conversations about sexual health and disease prevention, individuals practicing ENM can effectively manage risks while maintaining fulfilling intimate connections.

Chapter Highlights

- Most therapists in the United States have a monocentric point of view. Clinicians should not automatically assume that all relationship difficulties stem from being ethically non-monogamous.
- Therapists should explore common misconceptions about ENM involving religion, the law, what ENM does and doesn't promote and consist of, and other dynamics that are often misconstrued.
- Common misconceptions include the following:

  - ENM violates all religious tenets
  - ENM is against the law
  - ENM perpetuates child abuse and neglect
  - ENM promotes sex addiction
  - ENM indicates attachment disorders
  - ENM is cheating
  - ENM as a means to repair a marriage
  - ENM means never experiencing jealousy
  - ENM promotes STIs.

References

AASECT. (2016). *AASECT position on sex addiction: AASECT: American Association of Sexuality Educators, Counselors and Therapists.* Retrieved January 12, 2023, from https://www.aasect.org/position-sex-addiction

American Psychiatric Association. (2013). *Diagnostic and statistical manual of mental disorders (DSM-5®).* American Psychiatric Publishing.

Fern, J. (2020). *Polysecure: Attachment, trauma and consensual nonmonogamy.* Thorntree Press, LLC.

Focus on the Family. (2023, August 21). *Oral and anal sex: Biblical guidelines for intimacy in marriage.* Retrieved from https://www.focusonthefamily.com/family-qa/oral-and-anal-sex-biblical-guidelines-for-intimacy-in-marriage/

Haupert, M. L., Gesselman, A. N., Moors, A. C., Fisher, H. E., & Garcia, J. R. (2016). Prevalence of experiences with consensual non-monogamous relationships: Findings from two national samples of single Americans. *Journal of Sex & Marital Therapy, 43*(5), 424–440. 10.1080/0092623x.2016.1178675

Lehmiller, J. J. (2015). A comparison of sexual health history and practices among monogamous and consensually non-monogamous sexual partners. *The Journal of Sexual Medicine, 12*(10), 2022–2028. 10.1111/jsm.12987

Mark, K. P., Janssen, E., & Milhausen, R. R. (2011). Infidelity in heterosexual couples: Demographic, interpersonal, and personality-related predictors of extradyadic sex. *Archives of sexual behavior, 40*(5), 971–982.

Mogilski, J. K., Reeve, S. D., Nicolas, S. C., Donaldson, S. H., Mitchell, V. E., & Welling, L. L. (2019). Jealousy, consent, and compersion within monogamous and consensually non-monogamous romantic relationships. *Archives of Sexual Behavior, 48*(6), 1811–1828. 10.1007/s10508-018-1286-4

Moors, A. C., Ryan, W., & Chopik, W. J. (2019). Multiple loves: The effects of attachment with multiple concurrent romantic partners on relational functioning. *APA PsycInfo, 147*, 102–110. 10.1016/j.paid.2019.04.023

Murphy, P. A., Joel, S., & Muse, A. (2021). A prospective investigation of the decision to open up a romantic relationship – Annelise Parkes Murphy, Samantha Joel, Amy Muise, 2021. *Social Psychological and Personality Science, 12*(2), 194–201. https://journals.sagepub.com/doi/abs/10.1177/1948550 619897157?journalCode=sppa

Orion, R. (2018). *A therapist's guide to consensual nonmonogamy: Polyamory, swinging, and open marriage.* Routledge.

Sheff, E. (2014a). The relationship among polyamory, swinging, and open relationships in the United States. *Journal of Sex Research, 51*(6), 588–600.

Sheff, E. (2014b). *Religious attitudes towards polyamory.* Psychology Today. Retrieved January 12, 2023, from https://www.psychologytoday.com/us/blog/ the-polyamorists-next-door/201401/religious-attitudes-towards-polyamory

Sheff, E. (2015). *The polyamorists next door: Inside multiple-partner relationships and families.* Rowman & Littlefield.

Stein, E. (2019). Adultery and non-monogamy: A legal minefield. *Family Law Quarterly, 53*(1), 149–169.

The Conversation. (2023, April 24). Ethical non-monogamy: What to know about these often misunderstood relationships. Retrieved from https://theconversation. com/us/topics/ethical-non-monogamy-137516

Vigorito, A., Arial, M., & Cortoni, F. (2016). Beyond myth and towards a multidimensional understanding of hypersexuality. *Current Sexual Health Reports, 8*(4), 221–230.

Chapter 5

Ethical Clinical Practice with ENM

Ethical Clinical Practice with ENM

Governing institutions for mental health practitioners, such as professional associations, often have ethical codes highlighting the importance of cultural humility and competence when working with clients from diverse backgrounds or lifestyles (Duke, 2022). These codes emphasize the therapist's responsibility to provide effective and culturally appropriate care to all clients, regardless of their familiarity or experience with specific populations.

These codes' ethical principles and guidelines serve as a valuable resource for therapists to reference and refresh their knowledge of best practices. For example, the American Psychological Association (APA) provides a comprehensive code of ethics that addresses the importance of cultural competence and the need for ongoing education and awareness (APA, 2017). The National Association of Social Workers (NASW) also emphasizes cultural competence in its Code of Ethics (2021).

When working with clients in open or polyamorous relationships, therapists can consult these ethical codes to ensure they uphold their professional obligations and provide quality care. The Step 8: Managing Relationships section mentioned can guide therapists in navigating the dynamics of alternative relationships and utilizing the information discussed with clients appropriately and ethically.

By familiarizing themselves with the ethical codes and regularly reviewing the guidelines, therapists can ensure that they meet their professional obligations and provide culturally sensitive and competent care to all clients, including those in alternative relationships.

***

DOI: 10.4324/9781003464891-7

CLINICAL, SCHOOL, AND COUNSELING PSYCHOLOGY: AMERICAN PSYCHOLOGICAL ASSOCIATION (APA)

Principle A: Beneficence and Nonmaleficence

Psychologists strive to benefit those with whom they work and take care to do no harm. In their professional actions, psychologists seek to safeguard the welfare and rights of those with whom they interact professionally and other affected persons, and the welfare of animal subjects of research. When conflicts occur among psychologists' obligations or concerns, they attempt to resolve these conflicts in a responsible fashion that avoids or minimizes harm. Because psychologists' scientific and professional judgments and actions may affect the lives of others, they are alert to and guard against personal, financial, social, organizational, or political factors that might lead to misuse of their influence. Psychologists strive to be aware of the possible effect of their own physical and mental health on their ability to help those with whom they work.

Clinical Considerations

When working with ethical non-monogamous individuals, therapists can incorporate the principles of beneficence and nonmaleficence (doing good and avoiding harm) in the following ways:

1   Benefit the client.

- Therapists should focus on the well-being of their clients and provide them with interventions and strategies that support their mental health and relationship satisfaction. This may involve exploring communication skills, boundary-setting, and conflict-resolution techniques for ethical non-monogamous relationships.

2   Not harm.

- Therapists should ensure that their interventions and client interactions do not cause harm. They should be mindful of any personal biases, judgments, or assumptions they may hold about ethical non-monogamy and work toward creating a safe and non-judgmental therapeutic space.

3   Safeguard welfare and rights.

- Therapists should respect and uphold the rights and welfare of their clients in ethical non-monogamous relationships. This includes ensuring confidentiality, informed consent, and the client's autonomy in decision-making.

4 Resolve conflicts responsibly.

- Whenever conflicts arise between therapists' obligations or concerns, they should strive to find responsible and ethical resolutions that minimize harm. This may involve seeking consultation or supervision to navigate complex issues and prioritize the client's best interests.

5 Avoid misuse of influence.

- Therapists should be aware of and guard against personal, financial, social, organizational, or political factors that might compromise the ethical care they provide to ethical non-monogamous individuals. They should prioritize the client's needs and avoid actions that could exploit or misuse their professional influence.

6 Attend to their well-being.

- Recognizing that their own physical and mental health can impact their ability to provide adequate care, therapists should prioritize self-care and seek support or supervision as needed. This ensures they are in the best state to support and facilitate their clients' growth and well-being.

By incorporating the principles of beneficence and nonmaleficence, therapists can provide ethical and practical care to individuals in ethical non-monogamous relationships, fostering their personal growth and relationship satisfaction while maintaining professional integrity.

**

CLINICAL, SCHOOL, AND COUNSELING PSYCHOLOGY: AMERICAN PSYCHOLOGICAL ASSOCIATION (APA)

Principle E: Respect for People's Rights and Dignity

Psychologists respect the dignity and worth of all people and the rights of individuals to privacy, confidentiality, and self-determination. Psychologists know that special safeguards may be necessary to protect the rights and welfare of persons or communities whose vulnerabilities impair autonomous decision-making. Psychologists are aware of and respect cultural, individual, and role differences, including those based on age, gender, gender identity, race, ethnicity, culture, national origin, religion, sexual orientation, disability, language, and socioeconomic status, and consider these factors when working with members of such groups. Psychologists try to eliminate the effect on their work of biases based on those factors, and they do not knowingly participate in or condone the activities of others based upon such prejudices.

Clinical Considerations

Incorporating the principle of Respect for People's Rights and Dignity when working with ethical non-monogamous individuals, therapists can adopt the following practices:

1 Create a safe and non-judgmental space.

- Therapists should create an environment that is accepting, non-judgmental, and safe for ethical non-monogamous individuals to express themselves without fear of discrimination or prejudice.
- They should validate and respect the individuals' relationship choices, even if they differ from societal norms or personal beliefs.
- They should be knowledgeable about ethical non-monogamy and its various forms to understand these individuals' unique challenges and dynamics.

2 Cultural competence.

- Therapists should be aware of and respect individual and cultural differences when working with ethical non-monogamous individuals.
- They should understand how factors such as age, gender, gender identity, race, ethnicity, culture, religion, sexual orientation, disability, language, and socioeconomic status can influence individuals' lived experiences and challenges in ethical non-monogamous relationships.
- They should work to eliminate any biases based on these factors and ensure that their values or prejudices do not impact their therapeutic approach.

3 Validate autonomy and self-determination.

- Therapists should respect and support the autonomy and self-determination of their clients in ethical non-monogamous relationships.
- They should recognize that individuals can decide their relationship structures and define boundaries and rules.
- They should avoid imposing their values or judgments on their clients' choices and support them in finding their paths to fulfillment and well-being.

4   Protect privacy and confidentiality.

- Therapists should prioritize maintaining privacy and confidentiality for ethical non-monogamous individuals.
- They should be aware of the potential sensitivities around non-monogamy and keep their clients' personal information, relationship details, and identities confidential.
- They should follow ethical guidelines and legal regulations regarding confidentiality and take appropriate measures to protect their clients' privacy.

5   Avoid participating in prejudices.

- Therapists should not knowingly participate in or support activities that discriminate against or oppress individuals in ethical non-monogamous relationships.
- They should be proactive in recognizing and addressing their biases or prejudices, and they should actively seek to eliminate the impact of these biases on their work with their clients.
- They should advocate for the rights and well-being of ethical non-monogamous individuals and actively work toward societal acceptance and understanding of diverse relationship structures.

By incorporating these practices, therapists can uphold the Respect for People's Rights and Dignity when working with ethical non-monogamous individuals and create a therapeutic environment that fosters growth, understanding, and support.

***

CLINICAL, SCHOOL, AND COUNSELING PSYCHOLOGY: AMERICAN PSYCHOLOGICAL ASSOCIATION (APA)

2.01 Boundaries of Competence

a   Psychologists provide services, teach, and conduct research with populations and in areas only within the boundaries of their competence, based on their education, training, supervised experience, consultation, study, or professional experience.

b   Where scientific or professional knowledge in the discipline of psychology establishes that an understanding of factors associated with age, gender, gender identity, race, ethnicity, culture, national origin, religion, sexual orientation, disability, language, or socioeconomic status is essential for effective implementation of their services or research, psychologists have or obtain the training, experience, consultation, or supervision necessary to ensure the competence of their services, or they make appropriate referrals, except as provided in Standard 2.02, Providing Services in Emergencies.

c Psychologists planning to provide services, teach, or conduct research involving populations, areas, techniques, or technologies new to them undertake relevant education, training, supervised experience, consultation, or study.

d When psychologists are asked to provide services to individuals for whom appropriate mental health services are not available and for which psychologists have not obtained the competence necessary, psychologists with closely related prior training or experience may provide such services in order to ensure that services are not denied if they make a reasonable effort to obtain the competence required by using relevant research, training, consultation, or study.

Clinical Considerations

Incorporating the principle of Boundaries of Competence when working with ethical non-monogamous individuals, therapists can adopt the following practices:

1 Seeking education and training.

- Therapists should seek education and training to understand the unique challenges and dynamics of ethical non-monogamous relationships and incorporate this knowledge into their practice.
- They should seek out coursework, seminars, workshops, or supervised experience opportunities to learn about ethical non-monogamy.
- They should be knowledgeable about different types of ethical non-monogamous relationships and variations of non-monogamy to ensure competence in treating diverse clients.

2 Knowing limitations.

- Therapists should be aware of their limitations in treating ethical non-monogamous individuals and not provide services beyond the boundaries of their competence.
- They should recognize that ethical non-monogamy is a specialized area of practice. They should refer clients to other qualified professionals if they do not have the necessary education, training, or experience.
- They should be able to identify situations in which a referral to a specialist is necessary.

3 Staying current with research.

- Therapists should stay current with the most recent research and best practices regarding ethical non-monogamy.
- They should be aware of advancements in the field, such as new treatment modalities, research findings, and ethical guidelines, and integrate them into their practice.
- They should participate in continuing education or consultation to stay updated with advancements in the field.

4 Establishing limits.

- Therapists should establish limits in their practice when working with ethical non-monogamous individuals to maintain professional boundaries.
- They should recognize the potential for multiple relationships in the context of ethical non-monogamous individuals and maintain objectivity even when they have personal relationships with individuals involved in ethical non-monogamy.
- They should modify their role or withdraw from working with these individuals if conflicts of interest arise.

5 Taking steps in emergencies.

- In situations where appropriate mental health services are not available for ethical non-monogamous individuals, therapists with closely related prior training or experience may provide such services to ensure that services are not denied.
- Therapists should ensure that they make every effort to obtain the necessary competence required through research, training, consultation, or study to provide ethical non-monogamous individuals with appropriate mental health services.

By incorporating these practices, therapists can uphold the principle of Boundaries of Competence when working with ethical non-monogamous individuals and provide competent and ethical care that supports their clients' well-being.

***

CLINICAL, SCHOOL, AND COUNSELING PSYCHOLOGY: AMERICAN PSYCHOLOGICAL ASSOCIATION (APA)

2.03 Maintaining Competence

Psychologists undertake ongoing efforts to develop and maintain their competence.

Clinical Considerations

Incorporating the principle of Maintaining Competence when working with ethical non-monogamous individuals, therapists can adopt the following practices:

1   Continuing education.

    • Therapists should engage in ongoing professional development and continuing education to expand their knowledge and skills related to ethical non-monogamy.
    • They should attend workshops, conferences, or webinars focused on ethical non-monogamy and related topics to stay updated with the latest research and best practices.
    • They should seek relevant literature, articles, and books to deepen their understanding and maintain competence.

2   Consultation and supervision.

    • Therapists should seek consultation or supervision from experienced professionals to enhance their competence when working with ethical non-monogamous individuals.
    • They could reach out to experts in ethical non-monogamy or join peer consultation groups to discuss cases, receive feedback, and learn from others' experiences.
    • Regular consultation or supervision can help therapists reflect on their work, identify areas for growth, and ensure they are providing the highest quality of care.

3   Self-reflection and self-assessment.

    • Therapists should engage in self-reflection and self-assessment to identify their strengths and areas for improvement when working with ethical non-monogamous individuals.
    • They should critically evaluate their knowledge, skills, and attitudes to ensure competence in this specialized practice area.
    • They could set personal goals for professional growth, seek feedback from clients or colleagues, and engage in self-directed learning to address gaps in their competence.

4   Professional networks and communities.

    • Therapists should actively engage with professional networks and communities focused on ethical non-monogamy.
    • They can join online forums, social media groups, or professional organizations dedicated to ethical non-monogamy to connect with

other professionals and stay informed about the latest developments in the field.

- Collaborating and sharing knowledge with colleagues can support ongoing competence development and provide valuable opportunities for learning and growth.

5 Evaluation of effectiveness.

- Therapists should regularly evaluate the effectiveness of their interventions and approaches when working with ethical non-monogamous individuals.
- They should collect and analyze client feedback, track treatment outcomes, and assess their performance to ensure they provide effective and culturally sensitive care.
- This self-evaluation process enables therapists to identify areas for improvement, make necessary adjustments, and maintain their competence in working with ethical non-monogamous individuals.

By incorporating these practices, therapists can uphold the principle of Maintaining Competence when working with ethical non-monogamous individuals, ensuring they provide the most effective and ethical care possible.

***

CLINICAL, SCHOOL, AND COUNSELING PSYCHOLOGY: AMERICAN PSYCHOLOGICAL ASSOCIATION (APA)

3.04 Avoiding Harm

a Psychologists take reasonable steps to avoid harming their clients/patients, students, supervisees, research participants, organizational clients, and others with whom they work, and to minimize harm where it is foreseeable and unavoidable.

Clinical Considerations

When working with ethical non-monogamous individuals, psychologists must take reasonable steps to avoid harming their clients/patients, students, supervisees, research participants, organizational clients, and others with whom they work and minimize harm where it is foreseeable and unavoidable (APA, 2017).

Here are some examples of how therapists can incorporate this principle into their practice:

1   Assessing individual and relationship functioning.

- Therapists should assess each non-monogamous individual's and their partners' physical, mental, emotional, and social functioning levels to ensure the potential for harm is minimized.
- They should evaluate the relationship dynamics to identify and address any potential sources of harm.
- They should help clients develop communication skills and conflict resolution strategies to avoid or manage harm when conflicts arise.

2   Providing education and information.

- Therapists should provide accurate and non-judgmental information to clients about ethical non-monogamy, including associated risks and benefits.
- They should educate clients on sexually transmitted infections (STIs) and prevention, as risk factors for STIs can increase in non-monogamous relationships (Schrimshaw et al., 2013).
- They should discuss the importance of emotional safety and the impact of failure to maintain safe and consensual behaviors and agreements.

3   Fostering safety.

- Therapists should encourage non-monogamous individuals to establish agreed-upon boundaries and emotional safety guidelines concerning their relationships.
- They should support and encourage methods for establishing clarity and consent before adding new partners (e.g., checklist models) and continuing transparency in ongoing relationships (Moors & Schechinger, 2018).
- They should promote awareness of one's and partner(s)'s emotional states, preferences, and attitudes and foster honest and open communication, trust, and respect.

4   Treating trauma and promoting resiliency.

- Therapists should be prepared to address and treat issues that arise due to traumatic experiences that can occur in non-monogamous relationship contexts.
- They should support clients in developing protective factors, enhancing resilience in the face of harmful experiences, and developing coping strategies (Smith & Mattick, 2015).

By utilizing these approaches, therapists can reduce the potential for harm and foster healthy communication, integrity, and resilience in their non-monogamous clients.

***

CLINICAL, SCHOOL, AND COUNSELING PSYCHOLOGY: AMERICAN PSYCHOLOGICAL ASSOCIATION (APA)

3.05 Multiple Relationships

a Multiple relationships occur when a psychologist is in a professional role with a person and (1) at the same time is in another role with the same person, (2) at the same time is in a relationship with a person closely associated with or related to the person with whom the psychologist has the professional relationship, or (3) promises to enter into another relationship in the future with the person or a person closely associated with or related to the person. A psychologist refrains from entering into multiple relationships if the multiple relationships could reasonably be expected to impair the psychologist's objectivity, competence, or effectiveness in performing his or her functions as a psychologist or otherwise risks exploitation or harm to the person with whom the professional relationship exists. Multiple relationships that would not reasonably be expected to cause impairment or risk exploitation or harm are not unethical.

b If a psychologist finds that, due to unforeseen factors, a potentially harmful multiple relationship has arisen, the psychologist takes reasonable steps to resolve it with due regard for the best interests of the affected person and maximal compliance with the Ethics Code.

c When psychologists are required by law, institutional policy, or extraordinary circumstances to serve in more than one role in judicial or administrative proceedings, at the outset they clarify role expectations and the extent of confidentiality and thereafter as changes occur.

Clinical Considerations

When working with ethical non-monogamous individuals, therapists must adhere to the ethical principles outlined in Standard 3.05 of the American Psychological Association's Ethics Code, which addresses multiple relationships (2017).

Here are examples of how therapists can incorporate this principle into their practice:

1 Recognizing and avoiding multiple relationships.

   • Therapists should be aware of and identify any potential multiple relationships that may arise with non-monogamous clients, their partners, or closely associated individuals.

- They should refrain from entering into multiple relationships if it could impair their objectivity, competence, or effectiveness as a therapist or if it risks exploitation or harm to the person with whom the professional relationship exists.

  - For example, a therapist who is also a member of a non-monogamous community should not provide therapy to individuals within that community to avoid potential conflicts or biases.

2 Resolving potentially harmful multiple relationships.

- If a therapist finds that a potentially harmful multiple relationship has inadvertently developed, they should take reasonable steps to address and fix it.
- They should consider the best interests of the affected person and aim for maximal compliance with the Ethics Code when determining how to resolve the situation.
- This may involve referring the client to another therapist, terminating one of the relationships, or establishing clear boundaries and ethical guidelines to mitigate harm.

3 Clarifying roles and confidentiality in legal or administrative proceedings.

- When therapists are required to serve in more than one role in judicial or administrative proceedings involving non-monogamous clients, they should clarify role expectations and the extent of confidentiality from the outset.
- As changes occur in these proceedings, therapists should communicate any modifications to their roles and maintain confidentiality and ethical guidelines.

By following these examples, therapists can navigate multiple relationships effectively and ethically when working with ethical non-monogamous individuals.

***

CLINICAL, SCHOOL, AND COUNSELING PSYCHOLOGY: AMERICAN PSYCHOLOGICAL ASSOCIATION (APA)

4.01 Maintaining Confidentiality

Psychologists have a primary obligation and take reasonable precautions to protect confidential information obtained through or stored in any medium, recognizing that the extent and limits of confidentiality may be regulated by law or established by institutional rules or professional or scientific relationships.

Clinical Considerations

When working with ethical non-monogamous individuals, therapists must maintain confidentiality, as outlined in Standard 4.01 of the American Psychological Association's Ethics Code (2017).

Here are examples of how therapists can incorporate this principle into their practice:

1   Explain the limits of confidentiality.

  • At the outset of therapy, therapists should explain to non-monogamous individuals the extent and limits of confidentiality. This includes discussing any legal, institutional, or professional rules that may regulate the disclosure of confidential information.
  • Therapists can clearly explain how their confidential information will be protected and under what circumstances confidentiality may be breached (e.g., if there is a risk of harm to themselves or others).

2   Safeguard confidential information.

  • Therapists should take reasonable precautions to protect the confidentiality of the information obtained from non-monogamous individuals. This extends to data stored in any medium, including electronic records or paper files.

    • Examples of safeguarding confidentiality include using secure electronic record-keeping systems, keeping physical files in locked cabinets, and ensuring that only authorized individuals have access to confidential information.

3   Obtain informed consent for disclosure.

  • If there is a need to disclose confidential information from non-monogamous individuals, therapists should obtain their informed consent beforehand, when possible.
  • Therapists should explain the purpose and potential consequences of the disclosure and discuss any alternative ways to achieve the stated goal while minimizing the amount of disclosed information.

4   Consult with colleagues and professionals.

  • Therapists may seek consultation with colleagues or professionals if they have questions or concerns about maintaining confidentiality in their work with non-monogamous individuals.
  • Such consultations can help therapists ensure they take appropriate precautions and adhere to ethical guidelines.

By incorporating these examples, therapists can uphold the ethical principle of maintaining confidentiality when working with non-monogamous individuals, ensuring the privacy and trust of their clients.

***

CLINICAL, SCHOOL, AND COUNSELING PSYCHOLOGY: AMERICAN PSYCHOLOGICAL ASSOCIATION (APA)

10.02 Therapy Involving Couples or Families

a   When psychologists agree to provide services to several persons who have a relationship (such as spouses, significant others, or parents and children), they take reasonable steps to clarify at the outset (1) which of the individuals are clients/patients and (2) the relationship the psychologist will have with each person. This clarification includes the psychologist's role and the probable uses of the services provided or the information obtained. (See also Standard 4.02, Discussing the Limits of Confidentiality.)

b   If it becomes apparent that psychologists may be called on to perform potentially conflicting roles (such as family therapist and then witness for one party in divorce proceedings), psychologists take reasonable steps to clarify and modify, or withdraw from, roles appropriately. (See also Standard 3.05c, Multiple Relationships.)

Clinical Considerations

When working with ethical non-monogamous individuals, therapists must adhere to the ethical principles of therapy involving couples or families as outlined in Standard 10.02 of the American Psychological Association's Ethics Code (2017).

Here are examples of how therapists can incorporate this principle into their practice:

1   Clarify roles and relationships.

  • When providing services to non-monogamous individuals in a relationship, therapists should clarify which individuals are clients/patients and the relationship the therapist will have with each person from the outset.
  • This clarification should include the probable uses of the services provided, the information obtained, and the therapist's role in working with non-monogamous individuals.

- Examples of establishing these boundaries and relationships include providing individual sessions in addition to couples or group sessions or working with non-monogamous individuals to develop clear expectations for the therapeutic relationship.

2 Clarify and modify potentially conflicting roles.

- Suppose it becomes apparent that therapists may be called on to perform potentially conflicting roles with non-monogamous individuals (e.g., therapist and expert witness in divorce proceedings). They should take reasonable steps to clarify, modify, or withdraw from such roles appropriately.
- In cases where therapists need to modify or withdraw from their role, they should take steps to ensure the best interests of the non-monogamous individuals and minimize harm.

    - For example, a therapist who is also providing therapy to an individual involved in a non-monogamous relationship and who is also called upon to testify in a court proceeding should clarify the extent of their role and duty to the court and their existing clients.

By incorporating these examples, therapists can navigate therapy involving non-monogamous relationships efficiently and ethically, ensuring that transparent relationships and boundaries are established, and potentially conflicting roles are clarified and resolved.

***

CLINICAL, SCHOOL, AND COUNSELING PSYCHOLOGY: AMERICAN PSYCHOLOGICAL ASSOCIATION (APA)

10.03 Group Therapy

When psychologists provide services to several persons in a group setting, they describe at the outset the roles and responsibilities of all parties and the limits of confidentiality.

Clinical Considerations

When working with ethical non-monogamous individuals in a group therapy setting, therapists must adhere to the ethical principle of group therapy as outlined in Standard 10.03 of the American Psychological Association's Ethics Code (2017).

Here are examples of how therapists can incorporate this principle into their practice:

1 Describe roles and responsibilities.

- At the outset of the group therapy process, therapists should clearly describe the roles and responsibilities of all parties involved, including the therapist and the non-monogamous individuals participating in the group.
- This may include explaining the purpose and structure of group therapy, the expectations for participation, and the therapist's role in facilitating the group process.
- Therapists can provide information about the shared responsibility for creating a safe and supportive environment for all group members, including respecting confidentiality.

2 Discuss the limits of confidentiality.

- Therapists should discuss and set clear expectations regarding the limits of confidentiality in the group therapy setting.
- This discussion should cover what information will be kept confidential within the group and under what circumstances there may be a need to breach confidentiality (e.g., if there is a risk of harm to oneself or others).
- Therapists can facilitate a group discussion where participants can openly express their comfort levels and concerns about confidentiality.

3 Obtain informed consent for group therapy.

- Before starting group therapy, therapists should obtain informed consent from non-monogamous individuals who wish to participate.
- Informed consent includes discussing the purpose, format, and goals of the group therapy, as well as any potential risks, benefits, or limitations. This allows participants to make an informed decision about their involvement.

By incorporating these examples, therapists can ensure that non-monogamous individuals in group therapy are aware of their roles and responsibilities and clearly understand the limits of confidentiality within the group setting.

**

MARRIAGE AND FAMILY THERAPISTS: AMERICAN ASSOCIATION OF MARRIAGE AND FAMILY THERAPISTS (AAMFT)

1.3 Multiple Relationships

Marriage and family therapists are aware of their influential positions with respect to clients, and they avoid exploiting the trust and dependency of such persons. Therapists, therefore, make every effort to avoid conditions and multiple relationships with clients that could impair professional judgment or increase the risk of exploitation. Such relationships include, but are not limited to, business or close personal relationships with a client or the client's immediate family. When the risk of impairment or exploitation exists due to conditions or multiple roles, therapists document the appropriate precautions taken.

Clinical Considerations

When working with ethical non-monogamous individuals, therapists must adhere to the ethical principle of multiple relationships as outlined in Standard 1.3 of the American Association for Marriage and Family Therapy's Code of Ethics.

Here are examples of how therapists can incorporate this principle into their practice:

1 Avoid conditions and multiple relationships that could impair professional judgment.

- Therapists should be aware of their influential positions with their clients and take precautions to avoid situations where their professional judgment may be impaired.
- This includes avoiding business or close personal relationships with clients or their immediate family members that could compromise the therapeutic relationship or create conflicts of interest.

  - For example, suppose a therapist is providing therapy to a non-monogamous individual and is personally involved in a non-monogamous relationship with another person who is also the client's partner. In that case, the therapist must recognize the potential risk of impaired professional judgment and take appropriate precautions, such as referring the client to another therapist.

2 Document precautions taken in cases where risks of impairment or exploitation exist.

- When therapists recognize that there is a risk of impairment or exploitation due to conditions or multiple roles, they should document the precautions taken to mitigate these risks.
- This can include documenting the therapist's efforts to maintain professional boundaries, disclosing potential conflicts of interest, and obtaining informed consent from all parties involved in the therapy process.

- For example, therapists can document the steps they have taken to ensure impartiality, maintain confidentiality, and prevent any exploitation of the trust and dependency of their non-monogamous clients.

By incorporating these examples, therapists can uphold the ethical principle of multiple relationships when working with non-monogamous individuals, ensuring that professional judgment is not impaired and the risk of exploitation is minimized.

***

MARRIAGE AND FAMILY THERAPISTS: AMERICAN ASSOCIATION OF MARRIAGE AND FAMILY THERAPISTS (AAMFT)

1.7 Abuse of the Therapeutic Relationship

Marriage and family therapists do not abuse their power in therapeutic relationships.

Clinical Considerations

When working with ethical non-monogamous individuals, therapists must adhere to the ethical principle of avoiding abuse of the therapeutic relationship as outlined in Standard 1.7 of the American Association for Marriage and Family Therapy's Code of Ethics.

Here are examples of how therapists can incorporate this principle into their practice:

1 Maintain professional boundaries.

- Therapists should establish and maintain appropriate professional boundaries with non-monogamous individuals to avoid crossing into personal or exploitative territory.
- This includes refraining from engaging in any behavior or actions perceived as abusive, whether physical, emotional, or sexual.

  - For example, therapists should avoid engaging in any form of sexual or romantic relationship with clients, as it would constitute a clear violation of professional boundaries.

2 Be mindful of power dynamics.

- Therapists should be aware of the power dynamics inherent in the therapeutic relationship and take steps to mitigate the potential for abuse of that power.

- This includes being mindful of any power differentials between the therapist and non-monogamous individuals, such as differences in age, gender, social status, or other factors.
- Therapists should strive to create a safe and egalitarian therapeutic environment that empowers non-monogamous individuals to make choices and decisions for themselves.

3 Seek consultation and supervision when needed.

- If therapists find themselves in situations where they are unsure about the appropriateness of their actions or if they suspect they may be at risk of abusing their power, they should seek consultation and supervision from colleagues or mentors.
- Consulting with a trusted colleague or supervisor can provide valuable guidance and help therapists navigate any ethical dilemmas or challenges.

By incorporating these examples, therapists can uphold the ethical principle of avoiding abuse of the therapeutic relationship when working with non-monogamous individuals, ensuring that their power as therapists is not abused and that the therapy process remains safe and respectful.

***

MARRIAGE AND FAMILY THERAPISTS: AMERICAN ASSOCIATION OF MARRIAGE AND FAMILY THERAPISTS (AAMFT)

1.8 Client Autonomy in Decision Making

Marriage and family therapists respect the rights of clients to make decisions and help them understand the consequences of these decisions. Therapists clearly advise clients that clients have the responsibility to make decisions regarding relationships such as cohabitation, marriage, divorce, separation, reconciliation, custody, and visitation.

Clinical Considerations

When working with ethical non-monogamous individuals, therapists must adhere to the ethical principle of respecting client autonomy in decision-making as outlined in Standard 1.8 of the American Association for Marriage and Family Therapy's Code of Ethics.

Here are examples of how therapists can incorporate this principle when working with non-monogamous individuals:

1 Promote informed decision-making.

   - Therapists should provide non-monogamous clients with all the necessary information they need to make informed decisions regarding their relationships.
   - This includes discussing the potential consequences, risks, benefits, and alternatives related to decisions such as cohabitation, marriage, divorce, separation, reconciliation, custody, and visitation.
   - Therapists should ensure that clients understand the impact these decisions may have on their lives and relationships.

2 Clarify the responsibility of decision-making.

   - Therapists need to affirm and communicate to non-monogamous clients that they have the sole responsibility for making decisions about their relationships.
   - Therapists should emphasize that clients have the right to determine the course of their relationships based on their values, desires, and needs.
   - Encourage clients to consider their values, needs, and goals when making decisions rather than relying solely on external expectations or societal norms.

3 Provide support and guidance.

   - While clients have autonomy in decision-making, therapists can offer support, insight, and guidance.
   - Therapists can help non-monogamous individuals explore the various options available to them and assist them in understanding the potential implications of their decisions on their overall well-being and relationships.
   - Creating a safe space where clients feel comfortable sharing their concerns, fears, and hopes while respecting their ultimate decision-making authority is crucial.

By incorporating these examples, therapists can uphold the ethical principle of client autonomy in decision-making when working with non-monogamous individuals. This ensures that clients' rights to make decisions about their relationships are respected and that therapists provide the necessary support and guidance through the decision-making process.

***

MARRIAGE AND FAMILY THERAPISTS: AMERICAN ASSOCIATION OF MARRIAGE AND FAMILY THERAPISTS (AAMFT)

1.9 Relationship Beneficial to Client

Marriage and family therapists continue therapeutic relationships only so long as it is reasonably clear that clients are benefiting from the relationship.

Clinical Considerations

When working with ethical non-monogamous individuals, therapists must adhere to the ethical principle of maintaining therapeutic relationships only as long as it is reasonably clear that clients benefit from the relationship, as outlined in Standard 1.9 of the American Association for Marriage and Family Therapy's Code of Ethics.

Here are examples of how therapists can incorporate this principle into their practice:

1   Regularly assess client progress.

- Therapists should regularly assess the progress of non-monogamous clients throughout the therapeutic relationship.
- This includes evaluating whether clients are experiencing a positive change in their well-being, relationships, and overall functioning due to therapy.
- Therapists should use evidence-based assessment tools, client feedback, and ongoing communication to gauge how much clients benefit from the therapeutic process.

2   Openly discuss progress with clients.

- Therapists should share and discuss their observations and assessment of client progress with non-monogamous clients.
- This involves clearly understanding clients' positive outcomes and improvements they have achieved through therapy.
- Open communication about progress ensures that the therapist and the client are on the same page regarding the therapeutic goals and outcomes.

3 Re-evaluate therapy goals when necessary.

- Therapists should periodically re-evaluate therapy goals and treatment plans to ensure they align with the changing needs and progress of non-monogamous clients.
- If it becomes evident that the therapeutic relationship is no longer benefiting the client, therapists should discuss this with the client and explore alternative options.
- In cases where therapy may not be practical or appropriate, therapists should refer clients to other professionals or resources that may better meet their needs.

4 Seek consultation and supervision when needed.

- If therapists are uncertain about the efficacy or direction of therapy with non-monogamous clients, they should seek consultation or supervision from colleagues or mentors.
- Consulting with peers and supervisors can provide valuable insights and guidance for navigating any challenges or dilemmas during therapy.
- This helps ensure that therapists maintain an objective perspective in evaluating the benefits of therapy for clients.

By incorporating these examples, therapists can uphold the ethical principle of maintaining therapeutic relationships only if it is reasonably clear that clients benefit from the relationship. This supports the well-being and progress of non-monogamous clients and ensures the effectiveness of therapy.

***

MARRIAGE AND FAMILY THERAPISTS: AMERICAN ASSOCIATION OF MARRIAGE AND FAMILY THERAPISTS (AAMFT)

3.10 Scope of Competence

Marriage and family therapists do not diagnose, treat, or advise on problems outside the recognized boundaries of their competencies.

Clinical Considerations

When working with ethical non-monogamous individuals, therapists must adhere to the ethical principle of working within the recognized boundaries of their competencies, as outlined in Standard 3.10 of the American Association for Marriage and Family Therapy's Code of Ethics. Here are examples of how therapists can incorporate this principle into their practice:

1 Maintain competency in non-monogamous relationships.

- Therapists should actively seek training, supervision, and continuing education to develop and maintain competency in working with non-monogamous relationships.
- This includes staying updated on research, resources, and best practices related to ethical non-monogamy.
- Therapists should know the dynamics, challenges, and unique considerations that non-monogamous individuals may face in their relationships.

2 Recognize and refer out when necessary.

- Therapists should recognize their limitations and refer non-monogamous clients to colleagues or professionals who have specific expertise in non-monogamous relationships when appropriate.
- This may occur when the clients' complexity or specific needs exceed the therapist's level of competence.
- By recognizing the boundaries of their competencies, therapists ensure that clients receive the best possible care and support.

3 Collaborate with experts in related fields.

- Therapists can collaborate with experts in related fields, such as sex therapy, LGBTQ+ counseling, or relationship coaching, to provide comprehensive and specialized support to non-monogamous clients.
- This collaboration allows therapists to benefit from the knowledge and expertise of professionals in specific areas while still maintaining their focus on the therapeutic process.

4 Seek consultation when faced with ethical dilemmas.

- If therapists encounter ethical difficulties or situations beyond their scope of competence when working with non-monogamous clients, they should seek consultation from colleagues, supervision, or professional organizations.
- Consultation can guide therapists in navigating complex situations or dilemmas that may arise during the therapeutic process.
- This helps therapists ensure they deliver appropriate and competent care to non-monogamous individuals.

By incorporating these examples, therapists can uphold the ethical principle of working within the recognized boundaries of their competencies when working with non-monogamous individuals. This ensures that therapy is conducted competently and that clients receive appropriate care and support.

***

CLINICAL SOCIAL WORKERS: NATIONAL ASSOCIATION OF SOCIAL WORKERS (NASW)

Preamble

The primary mission of the social work profession is to enhance human well-being and help meet the basic human needs of all people, with particular attention to the needs and empowerment of people who are vulnerable, oppressed, and living in poverty. A historic and defining feature of social work is the profession's dual focus on individual well-being in a social context and the well-being of society. Fundamental to social work is attention to the environmental forces that create, contribute to, and address problems in living.

Social workers promote social justice and social change with and on behalf of clients. "Clients" is used inclusively to refer to individuals, families, groups, organizations, and communities. Social workers are sensitive to cultural and ethnic diversity and strive to end discrimination, oppression, poverty, and other forms of social injustice. These activities may be in the form of direct practice, community organizing, supervision, consultation, administration, advocacy, social and political action, policy development and implementation, education, and research and evaluation. Social workers seek to enhance the capacity of people to address their own needs. Social workers also seek to promote the responsiveness of organizations, communities, and other social institutions to individuals' needs and social problems.

The mission of the social work profession is rooted in a set of core values. These core values, embraced by social workers throughout the profession's history, are the foundation of social work's unique purpose and perspective:

• Service
• Social justice
• Dignity and worth of the person
• Importance of human relationships
• Integrity
• Competence.

This constellation of core values reflects what is unique to the social work profession. Core values, and the principles that flow from them, must be balanced within the context and complexity of the human experience.

Clinical Considerations

When working with ethical non-monogamous individuals, clinical social worker therapists can incorporate the core values and principles outlined by the NASW.

Here are examples of how therapists can integrate these values into their practice:

1   Embrace the core value of service.

- Therapists should prioritize the well-being and empowerment of their non-monogamous clients.
- This involves actively working to meet the basic human needs of clients and promoting their overall well-being.
- Therapists can provide a safe and supportive space for clients to explore their relationships and address any challenges they may face.

2   Advocate for social justice.

- Therapists should strive to address discrimination, oppression, and social injustices that non-monogamous individuals may encounter.
- This can be done through individual advocacy, community organizing, or social and political action to challenge societal norms and promote acceptance and understanding of ethical non-monogamy.
- Therapists can also assist clients in advocating for their rights within their relationships and larger society.

3   Respect the dignity and worth of the person.

- Therapists should approach non-monogamous individuals with respect, empathy, and a non-judgmental attitude.
- This involves recognizing and valuing clients' diverse lived experiences, values, and beliefs, including their choice to engage in ethical non-monogamy.
- Therapists should help clients develop a positive self-image, overcome stigma, and embrace their authentic selves.

4   Foster the importance of human relationships.

- Therapists should understand and support the importance of various types of relationships in the lives of non-monogamous individuals.
- This includes helping clients navigate and nurture their multiple relationships, establish healthy boundaries, and enhance communication and intimacy within their partnerships.
- Therapists can also assist clients in enhancing their support networks and building connections with others who understand and accept their lifestyle.

5 Uphold integrity and competence.

- Therapists should ensure their practice is grounded in ethical principles and maintain professional competence.
- This involves continually seeking supervision, consultation, and continuing education to enhance their knowledge and skills in working with non-monogamous individuals.
- Therapists should adhere to the NASW Code of Ethics and ethical guidelines specific to their jurisdictions.

By incorporating these examples, therapists working with ethical non-monogamous individuals can align their practice with the core values and principles of the NASW. This supports the well-being and empowerment of non-monogamous clients while working toward social justice and promoting acceptance of diverse relationship structures.

***

CLINICAL SOCIAL WORKERS: NATIONAL ASSOCIATION OF SOCIAL WORKERS (NASW)

Purpose of the NASW Code of Ethics

Professional ethics are at the core of social work. The profession has an obligation to articulate its basic values, ethical principles, and ethical standards. The NASW Code of Ethics sets forth these values, principles, and standards to guide social workers' conduct. The Code is relevant to all social workers and social work students, regardless of their professional functions, the settings in which they work, or the populations they serve.

The NASW Code of Ethics serves six purposes:

1 The Code identifies core values on which social work's mission is based.
2 The Code summarizes broad ethical principles that reflect the profession's core values and establishes a set of specific ethical standards that should be used to guide social work practice.
3 The Code is designed to help social workers identify relevant considerations when professional obligations conflict or ethical uncertainties arise.
4 The Code provides ethical standards to which the general public can hold the social work profession accountable.
5 The Code socializes practitioners new to the field to social work's mission, values, ethical principles, and ethical standards, and encourages all social workers to engage in self-care, ongoing

education, and other activities to ensure their commitment to those same core features of the profession.

6 The Code articulates standards that the social work profession itself can use to assess whether social workers have engaged in unethical conduct. NASW has formal procedures to adjudicate ethics complaints filed against its members.* In subscribing to this Code, social workers are required to cooperate in its implementation, participate in NASW adjudication proceedings, and abide by any NASW disciplinary rulings or sanctions based on it.

The Code offers a set of values, principles, and standards to guide decision-making and conduct when ethical issues arise. It does not provide a set of rules that prescribe how social workers should act in all situations. Specific applications of the Code must take into account the context in which it is being considered and the possibility of conflicts among the Code's values, principles, and standards. Ethical responsibilities flow from all human relationships, from the personal and familial to the social and professional.

Clinical Considerations

When working with ethical non-monogamous individuals, therapists can incorporate and apply the principles and standards outlined in the NASW Code of Ethics.

Here are examples of how therapists can do this:

1 Identify core values.

- The therapist should recognize and uphold the core values of social work, such as service, social justice, dignity and worth of the person, importance of human relationships, integrity, and competence.
- This involves understanding and respecting the diverse beliefs and values of ethical non-monogamous individuals and ensuring that therapeutic interventions align with these values.

2 Apply ethical principles.

- The therapist should utilize the broad ethical principles outlined in the Code to guide their practice.
- This includes principles such as respect for autonomy, promoting client self-determination, maintaining confidentiality, and avoiding conflicts of interest.

- The therapist can collaborate with ethical non-monogamous clients to ensure their autonomy and decision-making power within their relationships are respected and supported.

3   Manage ethical dilemmas.

- The therapist should be prepared to address ethical uncertainties and conflicts in working with ethical non-monogamous individuals.
- This involves using the Code as a resource to help navigate these dilemmas and make informed decisions that prioritize the well-being and autonomy of the clients.
- The therapist can seek consultation or supervision to address ethical considerations appropriately.

4   Accountability and self-care.

- The therapist should know that the Code holds the social work profession accountable to the general public.
- This means that the therapist should strive to maintain professional conduct and adhere to the ethical standards within their work with ethical non-monogamous individuals.
- The therapist should also engage in ongoing self-care and professional development to ensure continued commitment to the values and principles of the profession.

5   Adjudication and cooperation.

- The therapist should be familiar with the NASW's procedures for adjudicating ethics complaints and willing to cooperate to implement the Code.
- This involves participating in any proceedings related to ethics complaints and abiding by any disciplinary rulings or sanctions issued by the NASW, if applicable.

6   Contextual considerations.

- The therapist should recognize that specific applications of the Code must adapt to the client's unique context and the potential conflicts among the Code's values, principles, and standards.
- This requires the therapist to approach each ethical issue with sensitivity and flexibility, considering the individual, familial, social, and professional aspects of the client's life.

By incorporating these examples, therapists working with ethical non-monogamous individuals can ensure that their practice aligns with the NASW Code of Ethics. This will promote ethical decision-making, respect for client autonomy, and the overall well-being of their clients.

***

CLINICAL SOCIAL WORKERS: NATIONAL ASSOCIATION OF SOCIAL WORKERS (NASW)

1.04 Competence

a   Social workers should provide services and represent themselves as competent only within the boundaries of their education, training, license, certification, consultation received, supervised experience, or other relevant professional experience.
b   Social workers should provide services in substantive areas or use intervention techniques or approaches that are new to them only after engaging in appropriate study, training, consultation, and supervision from people who are competent in those interventions or techniques.
c   When generally recognized standards do not exist with respect to an emerging area of practice, social workers should exercise careful judgment and take responsible steps (including appropriate education, research, training, consultation, and supervision) to ensure the competence of their work and to protect clients from harm.
d   Social workers who use technology in the provision of social work services should ensure that they have the necessary knowledge and skills to provide such services competently. This includes an understanding of the special communication challenges when using technology and the ability to implement strategies to address these challenges.
e   Social workers who use technology in providing social work services should comply with the laws governing technology and social work practice in the jurisdiction in which they are regulated and located and, as applicable, in the jurisdiction in which the client is located.

Clinical Considerations

When working with ethical non-monogamous individuals, therapists can apply the competence standards outlined in the NASW Code of Ethics.

Here are examples of how therapists can incorporate these standards into their practice:

a   Boundaries of competence.

• Therapists should only provide services and represent themselves as competent within the boundaries of their education, training, license, certification, consultation received, supervised experience, or other relevant professional experience.

- This means therapists should have a solid understanding of ethical non-monogamy and individuals' unique needs and dynamics in these types of relationships before offering services in this area.

b Study, training, and supervision.

- Therapists should engage in appropriate study, training, consultation, and supervision when offering services in substantive areas related to ethical non-monogamy or using intervention techniques specific to these relationships.
- They should seek guidance and mentorship from professionals working with ethical non-monogamous individuals to ensure the highest standard of care.

c Emerging areas of practice.

- In practice areas still emerging, such as ethical non-monogamy, therapists should exercise careful judgment and take responsible steps to ensure competence and protect clients from harm.
- This may include engaging in ongoing education, conducting research, seeking training opportunities, consulting with experts, and maintaining supervision to stay up-to-date with best practices.

d Technology in practice.

- If therapists utilize technology in providing social work services to ethical non-monogamous individuals, they should ensure they have the necessary knowledge and skills to do so competently.
- This includes understanding the unique communication challenges that may arise when using technology and implementing strategies to address those challenges effectively.

e Compliance with laws.

- Therapists who incorporate technology into their practice with ethical non-monogamous individuals should comply with the laws governing technology and social work practice in their jurisdiction and the jurisdiction where the client is located.
- This ensures that ethical and legal standards are upheld and protects the well-being and confidentiality of the clients.

By applying these competence standards, therapists can ensure they provide knowledgeable and effective services to ethical non-monogamous individuals. This helps to establish trust and promote the well-being of their clients.

***

CLINICAL SOCIAL WORKERS: NATIONAL ASSOCIATION OF SOCIAL WORKERS (NASW)

1.05 Cultural Competence

a Social workers should demonstrate an understanding of culture and its function in human behavior and society, recognizing the strengths that exist in all cultures.

b Social workers should demonstrate knowledge that guides practice with clients of various cultures and be able to demonstrate skills in the provision of culturally informed services that empower marginalized individuals and groups. Social workers must take action against oppression, racism, discrimination, and inequities, and acknowledge personal privilege.

c Social workers should demonstrate awareness and cultural humility by engaging in critical self-reflection (understanding their own bias and engaging in self-correction), recognizing clients as experts of their own culture, committing to lifelong learning, and holding institutions accountable for advancing cultural humility.

d Social workers should obtain education about and demonstrate an understanding of the nature of social diversity and oppression with respect to race, ethnicity, national origin, color, sex, sexual orientation, gender identity or expression, age, marital status, political belief, religion, immigration status, and mental or physical ability.

e Social workers who provide electronic social work services should be aware of cultural and socioeconomic differences among clients' use of and access to electronic technology and seek to prevent such potential barriers. Social workers should assess cultural, environmental, economic, mental, or physical ability, linguistic, and other issues that may affect the delivery or use of these services.

Clinical Considerations

When working with ethical non-monogamous individuals, therapists can incorporate the cultural competence standards outlined in the NASW Code of Ethics.

Here are examples of how therapists can apply these standards in their practice:

a Understanding culture.

- Therapists should demonstrate an understanding of culture and its function in human behavior and society. This includes recognizing the strengths in all cultures, including those related to ethical non-monogamy.

b Culturally informed practice.

- Therapists should have knowledge that guides their practice with clients from various cultures, including those in ethical non-monogamous relationships.
- They should be able to demonstrate skills in providing culturally informed services that empower marginalized individuals and groups, taking action against oppression, racism, discrimination, and inequities.
- This includes acknowledging their privilege and addressing power imbalances within therapeutic relationships.

c Cultural humility.

- Therapists should demonstrate awareness and cultural humility by engaging in critical self-reflection, understanding their biases, and self-correction.
- They should recognize clients as experts in their own culture, commit to lifelong learning, and hold institutions accountable for advancing cultural humility.

d Diversity and oppression.

- Therapists should obtain education about and demonstrate an understanding of the nature of social diversity and oppression, including factors such as race, ethnicity, national origin, color, sex, sexual orientation, gender identity or expression, age, marital status, political belief, religion, immigration status, and mental or physical ability.
- This understanding helps therapists provide empathetic and inclusive care to clients from diverse backgrounds, including those in ethical non-monogamous relationships.

e Electronic social work services and cultural differences.

- Therapists providing electronic social work services should be aware of cultural and socioeconomic differences among clients' use of and access to electronic technology.
- They should strive to prevent potential barriers by assessing cultural, environmental, economic, mental or physical ability, linguistic, and other issues that may affect the delivery or use of these services.

- This ensures that therapists can provide equitable care to all clients, regardless of their cultural background or access to technology.

By incorporating these cultural competence standards, therapists can create a safe and inclusive environment for ethical non-monogamous individuals. This approach promotes cultural humility, addresses power imbalances, and fosters client empowerment.

***

CLINICAL SOCIAL WORKERS: NATIONAL ASSOCIATION OF SOCIAL WORKERS (NASW)

1.06 Conflicts of Interest

a Social workers should be alert to and avoid conflicts of interest that interfere with the exercise of professional discretion and impartial judgment. Social workers should inform clients when a real or potential conflict of interest arises and take reasonable steps to resolve the issue in a manner that makes the clients' interests primary and protects clients' interests to the greatest extent possible. In some cases, protecting clients' interests may require termination of the professional relationship with proper referral of the client.

b Social workers should not take unfair advantage of any professional relationship or exploit others to further their personal, religious, political, or business interests.

c Social workers should not engage in dual or multiple relationships with clients or former clients in which there is a risk of exploitation or potential harm to the client. In instances when dual or multiple relationships are unavoidable, social workers should take steps to protect clients and are responsible for setting clear, appropriate, and culturally sensitive boundaries. (Dual or multiple relationships occur when social workers relate to clients in more than one relationship, whether professional, social, or business. Dual or multiple relationships can occur simultaneously or consecutively.)

d When social workers provide services to two or more people who have a relationship with each other (e.g., couples, or family members), social workers should clarify with all parties which individuals will be considered clients and the nature of social workers' professional obligations to the various individuals who are receiving services. Social workers who anticipate a conflict of interest among the individuals' receiving services or who anticipate having to perform potentially conflicting roles (e.g., when a social worker is asked to testify in a child custody dispute or divorce proceedings involving clients) should clarify their role with the parties involved and take appropriate action to minimize any conflict of interest.

e Social workers should avoid communication with clients using technology (such as social networking sites, online chat, e-mail, text messages, telephone, and video) for personal or non-work-related purposes.

f Social workers should be aware that posting personal information on professional websites or other media might cause boundary confusion, inappropriate dual relationships, or harm to clients.

g Social workers should be aware that personal affiliations may increase the likelihood that clients may discover the social worker's presence on websites, social media, and other forms of technology. Social workers should be aware that involvement in electronic communication with groups based on race, ethnicity, language, sexual orientation, gender identity or expression, mental or physical ability, religion, immigration status, and other personal affiliations may affect their ability to work effectively with particular clients.

h Social workers should avoid accepting requests from or engaging in personal relationships with clients on social networking sites or other electronic media to prevent boundary confusion, inappropriate dual relationships, or harm to clients.

Clinical Considerations

When working with ethical non-monogamous individuals, therapists can incorporate the following guidelines based on the NASW Code of Ethics:

a Identifying and addressing conflicts of interest.

- Therapists should be vigilant in identifying and avoiding conflicts of interest that could impact their professional judgment and discretion.
- Suppose an actual or potential conflict of interest arises. In that case, therapists should inform their clients about it and take reasonable steps to resolve the issue to prioritize the client's interests and protect them to the greatest extent possible.
- Resolving conflicts of interest might sometimes require terminating the professional relationship with a proper referral for the client.

b Avoiding exploitation and personal interests.

- Therapists should not take unfair advantage of their professional relationships or exploit clients to further their personal, religious, political, or business interests.
- Therapists should maintain professional boundaries and avoid actions that could compromise the therapeutic relationship.

c Managing dual or multiple relationships.

- Therapists should not engage in dual or multiple relationships with clients or former clients if there is a risk of exploitation or potential harm.
- In situations where dual or multiple relationships are unavoidable, therapists should take steps to protect their clients and establish clear, appropriate, and culturally sensitive boundaries.
- Dual or multiple relationships can occur when therapists have relationships with clients that extend beyond the professional context, such as social or business relationships, and therapists should be mindful of the potential for conflicts and power dynamics.

d Clarifying professional obligations within multiple client relationships.

- When providing services to multiple clients with a relationship with each other (e.g., couples, family members), therapists should clarify with all parties which individuals will be considered clients and explain the nature of the therapist's professional obligations to each person.
- If a conflict of interest is anticipated among the individuals receiving services or if the therapist may have to fulfill potentially conflicting roles (e.g., testifying in a child custody dispute involving clients), the therapist should clarify their position with all involved parties and take appropriate action to minimize conflicts of interest.

(e)–(h) These additional guidelines pertain to the use of technology and online communication. While they do not directly relate to working with ethical non-monogamous individuals, therapists should be aware of best practices to maintain professional boundaries and avoid boundary confusion, inappropriate dual relationships, or harm to clients in the digital context.

By incorporating these ethical guidelines, therapists can ensure that they provide ethical and practical support to ethical non-monogamous individuals while maintaining professionalism and safeguarding the therapeutic relationship.

***

CLINICAL SOCIAL WORKERS: NATIONAL ASSOCIATION OF SOCIAL WORKERS (NASW)

1.09   Sexual Relationships

a   Social workers should under no circumstances engage in sexual activities, inappropriate sexual communications through the use of technology or in person, or sexual contact with current clients, whether such contact is consensual or forced.

b   Social workers should not engage in sexual activities or sexual contact with clients' relatives or other individuals with whom clients maintain a close personal relationship when there is a risk of exploitation or potential harm to the client. Sexual activity or sexual contact with clients' relatives or other individuals with whom clients maintain a personal relationship has the potential to be harmful to the client and may make it difficult for the social worker and client to maintain appropriate professional boundaries. Social workers—not their clients, their clients' relatives, or other individuals with whom the client maintains a personal relationship—assume the full burden for setting clear, appropriate, and culturally sensitive boundaries.

c   Social workers should not engage in sexual activities or sexual contact with former clients because of the potential for harm to the client. If social workers engage in conduct contrary to this prohibition or claim that an exception to this prohibition is warranted because of extraordinary circumstances, it is social workers—not their clients—who assume the full burden of demonstrating that the former client has not been exploited, coerced, or manipulated, intentionally or unintentionally.

d   Social workers should not provide clinical services to individuals with whom they have had a prior sexual relationship. Providing clinical services to a former sexual partner has the potential to be harmful to the individual and is likely to make it difficult for the social worker and individual to maintain appropriate professional boundaries.

Clinical Considerations

Therapists can ethically work with non-monogamous clients in ways that honor the relevant ethical guidelines. Social workers should not engage in sexual activities with their current or former clients or with individuals related to clients to prevent potential harm and maintain professional boundaries (2023). When working with non-monogamous clients, therapists should rely on healthy and effective communication practices that are culturally sensitive and based on consent, such as the three Cs: communication, consideration, and consent (Mogilski et al., 2021). Therapists can help clients explore and understand the challenges and advantages of ethical non-monogamous relationships while setting clear boundaries to maintain appropriate professional relationships.

Therapists should also be aware of potential biases and stigmatization toward non-monogamous relationships and make efforts to provide inclusive and accepting support for their clients. By doing so, therapists can support non-monogamous clients in their relationships while upholding ethical guidelines and providing effective therapeutic support.

Chapter Highlights

• The observance of ethical codes must be adhered to when counseling, regardless of the background and lifestyles of clients. (See Step 8 for information about ENM clients and the Code of Ethics.)
• Practitioners should strive not to harm.
• Clinicians should be privy to protection against personal, financial, social, organizational, or political factors that could lead to influence misuse.
• Effective therapists respect cultural, individual, and role differences, including those based on age, gender, gender identity, race, ethnicity, culture, national origin, religion, sexual orientation, disability, language, and socioeconomic status, and consider these factors when working with members of such groups.
• Clinicians should respect the nobility and value of all individuals. They must honor their clients' privacy, confidentiality, and self-determination rights.
• Therapists know that special safeguards may be necessary to protect the rights and welfare of individuals or communities whose susceptibilities weaken independent decision-making.
• Clinicians should only provide services, teach, and conduct research with populations and in areas only within the boundaries of their competence, based on their education, training, supervised experience, consultation, study, or professional experience.
• Practitioners must take reasonable steps to avoid harming their clients/patients, students, supervisees, research participants, organizational clients, and others with whom they work and to minimize harm where it is foreseeable and unavoidable.

- If a psychologist finds that, due to unforeseen factors, potentially harmful multiple relationships have arisen, the psychologist takes reasonable steps to resolve it with due regard for the best interests of the affected person and maximal compliance with the Ethics Code.
- Marriage and family therapists are aware of their influential positions concerning clients, and they avoid exploiting the trust and dependency of such persons. Therapists, therefore, make every effort to avoid conditions and multiple relationships with clients that could impair professional judgment or increase the risk of exploitation. Such relationships include but are not limited to business or close personal relationships with a client or the client's immediate family.
- Psychologists have a primary obligation and take reasonable precautions to protect confidential information obtained through or stored in any medium, recognizing that the extent and limits of confidentiality may be regulated by law or established by institutional rules or professional or scientific relationships.
- If it becomes apparent that psychologists may be called on to perform potentially conflicting roles (such as family therapist and then witness for one party in divorce proceedings), psychologists take reasonable steps to clarify, modify, or withdraw from roles appropriately.
- When psychologists provide services to several persons in a group setting, they describe at the outset the roles and responsibilities of all parties and the limits of confidentiality.
- Marriage and family therapists do not abuse their power in therapeutic relationships. Therapists advise clients that clients have the responsibility to make decisions regarding relationships such as cohabitation, marriage, divorce, separation, reconciliation, custody, and visitation.
- Marriage and family therapists do not diagnose, treat, or advise on problems outside the recognized boundaries of their competencies.
- If it becomes apparent that psychologists may be called on to perform potentially conflicting roles (such as family therapist and then witness for one party in divorce proceedings), psychologists take reasonable steps to clarify, modify, or withdraw from roles appropriately.
- The social work profession's mission is rooted in core values. These core values, embraced by social workers throughout the profession's history, are the foundation of social work's unique purpose and perspective:

  - Service
  - Social justice
  - Dignity and worth of the person
  - Importance of human relationships
  - Integrity
  - Competence.

References

American Association for Marriage and Family Therapy. (2015, January 1). *Code of ethics*. Retrieved January 12, 2023, from https://www.aamft.org/Legal_Ethics/Code_of_Ethics.aspx

American Psychological Association. (2017, January 1). *Ethical principles of psychologists and code of conduct*. American Psychological Association. Retrieved January 12, 2023, from https://www.apa.org/ethics/code

Duke, E. A. (2022). Ethical clinical practice with consensual non-monogamous clients. In M. D. Vaughan & T. R. Burnes (Eds.), *The handbook of consensual non-monogamy: Affirming mental health practice* (pp. 266–282). Essay, Rowman & Littlefield.

Mogilski, J., Rodrigues, D.L., Lehmiller, J.J., & Balzarini, R.N. (2021). Maintaining multi-partner relationships: Evolution, sexual ethics, and consensual non-monogamy.

Moors, A. C., & Schechinger, H. (2018). A checklist for sexual consent in non-monogamous relationships. *Sexual and Relationship Therapy*, *33*(3), 337–350. 10.1080/14681994.2018.1468255

National Association of Social Workers. (2021). *Read the code of ethics*. National Association of Social Workers. Retrieved January 12, 2023, from https://www.socialworkers.org/About/Ethics/Code-of-Ethics/Code-of-Ethics-English#:~:text=The%20NASW%20Code%20of%20Ethics,explicit%20guidance%20to%20social%20workers

Schrimshaw, E. W., Siegel, B. A., Downing Jr, M. J., & Parsons, J. T. (2013). Disclosure and concealment of sexual orientation and the mental health of non-gay-identified, behaviorally bisexual men. *Journal of Consulting and Clinical Psychology*, *81*(1), 141–153. 10.1037/a0029215

Smith, D. & Mattick, K. (2015). Resilience and psychological distress in a non-monogamous sample. *Journal of Sex Research*, *52*(4), 435–447. 10.1080/00224499.2013.876668

Part 2

Clinician's Guide and Treatment Plans

Step 1

Exploring Their Why and Uncovering Fears

Clinician's Guide and Treatment Plans

Now that you have gained a solid foundation of knowledge from the previous part, it's time to apply your newfound expertise. This part offers a comprehensive, step-by-step guide to helping ethical non-monogamy (ENM) couples and individuals begin their journey safely. As a seasoned practitioner, I encourage you to skip to the sections that pertain to your clients and make use of the activities, treatment plans, and homework that best suits their needs.

Keep in mind that each couple or individual has a unique journey, and some steps may not be relevant to their circumstances. Additionally, some couples or individuals may have skipped crucial aspects of the process, requiring them to revisit certain steps before moving forward successfully. Exercise expertise, sensitivity, and flexibility in adjusting your approach to meet the specific needs of your clients.

As the therapist, it is essential to fully evaluate the relationship's overall health before beginning this journey with the couple. There are several ways to accomplish this, and we will discuss assessment tools that work best for those wanting to enter ENM.

William Walter Waller, an American sociologist, was the first scientist to suggest that marriages that end in divorce could stem from the partners' disillusionment early in their relationship (1967). As the field of relationship study has progressed, more attention has been placed on non-heterosexual and unmarried romantic relationships; therefore, the modified tools can be fully utilized by therapists for couples in every relationship dynamic in the present day.

While the couple in your office is there for assistance in navigating the complexities of ENM, do they want to enter into this lifestyle to save their relationship from demise, or do they genuinely want to enhance their marriage moving forward?

DOI: 10.4324/9781003464891-9

Evaluation Tools for Identifying the Overall Health of the Relationship

Relationship Disillusionment Scale

The Marital Disillusionment Scale, developed by Sylvia Niehuis and Denise Bartell in 2006, is a self-reporting scale that measures disillusionment in marriage. Therapists use it to evaluate the current state of the

Relationship Disillusionment Scale

Circle the number that best represents how you agree or disagree with each statement, using the following scale:
1 = strong disagreement, 7 = strong agreement

	Disagree Agree
1. I am very disappointed in my relationship.	1 2 3 4 5 6 7
2. I am very disappointed in my partner.	1 2 3 4 5 6 7
3. My partner used to be my best friend, but now I sometimes don't like them as a person.	1 2 3 4 5 6 7
4. This relationship is not at all what I expected it to be; I feel very disappointed.	1 2 3 4 5 6 7
5. I used to think I was lucky to be with someone like my partner; now I'm not so sure I am lucky.	1 2 3 4 5 6 7
6. I used to love spending time with my partner, but now it's starting to feel like a chore.	1 2 3 4 5 6 7
7. I feel tricked, cheated, or deceived by love.	1 2 3 4 5 6 7
8. The relationship is not as enjoyable as I had expected it to be.	1 2 3 4 5 6 7
9. If I could go back in time, I would not have gotten involved with my partner.	1 2 3 4 5 6 7
10. My partner used to be on their best behavior while with me, but now they don't try to impress me.	1 2 3 4 5 6 7
11. My partner seems to be an entirely different person now.	1 2 3 4 5 6 7

Add up your responses. A score of 11 represents a lack of disillusionment, whereas a score of 77 represents the highest possible level of disillusionment.

SOURCE: Niehuis, S., & Bartell, D. (2006). The marital disillusionment scale: development and psychometric properties. North American Journal of Psychology, 8(1), 69–83.Copyright 2006. Reprinted and adapated with permission of the North American Journal of Pychology and the author.

Figure S1.1 Relationship Disillusionment Scale. Reprinted and adapted with permission of the North American Journal of Psychology.

relationship, further indicating if the couple wants to begin ENM for positive reasons and not a last-ditch effort to save the relationship.

The author has modified the original self-report questionnaire to reflect a more inclusive tool for the various relationship dynamics when working with individuals in ENM. Through the research conducted, the Relationship Disillusionment Scale highly correlates with assessing changes in (a) the feelings of love associated with their partner, (b) the display of affectionate behaviors toward the partner, (c) discernment of the partner's responsiveness, and (d) feelings of uncertainty toward the partner and the relationship.

The Couples Satisfaction Index

The Couples Satisfaction Index (CSI) was developed by Janette L. Funk and Rondald D. Rogge and used the item response theory to measure the individual's overall satisfaction in a relationship (2007). The CSI is a self-report questionnaire that can be used as a 32, 16, or 4-item scale depending on the intended application of the results. Jbilou et al. stated that "marital treatment studies benefit from the higher levels of precision and information offered by the 32-item scale, whereas the brevity of the 4-item scale is useful for national surveys" (2021). When using the 32-item scale, the scores can range from 0 to 161, with higher scores implying greater relationship satisfaction; however, scores falling below 104.5 propose great relationship dissatisfaction (Jbilou et al., 2021).

Gottman Relationship Checkup

Dr. John Gottman developed the Gottman Relationship Checkup from over 40 years of scientific research. The relationship assessment instrument "relies on intensive, detailed, and evidence-based information on why relationships succeed or fail" (Gottman website). This self-assessment can measure the general health of the relationship, the quality of friendship and intimacy, the nature of romance and passion, how the couple manages conflict, the overall trust and commitment, and more.

Upon completing the self-assessment by each partner, the therapist will have access to the results so they can evaluate the relationship and explore areas of concern with the couple before moving forward with ENM.

*To find the Gottman Relationship Checkup, visit: https://checkup.gottman.com/

Sexual History Intake

Taking a thorough sexual history from each partner is vital when determining areas of improvement for the couple and identifying trauma that might cause fractures in the relationship as they begin their journey into the ENM lifestyle. Unfortunately, sexual health is only one course of study when obtaining your degree in mental health counseling, resulting in many practitioners fumbling for the proper language or getting embarrassed by the conversation. The lack of training and fear of embarrassment often causes this significant topic to be skimmed over at best or ignored.

When conducting the sexual history intake, it is best to have each partner participate in an individual session in case the individual would like to discuss more delicate areas of concern (Metz et al., 2018). Traditionally, this is the second and third session when working with the couple. If information is presented regarding intense sexual trauma and you do not feel qualified to help the individual process the trauma, refer to a specialist for individual counseling. As the clinician, you have the decision to make:

1　Do you stop the program with the couple and begin again when you feel the sexual trauma has been processed, or
2　Continue with the program with the trauma partner in individual therapy. The sexual history intake is a discussion that will need to be had after the individual sexual history interviews have been concluded.

Here are some do's when conducting the sexual history intake:

1　Maintain eye contact, even if you get embarrassed.
2　Try to stay relaxed.
3　Use familiar terminology or the client's language in the session.
4　Ask detailed questions.
5　Maintain an open mind and non-judgmental attitude.
6　Be aware of your facial expressions, body language, and overall reactions when they detail your sexual preferences.

Here are some don'ts when conducting the sexual history intake:

1　Don't assume the client's sexuality. Ask for clarification.
2　Don't rush through the sexual history intake.
3　Don't act as if you know everything. It is acceptable to ask clarifying questions.
4　Don't assume you know what specific terms mean. Each individual has their meaning in particular terms, and you are encouraged to ask the client, "What does that term mean to you?"

Dr. Barry McCarthy is one of the leading advocates for sex therapy and has published 22 books on sex. During one of his many workshops, the author learned how to utilize his sexual history intake fully. Dr. McCarthy provided that the sexual history intake interview should be done individually, not together, and should be structured chronologically (Metz et al., 2018).

Per his instructions, "move from less anxious to more anxiety-provoking questions, be non-judgmental about atypical behavior, ask open-ended questions, probe for dysfunctional attitudes, behaviors, and emotions." Dr. McCarthy further suggests that the clinician should start by saying:

I want to understand your psychological, relational and sexual history both before and during this relationship. I want to hear all your strengths as well as vulnerabilities. I appreciate your being as forthcoming and blunt as possible. At the end, I'll ask if there is anything sensitive or secret that you do not want to share with your partner. (Metz et al., 2018)

Clinical Consideration: Due to working with the couple as a unit, many therapists disclose to their clients that they do not want to be the bearer of personal secrets; therefore, if the client does not want to share something with their partners, the therapist does not want to know.

Evaluate the Couple's ENM Foundational Education Level

Typically, couples that come to therapy wanting to explore ENM have researched the lifestyle minimally; however, you must know the extent of their knowledge, so you are speaking to them and not at them. In other words, you are not telling them things they already know. This is an excellent opportunity to clarify any misconceptions about ENM. Refer to Chapter 4 for a list of common misconceptions about ENM.

Here are some guiding questions to help facilitate your evaluation:

1   What does ENM mean to each of you?
2   What does the term commitment mean to each of you?
3   What constitutes cheating to each of you?

Activity for the Couple: Best Friend Fantasy

Have the couple close their eyes and imagine their partner being intimate with a close friend. Have the couple sit with that image for about 30 seconds. When they open their eyes, have them face each other and tell each other what they saw and how it made them feel.

1   The couple might say, "Oh, we are attracted to our best friends," or immediately react with, "Our best friends are off limits." That is not the point of this exercise. The point is to see how you feel about your partner sharing intimacy with someone who means something to you.
2   Their therapist notes their reactions when retelling their imagined scenario to their partner.

   a   Did you identify feelings of jealousy?
   b   Did you observe distress or animosity toward each other?

    c Was the couple comfortable fantasizing about this topic?
    d How was their behavior when telling their partner?
    e Did they seem embarrassed, or were they excited to tell each other?

Activity for the Couple: Exploring Your Why

Give the couple the handout, *Exploring Your Why*, and have them complete that before their session. They will need to bring the completed activity so the therapist can review it privately.

Explore Personal Fears, Validate, and Normalize

Everyone will have fears and hesitations about ENM due to the heteronormative scripts they learned during their formative years. The couple will have worries and uncertainties about how this would work for their relationship, and the beautiful aspect of ENM is that they can design their relationship any way they want to. There are no rules as long as they agree on their ethical boundaries as a couple and hold to their agreements. We will learn more about agreements in Step 5.

Addressing fears can sometimes be difficult for clients because they do not know what there is to be afraid of yet. Provide the couple with the handout, *Finding Your Fears,* and use it as a guide to help them identify their fears based on the most common fears experienced by others in ENM relationships.

1 This activity can be completed while in session.
2 Provide each of them with a copy of Finding Your Fears and ask them to identify common fears that spoke to them when reviewing the overall list.
3 You must remind the couple that their specific fears might not be listed and encourage them to write out their concern in the space provided.
4 Throughout the discussion about their fears, the therapist should normalize their feelings as much as possible. Also, remind them that if they had to write out their fear, that doesn't mean they are experiencing anxiety that no one else has ever experienced. It just means that it wasn't put on the list. The following are suggestions for leading that conversation:
    a "That is a very valid feeling. Can you tell me more about why you feel that way?
    b "It is very common for newbies to feel uncomfortable and overwhelmed. Can we explore those feelings together?
    c "You wrote down a specific fear. Would you like to read that so we can explore that as a group?
5 If they report that they don't have any fears yet, it is possible they haven't verbalized them yet. Please encourage them to keep this worksheet close so they can write down and process fears as they experience them.

Table S1.1 Creative Space

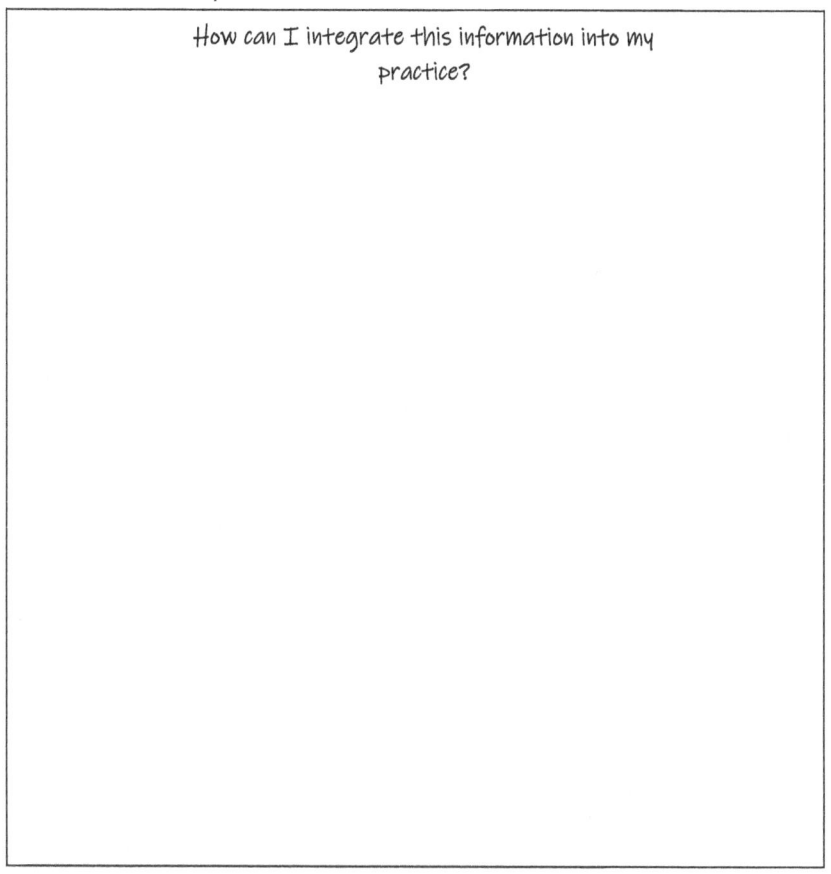

How can I integrate this information into my practice?

Source: Created by author.

Chapter Highlights

- Thoroughly evaluating the overall health of a relationship is of the utmost importance before beginning therapy with a couple.
- Valuable evaluation tools for identifying health in relationships include:
  - The Marital Disillusionment Scale
  - The CSI
  - Gottman Relationship Checkup and the Sexual History Intake.
- Evaluating the Couples' ENM Foundational Education Level is also imperative to the therapeutic process.
- Ask questions such as:

- What does ENM mean to each of you?
- What does the term commitment mean to each of you?
- What constitutes cheating to each of you?

- Utilize the *Exploring Your Why* treatment plan with the couple.

Treatment Plan: Exploring Their Why and Uncovering Fears

Behavioral Manifestations

1 The couple wants to explore what ENM would look like for their relationship.
2 One partner is unsure about ENM and would prefer to stay monogamous.
3 One or both partners need a clearer understanding of ENM.
4 One partner is not meeting all of the sexual needs of the other partner.
5 Considering ENM due to discontent or dissatisfaction with the current relationship.
6 One partner feels pressured or coerced to explore ENM.
7 Conflict resulting from the inability to deconstruct mononormative ideologies.
8 Conflict between partners stems from the cognitive dissonance of ENM and religious tenets.

Long-Term Client Goals

1 Resolve negative feelings and interpersonal conflicts created when ENM was introduced.
2 Acknowledge the need and/or desire to see other people removing the need to cheat and/or lie.
3 Commit to one partner staying monogamous while the other is ENM.
4 Each partner strives to maintain an open mindset when exploring their sexuality.
5 Respect their primary relationship while exploring aspects of their sexuality.
6 The couple explores their core values and identifies faulty beliefs that might negatively impact the primary relationship.
7 The couple understands that each ENM relationship is unique, and they can design their ENM relationship any way they choose.
8 The couple understands that ENM will not correct identified relationship issues.
9 Both partners equally agree to explore ENM together.
10 Partners escape the cognitive dissonance resulting from religious hypocrisy.

Short-Term Client Goals	Therapeutic Interventions
• Describe why ENM would be a good decision for the relationship.	• Evaluate the overall health of the relationship. • Ensure the couple does not want to open up about their relationship to save their relationship. • Determine if an ENM relationship dynamic is the best choice for the relationship.
• Build rapport with the couple while creating a therapeutic alliance.	• Gain an understanding of why the couple wants to pursue an ethical non-monogamous relationship. • Listen to their relationship narrative and conduct an oral history interview. Use the *"Intake ENM Interview"* guide in the resource section of this book during the intake session. • Utilize evaluation tools such as the Relationship Disillusionment Scale, The Couples Satisfaction Index (CSI), or the Gottman Relationship Checkup to identify areas of concern in the closed relationship that need to be addressed before opening up the relationship to ENM. • Educate the couple about how opening up about their relationship could highlight issues within the relationship they are trying to avoid.
• Provide an inclusive sexual history that details past experiences and current concerns that have influenced sexual behaviors and feelings.	• Obtain a thorough understanding of each partner's sexual history. • During the individual interviews, usually sessions 2 and 3, utilize Dr.Barry McCarthy's *"Sexual History Interview"* handout provided in the resource section of this book. • Verify that the partner is not feeling coerced or forced into an ENM relationship dynamic to save the relationship. • Normalize feelings of uncertainty and insecurity about ENM during the individual sessions. • Individually explore each partner's sexuality and encourage honest communication with their partner if they have not already done so. • Verbalize a basic understanding of ENM and provide fundamental insight into the comfortable relationship dynamics at this exploration stage. • Evaluate the couple's foundational knowledge regarding ethical non-monogamy. • Fill in knowledge gaps and clarify common misconceptions about ethical non-monogamy. • Ensure the clients understand that opening up their relationship healthily is a process and will take time.
• Openly discuss fears and hesitations about ENM.	• Explore personal fears and validate/normalize those feelings for the clients. • Ensure the couple understands the positive and negative aspects of pursuing an ethical non-monogamous dynamic. • Assign the couple with the homework *"Finding Your Fears."* from the resource section of this book.

(Continued)

Short-Term Client Goals	Therapeutic Interventions
• Understand the origin of traditional mononormative beliefs and how those beliefs affect the current relationship.	• Have the couple create a list of mononormative beliefs currently affecting their decision-making skills. • Explore the couple's beliefs about being able to love more than one person at a time. • Investigate the role sex plays in the relationship, the importance of sex in the relationship, and what being sexual in the relationship means for each partner. • Assess the couple's interpretation of the delicate balance between sex and love.
• Explore religious/spiritual beliefs that are contributing to cognitive dissonance.	• Each partner identifies how (or if) their religious/spiritual beliefs are causing cognitive dissonance. • Encourage each partner to explore their religious/spiritual framework's impact on their overall feelings about ENM. • Assist the couple in deconstructing purity culture and mononormative religious/spiritual beliefs about ENM.
• One partner wants to maintain monogamy, while the other wants to be ENM.	• Encourage each partner to explain why they choose their relationship orientation to the other. • Explore with the ENM partner their ability to provide time and space for the monogamous partner to process their feelings about them having outside relationships without resentment. • Have both partners evaluate if they can build a relationship that is respectful of all parties involved and not just each other.

References

Funk, J. L. & Rogge, R. D. (2007). Testing the ruler with item response theory: Increasing precision of measurement for relationship satisfaction with the Couples Satisfaction Index. *Journal of Family Psychology*, *21*, 572–583.

Jbilou, J., Charbonneau, A., Sonier, R.-P., Greenman, P. S., Levesque, N., Barriault, S., ... & Chomienne, M.-H. (2021). Canadian French translation of the couples satisfaction index: A pre-validation pilot study exploring men's perspective. *Research Square*. 10.21203/rs.3.rs-799178/v1

Metz, M., Epstein, N. & McCarthy, B. (2018). Cognitive-behavioral therapy for sexual dysfunction. Routledge, Taylor & Francis Group.

Niehuis, S., & Bartell, D. (2006). The marital disillusionment scale: Development and psychometric properties. *North American Journal of Psychology*, *8*(1), 69. https://link.gale.com/apps/doc/A159922637/AONE?u=anon~54783846&sid=googleScholar&xid=37fe1769

Waller, W. W. (1967). *The old love and the new: Divorce and readjustment*. Southern Illinois University Press.

Step 2

Communication

Communication Is Vital

Communication in ENM is paramount to the success of a relationship. ENM couples must communicate more than monogamous couples because there are more areas for misunderstandings, which can end a relationship before either partner realizes what has occurred. Healthy communication in ENM means having the courage to ask for what you want from your partners and being open to receiving communication from partners (Powell, 2018).

As a therapist, you are trained to provide effective communication strategies to clients, such as reflective listening, "I" Messages, intent vs. impact, and so much more. When working with ENM, couples are not different from monogamous couples in terms of *how* they effectively communicate with each other. Still, they present different challenges regarding *what* they are speaking to each other and future play partners (Orion, 2018). Orion further explains that "emotional safety requires each partner to have a certain level of self-esteem, skills in communicating needs and about practical issues, and the ability to compromise and share" (2018, p. 74).

Communication has two parts: how we receive the information and how we present the information. If Partner 1 is telling Partner 2 their needs and desires, but they don't feel heard, then deeper fractures in the relationship will present themselves. Consequently, if Partner 2 did not fully understand the request and did not ask clarifying questions, further ruptures could result.

Discover Healthy Communication Patterns

As mental health practitioners, we have had multiple courses throughout our educational journey highlighting the importance of effective communication and facilitating healthy communication with clients. When working with ENM clients, you will utilize those communication tools as well as help the clients learn WHAT to communicate about. Liz Powell, the author of *Building Open Relationships,* provided that "if we want our partners to give us

DOI: 10.4324/9781003464891-10

what we need, we have to ask for it," as well as "we have to get good at receiving the communication from our partners too" (2018, p. 71).

Receiving Communication Effectively

This is a skill that should be practiced often. In my private practice, I am constantly asking my clients if they are listening to their partners to understand their point of view better or for their partner to take a breath so they can jump right in and turn the conversation to where it is more favorable to them.

Exploring Listening Styles

According to Nichols (2020), there are different types of listening and other listening styles. Approximately 40% of people have more than one listening style that often corresponds to the specific listening situation.

Table S2.1 Different Types of Listening Styles

	Positive Characteristics	Negative Characteristics
People-Oriented	• Sensitive to people's feelings. • Needs to understand the thoughts and feelings of other people. • Focuses on emotions and appeals to emotion during arguments. • Appeal to emotion is when someone associates good feelings with being truthful; if X makes me feel good, then X must be true. If X makes me feel bad, then X must be false.	• Can become overly involved with others. • Unable to fault others. • Drawn to unhealthy relationships.
Content-Oriented	• Needs to know the details. • Concerned with what is said rather than who said it, testing others' credibility and truthfulness. • Looks for both the pros and cons during arguments.	• May reject some information because it lacks supporting evidence. • May ignore the ideas and wishes of their partner. • Has difficulty accepting "I don't know" as an answer.
Action-Oriented	• Interested in what will be done and what actions will occur. • They like structure and bullet points. • Thrive from a plan of action mentality.	• May be critical of their partner. • Have a hard time trusting others. • May not be a good listener.

(Continued)

Table S2.1 (Continued)

	Positive Characteristics	Negative Characteristics
Time- Oriented	• Want to know how long it will take to complete a request. • Does not like to waste time.	• Will try to listen while doing other tasks, not providing undivided attention to the partner. • Seek short, direct answers and to the point.

Source: The material in Table S2.1 has been adapted from "A Primer on Communication Studies" and is licensed under CC BY-NC-SA3.0.

How Well Do You Receive Communication?

Reflective listening is a grossly underdeveloped skill in our society that must be cultivated if a couple wants to enter an ENM lifestyle.

The couple will need to be proficient in one, if not all, of the techniques listed below:

1 Listen, reflect, then speak

   a Listen to the partner's concern, reflect on what they heard to ensure accuracy, and then speak about their feelings.

2 Listen, reflect, ask clarifying questions

   a Listen to the partner's concern, reflect on what they heard to ensure accuracy, and then ask clarifying questions.

3 Processing pause

   a Take a moment, approximately seven seconds, to gather your thoughts before speaking. Taking those seven seconds provides the brain processing time, so they are not speaking out of anger or saying something they did not mean.

4 Time-out

   a The boundaries around taking time-outs should be discussed in therapy or before the couple needs them.

   b The couple will need to agree on the following:

      i How do they call a time-out if needed?

      ii How long do they need to process their emotions?

      iii Determine what self-soothing techniques they will use during this time.

      iv When ready to resume the conversation, encourage them to use active listening skills.

Mastering Difficult Conversations

As a society, we are not taught how to conduct difficult conversations effectively, and our first line of defense is to shut down. This behavior will end an ethical non-monogamous relationship before they even have their first date with another couple. Communication is one of the most critical elements of ENM relationships.

Step 1: Determine the topic
Knowing what they will talk about BEFORE a problematic conversation will help clients enter into the discussion focused on the issue at hand, ensuring unnecessary details do not sidetrack them.

Step 2: Be solution-focused
After clients determine the topic, have them create a list of possible solutions they would like to explore with their partners. The speaker must be open to their partner's suggestions to address the issues adequately.

Step 3: Out of your head and down on paper
The client has their topic and has an idea about what they think they need swirling around in their heads, and now they need to phrase it in an easily understood way. This is a great place to have the client utilize the "I" Messages worksheet in the resources section of this book.

Step 4: Receiving negative feedback
Partner 1 might initiate a difficult conversation with Partner 2, but Partner 2 might have feedback they would like to share with Partner 1. This is not always easy, but it is necessary for relationship growth. Reassure the clients that they may not get the response they want and/or, throughout the conversation, they might find they were incorrect. Normalizing this will help the couple understand the benefits of holding difficult conversations.

Step 5: Mental preparation
The client is armed with their written "I" Message and ready to have the difficult conversation with their partner. Wrong! Factor in the nerves, the fear of rejection, and the judgment they have conjured in their head. They would rather do anything else but have this conversation, which is to be expected. Reassure the nervous partner and keep reminding them that their needs and desires are also critical.

Step 6: Take care of yourself and yours
The heightened emotional state that difficult conversations can evoke in clients can result in anxiety until the situation has been resolved. The couple needs to take care of themselves by participating in a self-care activity to relax and ensure they are attending to the relationship needs.

Explore Love Communication Styles

Gary Chapman, the author of *The 5 Love Languages,* explained that every individual has a "love language" and that couples can communicate their needs more effectively by understanding their partner's love language (2017). In the article by Tracey Anne Duncan, *Do Love Languages Matter? Psychologists Weigh In,* interviewee Stefani Goerlich, a Detroit-based clinical sexologist, "When I use the love languages concept with my clients, I explain to them that we have love languages that we 'speak' and love languages that we 'hear'" (Duncan, 2021).

While the five love languages concept is not an evidence-based practice, its popularity has spurred a few research studies. A research study conducted by Selena Bunt and Zoe J. Hazelwood in 2017, "Walking the walk, talking the talk: Love languages, self-regulation, and relationship satisfaction: Love languages, self-regulation, and satisfaction," suggests that utilizing the five love languages works best when both partners have adequate self-regulatory skills and are willing to change their behavior. Couples who are emotionally satisfied in their relationships tend to be in a mental headspace that can shake up their former dynamics by including ethical non-monogamy.

Erotic Communication Style

A person's erotic communication style is an erogenous map that provides insight into one's sexual style. The idea that we all have a unique map that leads to ultimate sexual pleasure was developed by somatic sexologist and educator Jaiya Ma (goop, 2022). Jaiya refers to them as tools for helping her clients identify their unique pathways to heightened arousal (Jaiya, 2023). Each person's erotic communication style considers what the individual finds pleasurable, the things that turn them on and those that turn them off, and what makes them achieve orgasm.

In my work with clients, I have them explore their erotic communication styles, and then we pair them with their Lust Language for enhanced foreplay that leads to mind-blowing sexual experiences. I explain that this is not a one-size-fits-all assessment; instead, it is an idea to help with sexual communication. There are five erotic communication styles, and encouraging your clients to explore their top two, primary and secondary, can be beneficial.

The primary erotic communication style embodies the most direct route to one's erotic pleasure. In contrast, the secondary erotic communication style works as a support system and adds flavor to one's pleasure. There is a blind spot that provides insight into those negative feelings that block people from fully experiencing erotic pleasure.

Jaiya has created a comprehensive website to accompany her book, *Your Blueprint for Pleasure,* that encourages couples to learn more about their erotic blueprint by visiting www.theblueprintbreakthrough.com where they can take a free version of the quiz or a more in-depth paid version (2023). This information can prove to be invaluable when helping clients learn how to sexually communicate with their partners.

Exploring Lust Languages

Similar to love languages, we all have lust languages. Our lust language dictates the sexy talk we prefer from our partners. If a couple does not understand their lust language, then what could have been a sexy conversation can turn quickly, limiting their partner's willingness to sext/text in the future. There are five broad lust languages; ambition, domination, sapiosexual, sensation, and transgression.

Ambition

If their partner has ambition as their lust language, then they enjoy talking about the intensity of sex. They want their partner to describe the pleasure they will receive in detail because hearing or reading helps them imagine their pleasure. These individuals will not be delighted with the dirty talk unless the sexting/sexy conversation reaches a climax.

If clients create an ambitious fantasy for their partner, they should begin with the end in mind and build it around how they imagine it is ending. These individuals receive pleasure from being teased, given small indications of their desire, and a slow build.

Example: "I will make you orgasm on my face!"

Domination

Those with domination as their lust language enjoy asserting control over their partner or being controlled by their lovers. In this dynamic, each partner has a specific role, dominant or submissive, and clearly understands the established rules. Being controlled or taking control is what turns on an individual with this lust language.

Example: "I'm going to make you beg for it!"

Sapiosexual

Those with a sapiosexual lust language are stimulated by high intellect and quick-witted banter. This lover finds intelligence arousing and is attracted to others who challenge them intellectually. According to Emily Morse, Ph.D., "the brain is the most powerful sex organ, and for sapiosexuals, this mind-body connection is crucial when it comes to arousal"; therefore, discussing deep, raw sexual desires and where they stem from "works well for sapiosexuals because the biggest turn on can be talking and listening about your turn-ons" (Daniel, 2022).

Sensation

This lust language focuses on the use of the physical senses. This person will get pleasure from the description of the sexual act itself and want as many sexy details as possible. Sensation seekers desire being told how their body smells and tastes to their partner, and their moans turn their partner on, and other descriptive languages.

Example: "Your touch makes me drunk!"

Transgression

Those who enjoy transgression as their lust language often associate sex with being dirty, kinky, and naughty. Transgression seekers prefer role-playing situations where they are being inappropriate, such as having an affair, participating in a tryst with their boss, and/or having sex in public. Due to transgression-based sexting, this lustful language could overwhelm someone who does not receive pleasure from this type of talk. This lust language is about finding out what their partner feels is "wrong" or "naughty" and then leaning into those experiences through sexy chat.

Example: "I want to make you orgasm while we are having dinner tonight with your parents!"

Respecting Off-Limit Topics

When working with ENM couples, understand they are not different from monogamous couples in terms of *how* they effectively communicate with each other. Still, they present different challenges regarding *what* they speak to each other and future play partners about (Orion, 2018). Partners must trust that they will not share intimate details about their relationship and life that could damage the primary relationship or individual reputations.

As the therapist, you must explore this with those involved and have them create boundaries around respecting topics that are more personal than others. Also, the couple must explore what information they will disclose after playing outside the primary relationship. Some partners want to know everything in detail, while others do not want to know anything. Knowing the specific information is a personal choice that needs to be addressed in the session. There is also a handout for the couple in the resource section of this chapter.

Here are a few guiding questions to ask the couple:

1   What information are you uncomfortable sharing with others?
2   How much information do you comfortably communicate with your friends and family outside of the lifestyle?
3   If you are not playing together, how much information do you want to receive about your significant other's experience with an outside partner?

Chapter Highlights

* Communication is paramount to a relationship's success.
* Therapists should provide effective communication strategies to their clients.
* Review Negative Communication Patterns and their alternatives

  * Blame vs. Seek Cooperation
  * Disdain/Disrespect vs. Positive Recognition
  * Hypersensitivity vs. Be Accountable
  * Disengaging vs. Rebalance and Refocus

* Encourage the couple to evaluate their listening styles and compare theirs to their partners to ensure they effectively listen to each other.
* Mastering difficult conversations creates a foundation for couples to use during critical times of communication:

  * Determine the topic
  * Be solution-focused
  * Out of your head and down on paper
  * Receiving negative feedback
  * Mental preparation
  * Take care of yourself and yours

* These strategies include "I" Messages, intent vs. impact, exploring love and lust languages, discovering healthy communication patterns, maneuvering through difficult conversations, and teaching couples how to respect off-limit topics.
* Erotic Communication Styles are erogenous maps that provide insight into one's sexual style enhancing their sexual experience.
* Lust Languages indicates the sexy talk we prefer from our partners

  * Ambition
  * Domination
  * Sapiosexual
  * Sensation
  * Transgression

- Ensure the couple is exploring and respecting off-limit topics with others outside the primary relationship.
- Incorporate the Communication treatment plan with couples.

***

Treatment Plan: Communication

Behavioral Manifestations

1   Unable to listen for understanding.
2   Evidence of the Four Horsemen; criticism, contempt, defensiveness, and stonewalling.
3   Hesitant or uncomfortable sharing their needs and desires due to fear of how their partner will receive the information.
4   When communicating about essential topics, one partner gets defensive and shuts down.
5   Unable to have difficult conversations without escalating hostility.
6   Difficult conversations escalate quickly and end unresolved.
7   One partner often feels criticized by the other partner.
8   One partner discusses topics with outside partners outside their primary partner's comfort level.

Long-Term Client Goals

1   Actively listen to each other.
2   Reduce and/or eliminate ineffective patterns of communication.
3   Partners communicate their needs and desires without escalating negative feelings.
4   While one partner speaks, the other listens and then reflects on what they heard before responding.
5   Disagreements no longer feel like unmanageable, overwhelming events as each partner learns to reflect on what they heard and ask clarifying questions.
6   Implement "time-out" breaks for emotional regulation when needed.
7   Each partner acknowledges and verbalizes an appreciation to the other when they feel heard and understood.
8   Using a Behavior Change Request when necessary to understand each partner's needs is essential.
9   Conduct difficult conversations without escalating emotions.
10   Agree on topics of conversation with partners outside the primary relationship.
11   Communicate the identified Love Language for their partner.
12   Communicate the identified Lust Language with their partner.

Short-Term Client Goals	Therapeutic Interventions
• Identify negative communication patterns.	• Evaluate how each partner receives communication when discussing difficult topics. • Encourage the couple to solve a significant problem as the therapist observes quietly, notating positive and negative elements of their communication style. • Educate the couple about Gottman's The Four Horseman and provide the antidotes. Visit www.gottman.com for more information and recommended use. • Provide feedback for positive areas of their communication style and feedback about areas of concern.
• Practice active listening during conversations with your partner.	• Have the partners practice active listening skills using "I" messages in the session. Use the *"I" Messages* handout provided in the resource section of this book. • Teach the couple active listening skills by having Partner 1 discuss their desires and needs while Partner 2 listens. Partner 2 summarizes what they heard and asks Partner 1 if what they heard was correct. If Partner 2 reflects back incorrect information, then Partner 1 clarifies, ensuring they feel heard before moving on in the discussion.
• Partners utilize assertive statements to communicate their needs and desires to the other partner in a non-blaming way.	• Encourage the couple to share thoughts, needs, and desires in a way that deepens their intimacy. • Have the partners practice assertive statements using "I" messages in the session. Use the *"Behavior Change Request"* handout provided in the resource section of this book. • Explore how disagreements and conflicts are frequently avoided because of an irrational fear of their partner's reaction, shame, and/or guilt. • Reinforce that disagreements are not avoidable and provide conflict resolution techniques to help mitigate the negative impact of differences. • Reinforce that relationship growth and development come from conflict and are sometimes necessary. • Determine irrational thoughts regarding conflict, rejection, judgment, shame, and guilt that contribute to effective communication. • Educate the couple about the evolution of guilt and prove that guilt is often self-inflicted.
• Practice taking a "time-out" during times of emotional flooding.	• Educate the couple about taking a "time out" when flooded with emotions during difficult conversations. Ensure they understand the importance of providing a time to return. • Demonstrate an understanding of when to use a "time out properly" and how to return to the conversation when they are not flooded with emotion. • Ensure the couple understands the importance of establishing a time to return to the conversation after practicing self-soothing exercises.

(Continued)

Short-Term Client Goals	Therapeutic Interventions
	• Have each partner identify a self-soothing exercise they could utilize during the "time-out."
• Effectively request a change in behavior from your partner.	• Inquire about common reactions from each partner when receiving challenging feedback. Ask them to write down short answers to the following questions: "How do you receive requests for a behavior change?" "Do you need to take time to process the received information?" • Help the partners identify the more profound issues hidden underneath their nagging tendencies when annoyed with their partner's behavior. • While in a session, have the partners select one behavior their partner does that they would like to see changed and practice requesting a behavior change request. Use the *"Behavior Change Request"* activity in the resource section of this book.
• Effectively have difficult conversations without quickly escalating to anger and shutting down.	• Each partner understands the rules of engagement when having difficult conversations; 1) determine the topic of conversation, 2) conceptualize the solutions to the discussion topic, 3) determine exactly what you want to say, ensuring your message is well received, 4) mentally prepare for the conversation, 5) create a plan-of-action for receiving challenging feedback from the partner, and 6) ensure to practice relationship care after the difficult conversation. • Ask the partners to determine the intent vs. the impact of their statements when they are finding the words to express their feelings (or assign *"Difficult Conversations"* in the resource section of this book).
• Partners agree on the topic of discussions acceptable to share with outside partners.	• Encourage the couple to explore what they are comfortable with those outside of the primary relationship, knowing about your dynamics. For example, are there details they only want to keep between themselves? Assign *"Off-Limit Topics"* from the resource section of this book. • When discussing topics not to be shared with others, have the partner fully explain why they feel this way and what it would be like for them emotionally if that information were shared with others outside of the primary relationship.
• Partners commit to speaking their partner's Love Language to foster feelings of love and appreciation.	• Have the couple complete Gary Chapman's *5 Love Language* quiz to identify what speaks love to them; word of affirmation, gifts, physical touch, quality time, or acts of service. • Have the couple explore how their partner can express love using their identified love language.

(Continued)

Short-Term Client Goals	Therapeutic Interventions
• Partners commit to speaking their partner's Lust Language to foster feelings of love and appreciation.	• Have the couple complete the *"Lust Languages"* activity found in the resource section of this book and review while in session. • Have the couple explore specific ways to use their partner's identified Lust Language to promote intimacy.

References

Bunt, S., & Hazelwood, Z. J. (2017). Walking the walk, talking the talk: Love languages, self-regulation, and relationship satisfaction. *Personal Relationships, 24*(2), 280–290. 10.1111/pere.12182

Chapman, G. D. (2017). *The 5 love languages: Singles edition.* Northfield Publishing.

Daniel, F. (2022, December 28). *Intellectual foreplay is a thing: 16 ways to turn on a sapiosexual.* mindbodygreen. https://www.mindbodygreen.com/articles/how-to-turn-on-sapiosexual-people#:~:text=Orate%20your%20foreplay&text=That's%20why%20deeply%20discussing%20both,about%20your%20turn%2Dons.%22

Duncan, T. A. (2021, May 21). *Do love languages actually matter? psychologists weigh in.* Mic. Retrieved January 12, 2023, from https://www.mic.com/life/do-love-languages-actually-matter-psychologists-weigh-in-18799908

goop (Ed.). (2022, July 26). *What's your erotic communication style type?* goop. Retrieved January 13, 2023, from https://goop.com/wellness/sexual-health/how-to-find-your-erotic-communicationstyle/

Jaiya. (2023). *Your blueprint for pleasure.* Sterling.

Nichols, A. O. (2020, August 17). *Listening styles.* Making Conflict Suck Less the Basics. Retrieved January 12, 2023, from https://boisestate.pressbooks.pub/makingconflictsuckless/chapter/listening-styles/#:~:text=People%2Doriented%20listeners%20are%20concerned%20about%20the%20emotional%20states%20of,who%20are%20caring%20and%20understanding

Orion, R. (2018). *A therapist's guide to consensual nonmonogamy: Polyamory, swinging, and open marriage.* Routledge.

Powell, D. L. (2018). *Building open relationships: Your hands on guide to swinging, polyamory, and beyond!* Dr. Liz Powell.

Step 3

Attachment Styles

Attachment Styles

Cultivating secure attachment while having multiple partners is possible and necessary for a successful ethical non-monogamy (ENM; Fern, 2020). Practicing secure attachment in ENM relationships requires that the partners communicate effectively, maintain trust in each other, adhere to their agreements, and honestly communicate about desired changes in the relationship. While they still have jealousy, there is an increased level of compassion for their partners, there is respect for their metamours, and they are supported when jealousy does occur.

As the therapist, you must understand that most attachment literature is mononormative. For example, "behaviors such as casual sex, one-night stands, sex outside of marriage, multiple sexual partners, partaking in bondage, voyeurism, exhibitionism, and even sexting are all associated with insecure attachment" (Fern, 2020, p. 118). The current research for attachment in ENM relationships does not support the narrative above. However, many therapists still believe that ENM relationships are a declaration of insecure attachment and characterize the client(s) as psychologically abnormal because of their lifestyle. In cases like those described above, a therapist should differentiate between the clients' purpose for specific sexual conduct, avoiding observing the sex act independently.

In the research survey, *Attached to Monogamy? Avoidance Predicts Willingness to Engage (But Not Actual Engagement) in Consensual Non-Monogamy,* researchers found no difference in the attachment styles for those who practice monogamy vs. those who practice ENM (Moors et al., 2014). There was also strong evidence that those in ENM relationships had lower attachment avoidance than those who practiced monogamy.

Furthermore, in the research study, *Multiple Loves: The Effects of Attachment with Multiple Concurrent Romantic Partners on Relational Functioning,* it was discovered that those living a polyamorous lifestyle treat each relationship as distinct and independent (Moors et al., 2019). They

DOI: 10.4324/9781003464891-11

form attachments with specific partners based on the characteristics of that relationship. If they have an insecure attachment with one partner, that does not affect the attachment in their other relationships (Moors et al., 2019).

Attachment Styles and Ethical Non-Monogamy

Anxious Attachment Style

Regarding the attachment theory, those with anxious attachment seem to be the least likely to succeed within an ENM relationship. However, conflicting evidence supports this; therefore, research cannot support that inference. In a 2020 doctoral dissertation, psychotherapist and researcher, Dr. Meara Thombre, found that those with anxious attachment styles have a less favorable view of ENM and are more likely to experience dissatisfaction than those with secure or avoidant attachment due to insecurity and jealous feelings surrounding sharing their partner(s) with others.

Those with an anxious attachment style may agree to participate in ENM because they need to please others, especially romantic partners. They persistently seek approval and affection from romantic partners and possibly gain more attention from outside romantic partners. Abandonment is the prevailing fear of an anxious attacher; therefore, if they feel this will make their partner happy and keep them in the anxious attacher's life, they are more likely to agree to ENM. However, those with anxious attachments might benefit from having multiple partners to address their emotions.

Additionally, Katz and Katz (2022) posited that those with anxious attachment styles are hyper-aware of their feelings and those close to them, resulting in frequent communication about needs. Consequently, communication is imperative for ENM. Suppose the anxious attacher works on identifying their attachment triggers and creating a plan of action for navigating them when they arise. In that case, they might have what it takes to be in a successful ENM relationship.

Avoidant Attachment Style

Due to avoidant attachers preferring to keep their emotions to themselves, there is a preconceived notion that they would be drawn to ENM. However, there is no research to support this notion, but there is research that supports avoidant attachers having a more positive sentiment toward ENM (Thombre, 2020). Research indicates that avoidant attachers possess positive regard for ENM.

Individuals with avoidant attachment in relationships tend to have difficulty depending on others and openly displaying their vulnerability. These qualities tend to be unhelpful when creating connections with multiple people. Katz and Katz (2022) posited that participating in polyamory would not be advantageous for avoidant individuals due to the magnitude of emotional intimacy and vulnerability required for prosperous and healthy polyamorous relationships. By understanding the two most common triggers for an avoidant attacher, emotional intimacy and vulnerability, and creating a plan of action to implement when triggered, avoidant attachers can have a successful and healthy ENM relationship.

Disorganized Attachment Style

Research specifically on disorganized attachment styles and ENM is scarce. Based on existing research, there can be assumptions that include individuals who report high attachment avoidance and anxiety. One study explored the difference between hierarchical and non-hierarchical ENM relationships and found that those in a hierarchical ENM relationship encounter less attachment avoidance and disquietude with their primary partner compared to those relationships with secondary partners (Flicker et al., 2021). The fear of abandonment and intimacy held by those with disorganized attachment would benefit more from having a hierarchical relationship structure due to having their primary partner available when needed.

Sharing can be difficult for disorganized attachers because they need closeness and space to feel supported but not overwhelmed by having multiple partners. Thankfully, those who practice ENM can have different attachment styles with their partners; therefore, one can conceivably work toward thriving attachment with each partner.

Secure Attachment Style

Many studies indicate that those participating in ENM relationships garner benefits similar to secure attachers in secure connections (Smith, 2021). Research also suggests that a more significant percentage of those in polyamorous relationships have more secure attachments than those in monogamous relationships (Katz & Katz, 2022). ENM relationships and secure attachment have many similarities, such as greater trust, intimacy, fewer bouts of jealousy, honesty, and significant friendships.

Dimensions of Attachment

Researchers have suggested that instead of categorizing people into one of the four categories—secure, preoccupied, dismissive-avoidant, and fearful-avoidant—clinicians view attachment using the two dimensions of anxiety and dismissive/avoidant (Mikulincer & Shaver, 2016).

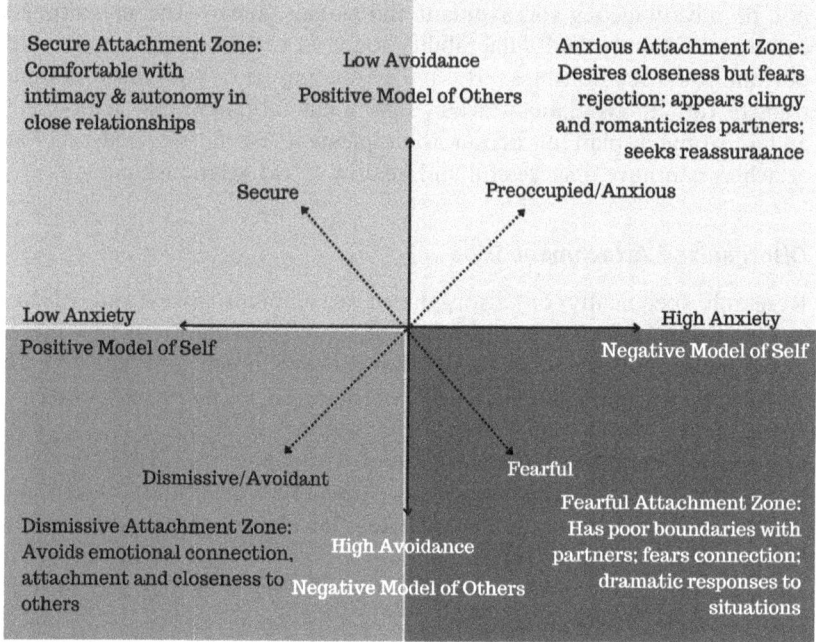

Figure S3.1 Dimensions of Attachment.

Source: Adapted from *Polyscecure,* by Jessica Fern (2020).

The four quadrants allow clinicians to see behaviors nuancedly according to where they fall along the axis instead of trying to fit attachments in one box. Fern suggested that "we also need to hold these categorical descriptions with some flexibility" (2020, p. 60). Patterns of attachment can exist on a continuum, and while understanding the negative is essential, being able to realize that each attachment style brings along their positives and strengths (Fern, 2020).

The Attachment and Trauma Integration Model

Using the nested model of attachment and trauma, polyamorous psycho-therapist Jessica Fern encourages us to open our minds to how emotional experiences influence significant relationships. In her book, *Polysecure,* Jessica Fern explained that "trauma and attachment wounds are not just an individual or relational experience … they also stem from the world we are in" (2020, p. 76). As explained by Fern, there are different dimensions or levels of human experience that are all interconnected and influence the decisions we make throughout our lives. The nested model of attachment

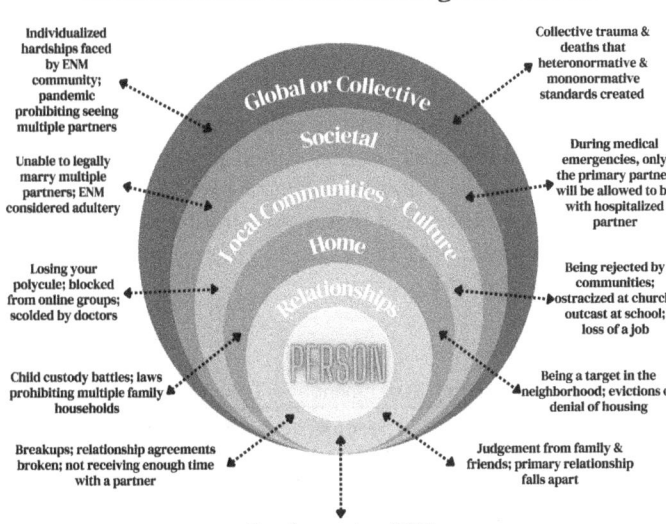

The Attachment & Trauma Integration Model

Individualized hardships faced by ENM community; pandemic prohibiting seeing multiple partners

Unable to legally marry multiple partners; ENM considered adultery

Losing your polycule; blocked from online groups; scolded by doctors

Child custody battles; laws prohibiting multiple family households

Breakups; relationship agreements broken; not receiving enough time with a partner

Collective trauma & deaths that heteronormative & mononormative standards created

During medical emergencies, only the primary partner will be allowed to be with hospitalized partner

Being rejected by communities; ostracized at church; outcast at school; loss of a job

Being a target in the neighborhood; evictions or denial of housing

Judgement from family & friends; primary relationship falls apart

Global or Collective

Societal

Local Communities   Culture

Home

Relationships

PERSON

Coming out as ENM

Coming out as ethically non-monogamous involves embracing your personal identity, understanding how multiple relationships align with your values, and addressing any internalized shame or negative beliefs associated with nonmonogamy.

Adapted from *Polysecure*, by Jessica Fern, 2020.

Figure S3.2 The Attachment and Trauma Integration Model.

Source: Adapted from *Polyscecure*, by Jessica Fern (2020).

and trauma provides the structure for identifying these differences and the effects they can cause within the various levels.

Self Level

Those embracing their ENM orientation or lifestyle have the same process and experience of coming out just as those who identify as LGBTQIA+. Society has taught us that heterosexual, monogamous relationships are the only acceptable dynamic; therefore, deconstructing monogamy can be difficult.

As their therapist, you must evaluate your personal biases and not project those on the client who has come to you for assistance in their journey. It is common for those exploring their new self and the faulty core beliefs they internalized throughout their life to question their identity. They can quickly become overwhelmed when designing the specific elements of their new orientation or new lifestyle choice that feels ethical and consensual to them personally. There is not one set way to "DO" ENM. It depends on what feels suitable to the client and the other partners involved.

Relationship Level

Relationship ruptures can occur for various reasons, so the client(s) must understand the possibilities early in their ENM journey to create a plan for when they arise. This table below is not meant to be an exhaustive list of possible relationship ruptures and therapeutic interventions. Still, these are some of the most common ones I have seen in my office while working with clients beginning their ENM journey.

Table S3.1 The Nested Model of Attachment and Trauma—Relationship Level

Possible Relationship Rupture *As Described in* Polysecure *by Jessica Fern (2020)*	Therapeutic Intervention *Developed by the Author for Use in ENM Dynamics*
Primary relationships/marriages might begin to fall apart; ENM is open to anyone, but it's not for everyone, and that is OK.	1 Have the couple revisit why ENM was the right choice for their relationship when they began their journey. 2 It might be an excellent decision to have the primary couple take a break from the other relationships and reconnect with their partner. 3 Complete a cost-benefit analysis of maintaining ENM.
Criticized, judged, and/or rejected by friends and family for choosing an ENM orientation or lifestyle choice.	1 Evaluate the client for Rejection Sensitivity Dysphoria. 2 Encourage the couple to build a new tribe of like-minded individuals who accept their decisions.
Friends and family might not want them around or alone with their children now that they are ENM.	1 Normalize this for the couple. People fear what they do not understand and encourage the couple to converse with their adult friends and answer any questions they might have. 2 Have the client suggest that the family member or friend read *When Someone You Love is Polyamorous* by Dr. Eli Sheff.
Interventions from friends and family.	1 Normalize this and assure the clients there is nothing pathologically wrong with them. 2 Remind the client that deconstructing monogamy is not easy but to keep having open conversations and answer any questions their loved ones might have.
They were no longer the initial primary partner's main focus of their time and attention.	1 Have the couple complete the *Rituals Of Connection* activity from the Gottman Institute.

(Continued)

Table S3.1 (Continued)

Possible Relationship Rupture As Described in Polysecure by Jessica Fern (2020)	Therapeutic Intervention Developed by the Author for Use in ENM Dynamics
	2 Have the neglected partner brainstorm things they can do with their former primary partner that make them feel special in the relationship.
Falling in love with a partner only to abruptly end the relationship due to factors beyond the affected partner's control.	1 Educate the couple about the grieving process and encourage the unaffected partner to support their partner's healing journey. 2 Encourage forgiveness and have the grieving partner explore their emotional dysregulation in the session.
Broken relationship agreements and/or safe sex agreements that put one partner at a higher risk.	1 Use "I" Messages to express their feelings about the agreement breach to their partner. 2 Reevaluate the relationship agreements and identify the areas that might need to be modified or adjusted so there are no future ruptures.
Not being included in decisions made to change relationship dynamics.	1 Use "I" Messages to express their feelings to their partner about how being left out of decision-making discussions makes them feel. 2 Explore realistic expectations for effective communication so everyone within the dynamic is included in the decision-making process.
Metamours have an equal voice in the relationship as the initial primary partner.	1 Explore with the partners what equality looks like for the relationship and identify areas of concern for the partner. 2 Discuss if these feelings are lingering from a mononormative mindset instead of ENM, and create realistic expectations.

Source: Adapted from *Polyscecure*, by Jessica Fern (2020).

Home Level

Many people will never understand ENM, nor will they take the time to educate themselves; therefore, they force their ideologies on others, demanding confirmation of their lifestyle dynamics. Those who choose ENM as a lifestyle or orientation will face many objections, especially those closest to them. Trauma can arise from being targeted by neighbors, landlords, and/or homeowner associations due to ENM. Being an outcast of the community is very difficult for those who want to live on their own terms. ENM family units are often evicted or denied housing, and few laws protect them.

Natasha Aggarwal, LLM., a clinical student in the LGBTQ+ Advocacy Clinic at the WilmerHale Legal Services Center of Harvard Law School, stated, "people have been fired from work because their boss discovered they were polyamorous ... It's a problem for health insurance, for living arrangements such as leases and deeds," she says, naming "a few of the areas that need legal protection" (McArdle, 2021). In 2020 and 2021, the Polyamory Legal Advocacy Coalition (PLAC) worked with the city of Cambridge and the town of Arlington to broaden the legal definition of domestic partnerships to include polyamorous relationships (McArdle, 2021).

On top of housing concerns, child custody battles where child protective services remove children from healthy, loving homes due to parental figures being polyamorous or in ENM relationships cause distress when practicing ENM. Dr. Eli Sheff, the leading academic expert on polyamorous families with children, conducted a 15-year study of polyamorous families with children and found that the three primary sources of challenges for custody are the other biological (or legal) parent, grandparents who don't believe in multiple partners, and State agencies such as CPS and religious institutions (Sheff, 2017).

Culture and Communities Level

There will be couples engaging in ENM that come to see therapists to help process the rejection they have experienced from the social group they once embraced before announcing they were ENM. A 2003 experiment by Naomi Eisenberger and colleagues posited that the brain does not distinguish between a broken bone and an aching heart. Due to these findings, rejection hurts (Sheff, 2017). Being rejected by social groups, church congregations, or general health providers can be physically and mentally painful.

Common Culture and Communities Ruptures:

- Rejected by social groups that were once a safe place
- Religious Affiliation abandonment
- Blocked from online groups or being blocked by friends and family
- Ostracized at school
- Job loss
- Fracture or break up within a polycule or ENM community
- Men (predominantly Caucasian and cis-gendered) are not afforded certain privileges as previously granted.

  - Jessica Fern stated, "while men (especially Caucasian and/or cis-gender) need to face the power dynamics that they have participated in and benefited from, the experience of going through a privilege flip can be disorienting, painful, and even traumatic" (p. 155).

- Scolded and/or misinformed by primary care physician or gynecologist
- Denied visitation with unwed partners who are in a care facility.

Rejection can have short- and long-term repercussions on the brain. Therapists are encouraged to assist clients in developing an awareness of their fear of rejection and possible connections to past rejection, perceived or real, and promote the use of self-acceptance statements.

Societal Level

There is an overlap between the culture, communities, and societal levels in that those practicing ENM are not legally protected in the United States or most other countries. I have had a client who marked themselves as having an "open relationship" on a dating app; their relationship status got back to their boss, and they were fired. Being unjustly fired from their employment was highly traumatic for the client.

Several judges have decided (without supporting evidence) that those who participate in an ENM relationship are less moral, less capable of caring for their children, and less stable than their monogamous counterparts. An example of this occurring is the case V.B. and C.B. v. J.E.B. and C.C. in 2012, where a polyamorous family was accused of child abuse, and the children were temporarily awarded to their maternal grandparents while an investigation was being conducted (Rosen, 2013). The investigation returned no evidence of abuse, and the children were returned to their partners; however, the grandparents were unsatisfied with being granted partial custody; they filed for full custody, and the trial court concurred. Thankfully, the Superior Court overturned that verdict, citing that the trial court instilled its view of morality, ignoring the evidence stating the parents were competent and ready for their parental duties.

Those who are serving our country in the U.S. Military can be charged with adultery in violation of Article 134 of the Uniform Code of Military Justice (UCMJ) (*10 U.S. Code § 934 - Art. 134. General Article | U.S. Code | US Law | LII | Legal Information Institute*, 1956). Extramarital sexual conduct was criminalized in the military to maintain "good order and discipline within the military." In 2019, the specific crime of "Adultery" was replaced with a more general term of "Extramarital sexual conduct" (Healy Law Group, LLC, 2019).

To be punished under Article 134, UCMJ, Government officials must prove the following:

1   The accused military personnel illicitly participated in extramarital activities with a specific person;

2 At the time of the extramarital conduct, the accused military personnel participated in the sexual activities knowing they, or the other party, were married to someone else; and

3 Under the circumstances, the accused military personnel's conduct was either:

a "to the prejudice of good order and discipline in the armed forces";

b "was of a nature to bring discredit upon the armed forces"; or

c "to the prejudice of good order and discipline in the armed forces and of a nature to bring discredit upon the armed forces."

(Healy Law Group, LLC, 2019)

Global Level

On the global level, ruptures can occur when heterosexual and mono-normative monogamous criteria have been actualized. For example, "an idealized form of intimacy was codified in cultural products such as television and mass advertising as the union of two individuals of different sexes, married and monogamous, actively procreating and raising a social unit as a contained, nuclear family" (Hammack et al., 2018). Families are susceptible to traumas and deadly situations when they do not fit the accepted mold.

Helping clients identify where their trauma stems from using the nested model of attachment and trauma will allow the client to grow past their trauma achieving post-traumatic growth. As Jessica Fern stated, "non-monogamy can be a pressure cooker for growth." When individuals identify old attachment wounds, process the attachment changes brought about by opening up the relationship, and heal insecurities formed from relationships founded on structural security instead of relational security, ENM is achievable.

Chapter Highlights

- Developing attachment while having multiple partners is feasible and necessary in successful ENM relationships.
- Research shows that those living in polyamorous lifestyles treat each relationship as independent.
- Attachment styles include:
  - Anxious Attachment Style
  - Avoidant Attachment Style
  - Disorganized Attachment Style
  - Secure Attachment Style.

- Rather than categorizing people in one of the aforementioned categories, clinicians should view attachment using two dimensions: anxiety and dismissive/avoidant.
- The Nested Model of Attachment and Trauma encourages therapists to explore how emotional experiences influence significant relationships.
- Therapists should focus on themselves and their own beliefs and possible biases and help couples navigate through possible relationship ruptures and issues that can occur on the home front in society, such as backlash, rejection, family judgment, job loss, etc.

Treatment Plan: Attachment Styles

Behavioral Manifestations

1 One or both partner(s) derive their worth from receiving positive feedback from the other resulting in constant pressure for feedback.
2 Perceived fears of abandonment by partner(s).
3 Feelings of jealousy when a primary partner spends time with outside partners.
4 Displays impulsive behaviors and frequent emotional dysregulation.
5 One partner frequently places blame on the other for issues within the relationship and overall relationship unhappiness.
6 Overwhelming feelings of helplessness.
7 Employs passive-aggressive behavior patterns to express dissatisfaction with their partner.

Long-Term Client Goals

1 Attain a healthy and realistic balance between independence and dependence.
2 Express dissatisfaction in a controlled and respectful way.
3 Eliminate or reduce the frequency of negative comments and behaviors that often occur when one partner is blaming another.
4 Reduce the frequency of contacting their partner during working hours or when they are with play partners.
5 Learn to make decisions without the influence of their partner.
6 Reevaluate current boundaries and make adjustments as needed to encourage healthy coping skills.
7 Explore interpersonal ways the partners can meet their personal needs by decreasing their absolute reliance on their partner(s).
8 Verbalize confidence and trust, eliminating allegations of dishonesty and disloyalty.

Short-Term Client Goals	Therapeutic Interventions
• Demonstrate an understanding of how the attachment style affects emotional safety, regulation of stress, ability to adapt, and resilience.	• Explore individual attachment styles to uncover patterns of behavior that cause challenges in the primary relationship. • Assist each partner in determining their primary caregiver as a child and how those early interactions with their attachment figure impact their relationship with their primary partner. • Help the partners identify how they derive their self-worth from their primary partner's positive feedback. • Help the partners identify how their attachment style contributes to their ability, or lack thereof, to trust their primary partner, offer forgiveness, and respond with constructive behavior instead of impulsive behavior.
• Verbalize an understanding of the attachment theory as being mononormative in nature. • Explore attachment styles to uncover patterns of emotional dependence in relationships. • Explore each partner's past experiences with emotional dependency spanning their lifetime.	• Educate the partners about the importance of distinguishing between the intentions of sexual behaviors and insecure attachment style. • Learn and apply skills that facilitate trust in significant others and find peace when not in their immediate presence. • Encourage the partners to create a timeline of important events in their individual and relationship developmental history that could contribute to their current relationship. • Explore the circumstances where each partner's developmental history, individual and relationship, has positively or negatively impacted their current functioning.
• Use assertive communication techniques to communicate angry thoughts and feelings constructively. • Accept that the pattern of insecure attachment, eagerness to please partner(s), need for constant reassurance, fear of abandonment, and loss of boundaries extend past the current relationship beginning in childhood.	• Have the partners practice "I" Messages while in the session. Use the *"I" Messages* handout provided in the resource section of this book. • Discuss and process feelings of abandonment resulting from the dependent partner's family or origin and past relationships. "Are there past experiences contributing to your current feelings and fears of abandonment?" • Explore if the dependent partner's difficulties with boundaries extend past their primary partner and into non-intimate relationships (coworkers, extended family, friends) and identify the need for a behavior change across all relationships if needed.
• Create and implement a plan of action for addressing anger-evoking situations.	• Educate the clients on creating and utilizing a Behavior Change POA effectively. Use the *"Behavior Change POA"* activity in the resource section of this book.

(Continued)

Short-Term Client Goals	Therapeutic Interventions
• Verbally agree to eliminate the primary relationship's explicit and/or implicit expectations that have resulted in disruption, mistakes, and anger.	• Motivate the client to explore alternative explanations for their partner's behavior instead of jumping to conclusions and assuming malicious intent. • Each partner agrees to evaluate their expectations that have resulted in disruption, mistakes, and anger and create realistic expectations to help discourage negative feelings in a relationship for their attachment and security needs instead of the emotional experience. • Help the partners identify ways to allow their direct experiences with partners to increase their emotional security in the relationship. • Explore how the dynamics in the relationship would change if they were to have casual, less entwined ENM relationships. • Ask each partner to explore what relationship security looks like for them. • Encourage the partners to identify behaviors that indicate they depend on the structure of the relationship.
• Identify how the partners can experience anxiety, emotional trauma, and attachment fractures when practicing ENM.	• Encourage the partners to explore how they have internalized mono-romantic beliefs and evaluate how these ideas have influenced their behaviors and choices using *The Nested Model of Attachment.*
• Compare and contrast attachment-based partners and non-attachment-based partners. • Highlight specific challenges that often present when transitioning from monogamy to ethical non-monogamy.	• Explore how the dynamics in the relationship would change if they were to practice attachment-based ENM. • Explore each challenge with the couple: resistance to the dynamics shift; underdeveloped relationship skills; being entangled with a primary partner; mismatched orientation; awakening of the self; and attachment crisis.
• Discuss and process primal attachment panic.	• Ask the partners to describe how attachment panic is a primal response that can be mislabeled as jealousy and write a plan highlighting alternatives to jealousy. Primal attachment panic: the overwhelming sense of grave danger when an attachment figure cannot be depended on (perceived or actual).
• Acknowledge and report instances of attachment anxiety.	• Ask the dependent partner to list any specific attachment anxiety they are experiencing;

(Continued)

Short-Term Client Goals	Therapeutic Interventions
	educate the non-dependent partner on how mixed signals affect the dependent client; explore the areas where the dependent partner feels inconsistency in their partner's responsiveness, support, and/or availability.
• A dependent partner explores whether they expect their partner to be an attachment figure.	• Assist the dependent partner in assessing what an attachment figure looks like in their life; have the non-dependent partner explore if they want to be an attachment figure for their partner; does the non-dependent partner have enough time, emotional space, and energy in their life to be the attachment figure for the partner at the level they need to be secure in their relationship. Provide *Dimensions of Attachment* from the resource section of this book.

References

Fern, J. (2020). *Polysecure: Attachment, trauma and consensual nonmonogamy.* Thorntree Press, LLC.

Flicker, S. M., Sancier-Barbosa, F., Moors, A. C., & Brown, L. (2021). A closer look at relationship structures: Relationship satisfaction and attachment among people who practice hierarchical and non-hierarchical polyamory. *Archives of Sexual Behavior, 50,* 1401–1417.

Hammack, P. L., Frost, D. M., & Hughes, S. D. (2018). Queer Intimacies: A new paradigm for the study of Relationship Diversity. *The Journal of Sex Research, 56*(4–5), 556–592. 10.1080/00224499.2018.1531281

Healy Law Group, LLC. (2019, October 1). *Understanding Article 134, UCMJ – extramarital sexual conduct.* Military Justice Attorneys. Retrieved October 13, 2022, from https://www.militaryjusticeattorneys.com/blog/article-134-umcj-extramarital-sexual-conduct/

Katz, M., & Katz, E. (2022). Reconceptualizing attachment theory through the lens of polyamory. *Sexuality and Culture, 26*(2), 792–809. 10.1007/s12119-021-09902-0

McArdle, E. (2021, August 3). *Polyamory and the law.* Harvard Law School. Retrieved August 27, 2022, from https://hls.harvard.edu/today/polyamory-and-the-law/

Mikulincer, M., & Shaver, P. R. (2016). *Attachment in adulthood, second edition: structure, dynamics, and change.* Guilford Publications.

Moors, A. C., Ryan, W., & Chopik, W. J. (2019). Multiple loves: The effects of attachment with multiple concurrent romantic partners on relational functioning. *APA PsycInfo, 147,* 102–110. 10.1016/j.paid.2019.04.023

Moors, A. C., & Schechinger, H. (2014, July 30). *Understanding sexuality: Implications of Rubin for relationship research and clinical practice.* Taylor & Francis Online. Retrieved October 12, 2022, from https://www.tandfonline.com/doi/abs/10.1080/14681994.2014.941347

Rosen, A. (2013, April 22). Case notes: Does a polyamorous relationship take away custody? [web log]. Retrieved August 27, 2022, from https://www.avramrosen. com/blog/2013/april/case-notes-does-a-polyamorous-relationship-take-/

Sheff, E. (2017, May 22). *Child custody issues for polyamorous families*. Psychology Today. Retrieved August 27, 2022, from https://www.psychologytoday.com/us/ blog/the-polyamorists-next-door/201705/child-custody-issues-polyamorous-families

Smith, J. A. (2021, March 26). *What polyamory can teach us about secure attachment*. Greater Good Science Center. Retrieved October 13, 2022, from https://greatergood.berkeley.edu/article/item/what_polyamory_can_teach_us_ about_secure_attachment

Thombre, M. (2020). Effects of choice orientation and consensual non-monogamy on relationship quality. *Doctoral dissertation, University of North Dakota*.

U.S. Congress. (1958). United States Code: Uniform Code of Military Justice, 10 U.S.C. §§ 801–940.

Step 4

Risks, Stigma and Sexual Orientation

Risks, Stigma, and Sexual Orientation

When couples first start exploring ENM, they often jump straight to the risks of the lifestyle. They question each other about sexually transmitted infections: What if one partner leaves the other or their family disowns them? These questions are valid; however, they should not stop a couple from exploring what ethical non-monogamy might look like for their relationship. As their therapist, you will need to explore all their questions about the risks that immediately come to mind and the risks they haven't thought about yet.

Liz Powell, Ph.D., stated that humans are biologically encouraged to over-perceive risk, especially in novel situations (Powell, 2018). The ability to perceive risks requires an individual to differentiate between a certain amount of risk and an individual's ability to accept a certain amount of risk.

When beginning something new, humans perceive higher risks than realistically presented, and our brains will send warning signals even if the presence of danger is not valid. Like all other activities in our lives, from driving to relationships, there is no risk-free road for ENM, but great rewards come with the risks.

Emotional Risks and Stigma

All relationships have emotional risks that must be weighed. Still, for those in ENM relationships, the risk potential increases dramatically because of the number of people added to the mix, along with their issues and baggage (Taormino, 2008). ENM provokes some common emotions, including jealousy, resentment, and fear of abandonment for participants, and by taking a deep look at oneself, those emotions and fears can be conquered.

This section will explore the origins and limitations of fear of abandonment and resentment. Still, due to the sheer magnitude of jealousy, we will dedicate an entire chapter to the roots and constraints of the green-eyed monster.

DOI: 10.4324/9781003464891-12

"Nothing builds intimacy like shared vulnerability," as stated by Hardy and Easton in their book *The Ethical Slut* (Hardy & Easton, 2017). Emotional risks can appear when we allow ourselves to be vulnerable; however, by expressing vulnerability, partners can break through previously established negative patterns (Wenzel, 2019).

Distinguished author and research professor at the University of Houston, Dr. Brené Brown defines vulnerability:

> I define vulnerability as uncertainty, risk, and emotional exposure. With that definition in mind, let's think about love. Waking up every day and loving someone who may or may not love us back, whose safety we can't ensure, who may stay in our lives or may leave without a moment's notice, who may be loyal to the day they die or betray us tomorrow— that's vulnerability.
>
> (Brown, 2012)

Steps for Vulnerability in ENM

"We can resist being vulnerable as a coping mechanism and means of emotional protection," says Shelley Sommerfeldt, PsyD, clinical psychologist and founder of the Loving Roots Project (Sommerfeldt, 2019). When individuals shut down, consciously or unconsciously, they feel they are protecting themselves; therefore, encouraging our clients to explore their ability to be vulnerable is imperative. Let's examine five ways you can assist your clients in becoming more open.

Mirror, Mirror on the Wall

Unfortunately, many humans have difficulty checking in with themselves because they fear what they will find. As you would practice with any client regardless of their relationship preferences, encourage the client to take a deep look inside themselves and uncover those faulty thought patterns and destructive self-talk. Faulty thought patterns can significantly impact intimate relationships by creating negative beliefs and perceptions, leading to misunderstandings, conflict, and emotional distress.

Here are some ways in which faulty thought patterns can harm intimate relationships:

- **Negative interpretations**
  - Faulty thought patterns often involve negative interpretations of one's partner's behavior or intentions. For example, someone may assume their partner intentionally tries to hurt them when they

forget to do a simple task. These negative interpretations can lead to resentment, anger, and distrust, damaging the emotional bond between partners.

- **Catastrophizing**

  - Faulty thought patterns can involve catastrophizing, which means exaggerating the negative consequences of a situation. For instance, someone may believe that a minor disagreement with their partner indicates a fundamental flaw in the relationship and that it is doomed to fail. This thinking can lead to excessive worry, emotional instability, and a lack of trust in the relationship.

- **Mind-reading**

  - Faulty thought patterns often involve mind-reading, where one assumes they know what their partner is thinking or feeling without evidence. This can lead to misunderstandings and miscommunications, as assumptions about the other person's thoughts and intentions are not always accurate. This can create a cycle of mistrust and frustration, as partners may feel misunderstood and unheard.

- **All-or-nothing thinking**

  - Faulty thought patterns often involve all-or-nothing thinking, where one sees situations and relationships as completely good or bad. This black-and-white thinking can prevent partners from seeing the nuances and complexities of the relationship, leading to unrealistic expectations, disappointment, and an inability to find common ground in disagreements.

- **Blaming and defensiveness**

  - Faulty thought patterns can contribute to blaming and defensiveness in the relationship. When individuals engage in wrong thinking, they may be more likely to blame their partner for relationship problems or become defensive when their actions are questioned. This cycle of blame and defensiveness can prevent open and constructive communication, leading to increased conflict and resentment.

Challenging and addressing these faulty thought patterns is essential to promote healthier and more fulfilling intimate relationships. Cognitive-behavioral therapy, including cognitive restructuring techniques, can help individuals identify and replace these negative thought patterns with more rational and balanced thinking. Couples therapy can also be beneficial in addressing these patterns and improving communication and understanding between partners.

Cognitive Restructuring in ENM

The American Psychological Association provided that cognitive behavioral therapy (CBT) "assumes that cognitive, emotional, and behavioral variables are functionally interrelated" and that those experiencing psychological issues can "learn better ways of coping with them" drastically improving the quality of their life and relationships (Bright & Bandura, 2004).

Identify Distressing Situation

I am not enough for my partner so they want other partners.

Cognitive Restructuring

My partner wants us to grow as a couple and expand our sexual horizons.

Identify Equivalent Feeling

~ Fear & Anxiety
~ Sadness & Depression
~ Guilt & Shame
~ Anger   ~ Jealousy

• Pick the strongest prevailing feeling first, i.e. guilt & shame, for this situation & complete the remaining steps.

• Process the next feeling, i.e. fear & anxiety, using the steps and so on if you feel the need.

Flooded With Thoughts

There may be several upsetting thoughts, identify as many as possible, here are guiding questions to ask:

~ What would it mean to you if XX happened?

~ If XX happened, what would happen then?

~ What would be so bad about XX happening?

Processing The Thoughts

Step 1: Analyze the accuracy of the identified thoughts thoroughly: what evidence supports this thought?

Step 2: List evidence that DOESN'T support the thought?

Guiding Questions:
~ Is there another way of looking at the situation?
~ Is my concern based more on feelings than the actual facts?

Make A Decision

☐ *NO, there is not evidence to support my thought?*
• Create an accurate thought that is supported by your evidence.
••••••••••••••••••••••••••
☐ *YES, there is evidence to support my thought?*
• Brainstorm & select best option
• Create a plan to execute best option
• Follow the plan & review for efficacy frequently

Figure S4.1 Cognitive Restructuring in ENM. Created by the Author.

Uncovering emotional insights can significantly impact intimate relationships by promoting understanding, empathy, and deeper connections between partners (Makinen & Johnson, 2006). When individuals recognize and understand their own emotions and those of their partner, it can lead to more effective communication, increased intimacy, and the ability to navigate challenges healthier (Wiebe et al., 2019).

Sue Johnson's Emotionally Focused Therapy (EFT) is a prominent approach that focuses on the role of emotions in relationships (Johnson, 2019). EFT emphasizes the importance of understanding and expressing emotions within a safe and secure attachment bond. By helping partners identify and explore their deeper feelings, EFT aims to create a stronger emotional connection and responsiveness between partners (Wiebe et al., 2020).

In EFT, the concept of "demon dialogues" is often utilized. Demon dialogues refer to repetitive negative cycles of interaction that couples get caught in, which are driven by underlying emotions and attachment needs (Johnson, 2019). These negative patterns can include blame, withdrawal, criticism, or defensiveness. By uncovering the emotions underneath these negative interactions, couples can gain insight into their needs, triggers, and partners (Johnson et al., 2001). This insight can help shift the relationship's dynamic from a negative cycle to a more positive and healthy interaction.

By uncovering emotional insights, couples can experience several positive effects in their relationship:

- **Increased empathy**
  - When partners can understand and empathize with each other's emotions, it fosters a more profound sense of connection and validation. This can lead to excellent emotional safety and security within the relationship.

- **Enhanced communication**
  - Uncovering emotional insights helps partners express their needs, fears, and vulnerabilities more effectively. This can improve communication, as couples can better express themselves and understand each other's perspectives.

- **Strengthened bond**
  - Understanding and exploring deeper emotions can foster a stronger emotional bond between partners. This increased emotional connection can lead to a greater sense of intimacy, trust, and overall relationship satisfaction.

Destructive Communication Patterns in ENM

'Demon Dialogue' is a term coined by Dr. Sue Johnson, co-founder of Emotion-Focused Therapy. The term is utilized to characterize the destructive cycles of conflict experienced within intimate relationships that results in feelings of being emotionally disconnected from their partner (Johnson, 2008). When there are multiple relationships in the mix Demon Dialogues can become overwhelming and negatively effect all relationships.

Which Demon is destroying your relationships?

"To name is to begin to tame."

~Dr. Sue Johnson

Tit-For-Tat Arguments

~ Back and forth verbal attacks

~ Clash of opinions!

~ Reactive & defensive nature of a verbal exchange

Core Message

""I refuse to let you control me. I'll show you."

Engage & Disengage

~ One partner irritates and finds fault

~ The other partner protects and withdraws

Core Message

As one partner protests and attacks more, the other partner responds by shutting down and distancing themselves at an accelerated rate.

Negative Spriraling

~ Stuck in "Tit-For-Tat" and/or "Engage & Disengage" for so long distance occurs.

~ Shutting down & Avoidance

~ Emotional Isolation

Core Message

"I'm hurting and scared. I'll withdraw and let us drift apart."

Johnson, S. (2008). Hold me tight: Seven 7 conversations for a lifetime of Love. Little, Brown.

Figure S4.2 Destructive Communication Patterns in ENM. Adapted from *Hold Me Tight* by Sue Johnson, 2008.

Self-Soothing

Practicing self-soothing techniques is vital for allowing the body's stimulated systems to reset and relax, especially when engaging in ENM, where there may be various opportunities for emotional overwhelm (Davis, 2023).

In her work, Sommerfeldt emphasizes that self-soothing involves comforting oneself to achieve emotional stability and balance (2018). It is a way to respond to emotional flooding and find inner calmness.

To support clients in exploring self-soothing techniques that work for them, a list of suggestions adapted from "The Empath's Survival Guide: Life Strategies for Sensitive People" by Dr. Judith Orloff can be helpful (Orloff, 2020):

- **Practice conscious breathing:** Focusing on slow, deep breaths can help calm the mind and relax the body.
- **Employ positive self-talk:** Use uplifting and affirming statements to counteract negative thoughts or self-doubt.
- **Develop a soothing mantra:** Create a personal mantra that resonates with you, such as "I am greater than my anxiety," and repeat it during distress.
- **Remember that you are not solely responsible for your fate or karma:** Emphasize that you are not in control of everything and release the burden of taking full responsibility for every outcome.
- **Engage endorphins:** Participate in activities that release endorphins, such as listening to a favorite song, placing a hand over the heart, or engaging in sexual intimacy.
- **Create compassion for oneself:** Cultivate self-compassion by treating oneself with kindness, understanding, and acceptance.

Individuals must explore and discover which self-soothing techniques resonate most with them and incorporate them into their self-care practices.

Pencil-in Check-ins

Regular reality checks are crucial for ethical non-monogamy (ENM) couples, as they allow for open communication and maintain emotional well-being (Baker & Langdridge, 2017). However, individuals in multiple relationships need to allow adequate processing time between each emotional conversation to avoid feeling overwhelmed (Veaux et al., 2014).

Regular check-ins allow couples to connect, share emotions, and ensure that everyone's needs are being met. However, it is essential to note that even positive conversations can incite a significant release of emotions, as vulnerability is a crucial aspect of check-ins (McGarey, 2018).

To maintain emotional balance during check-ins, it is recommended that individuals practice self-soothing techniques before, during, and after these conversations. Taking time for self-reflection, deep breathing exercises, or other calming activities can help individuals process and manage their emotions effectively.

Here is a list of guiding questions your clients can use to help them get started:

1   "What do you need more of from me?"
2   "What would you like us to accomplish together within the next three months?"
3   "Is there anything sexual you would like to try or experience that I can help with?"
4   "How can I help you feel more appreciated?"
5   "What do we disagree about, and how can we resolve it?"
6   "Is there anything you would like for me to do differently?"

Expand Comfort Zone

Engaging in hard conversations is crucial in any relationship, but it becomes even more critical when maintaining multiple relationships simultaneously in ethical non-monogamy (ENM). These conversations push emotional boundaries and allow couples to create new homeostasis and understanding after each discussion (Mitchell, 2019).

Having hard conversations in ENM can involve discussing boundaries, needs, desires, and potential challenges from engaging in multiple relationships. It requires open, honest, and vulnerable communication between all parties involved (Barker & Langdridge, 2017).

However, it is essential to acknowledge that these conversations can be emotionally overwhelming for individuals. If someone becomes flooded with emotions during a conversation, practicing self-soothing techniques and taking a break is advisable. This allows time for regulating emotions and prevents further escalation or damage in the discussion (Veaux et al., 2014).

Clients should be reminded of the importance of self-soothing and offered resources or guidance on techniques such as deep breathing, mindfulness, or engaging in activities that bring comfort and relaxation.

Returning to the conversation when emotions are regulated ensures that both individuals are better mentally and emotionally able to engage constructively and find resolution.

Practice Active Listening

Creating conversation agreements before engaging in intimate conversations is a valuable strategy to set couples up to successfully maintain open and vulnerable communication in ENM (Mitchell, 2019). These agreements establish a framework for how the conversation will unfold and help to create a safe and supportive environment for both individuals (Veaux et al., 2014).

A critical aspect of these conversation agreements is the commitment to being present for each other. This means actively listening, providing undivided attention, and avoiding distractions that can split attention and hinder effective communication (Gottman & Silver, 2015).

To enable couples to limit distractions before the conversation, it can be helpful to establish a ritual or routine that allows them to transition into a focused and present state of mind. This might involve setting aside specific time and space for the conversation, turning off electronic devices, and creating an environment of mutual respect and attentiveness (Barker & Langdridge, 2017).

By eliminating potential distractions, couples can fully engage in the conversation and give each other the attention and validation they deserve. This can contribute to a deeper connection and understanding between partners in ENM relationships.

Conversations Agreement Suggestions

1   No cell phones!
2   Turn off the TV.
3   Ensure kids are tended to and not creating distractions.
4   Turn toward each other.
5   Make eye contact.
6   Listen to understand; don't listen to respond.
7   If either person feels emotionally dysregulated, they can request a time-out.
8   During time-outs, come back to check-in with each other after 30 minutes. If more time is required, request it at this time.

Fear of Abandonment

Fear of the unknown is a powerful emotion and fuels jealousy and insecurities. Due to society's mononormative ideologies, we are imbued with the ethos that there can only be one perfect mate for us who will provide for our needs. When exploring ENM, many will begin their journey with fears that their partner will leave them for someone else, be replaced as the primary in their partner's life, and be alone when everything falls apart.

Those who enter an ENM lifestyle don't pass through a magical passageway where all their fears dissipate into a rainbow cloud driven by a Carebear, but many believe this is supposed to happen. If they decide to evaluate themselves and explore ENM, their hesitations, relationship narratives, and mononormative upbringing fade away.

The fear of abandonment can give rise to counterdependency, an internal belief that you don't require anyone and that depending on others is unwise. This counterdependency, in turn, leads to feelings of loneliness, distancing you from the reality that we, as humans, fundamentally need each other while also needing to cultivate self-trust (Jacobson, 2022).

Emotional indicators of fear of abandonment:

- Anxiety about being alone or panicking when not in a relationship.
- Rejection sensitivity.
- Shame, guilt, and self-blame when issues arise in the relationship.
- Apprehensive of intimacy.
- Fear the relationship is "going too well" and constantly waiting for the "shoe to drop."
- Distrust of others can cause emotional damage.

When a client's fear of abandonment overpowers their enthusiasm for ENM, clinicians have to guide them through the reality of the situation. Psychotherapist Susan Anderson stated, "transforming abandonment fear into emotional self-reliance involves radical acceptance of your separateness as an individual" (Anderson, 2020).

Many of the elements of overcoming a fear of abandonment are naturally built into ENM, including:

- **Communication:** Owning your fears and insecurities by openly communicating them to your partner, creating an emotionally secure environment where honesty is vital, and asking for or providing reassurance as needed.
- **Intentionality:** Scheduling specific moments to regularly explore each partner's needs, wants, and thoughts.
- **Specificity:** Identify where the fear is coming from and face it head-on. Feelings override logic when faced with fear. Identifying what triggered the fear for one partner can decrease the time feelings override logic, allowing reason to appear.
- **Responsibility:** Partners are not responsible for their significant other's feelings. Taking ownership of fear and realizing it is not your partner's responsibility to make you feel secure can be powerful.
- **Acceptance:** Fear of abandonment is an unconscious reflex from

childhood experiences. One does not register for this type of fear. This fear found them.

Resentment

Resentment does not spontaneously appear in relationships. It builds, creating negative sentiment override. Negative sentiment override is a build-up of everyday annoyances and frustrations that result in one partner feeling as if they no longer love each other (Rajendrakumar, 2022).

> Sentiment override refers to the couple's overall perspective on each other and the relationship which they carry with them into each interaction they have [...]. Their perspective on each other stems from the quality of their relationship friendship.
>
> (Keelan, 2022)

ENM can be a petri dish for resentment due to the many opportunities for insecurities to be unmasked. When partners feel unimportant, they don't feel like a priority, feel unheard and/or smothered by unrealistic expectations, and begin to develop anger towards their partner. In ENM, clinicians can recognize resentment building when one partner goes along with another and agrees to do something they weren't entirely comfortable with. Unspoken anger and resentment will create distance between the two partners, ineffective communication, and negative sentiment override.

> The key to avoiding resentment is to express your feelings, even if they are difficult to talk about, like anger, hurt, or betrayal. Even if you know the feelings are irrational, you must still honor them and communicate them.
>
> (Taormino, 2008)

Physical Risks and Stigma

Yes, sex can be dirty in various ways, and yes, sex can be dangerous, but what if you love multiple people? Sex is used to sell everything from toilet paper to lawn equipment, but openly communicating about sex is forbidden. Despite the many negative messages society pushes on us about sex, everyone has questions, and many want to experience more pleasure than they are receiving. Still, they are paralyzed by the fear of potential sexually transmitted infections (STIs), so they never explore their options.

Due to me being in an ENM relationship, studying ENM, and actively working with clients in ENM relationships, everyone in my life knows that I am open. The main question I get from those exploring ENM or detesting ENM is, "Aren't you afraid of diseases?" In our sex-negative world, "most people have stronger fears about, and aversions to infections that have decided are STIs than to other types of infections" (Powell, 2018, p. 97). The Centers for Disease Control and Prevention define sexually transmitted diseases (STDs) as

Sexually transmitted diseases (STDs), also known as sexually transmitted infections (STIs), are very common. STDs are diseases passed from one person to another through sexual contact.
(Centers for Disease Control and Prevention [CDC], 2022)

If we go by the CDC definition of STIs, wouldn't the common cold, COVID-19, the flu, or mononucleosis (mono) all be considered STIs? All of those can be passed from one person to another through kissing and sharing saliva during sexual contact. Yes, sexually transmitted diseases and infections should be considered when having sex with multiple people. Still, the shame and stigma that many internalize about STDs and STIs should be examined.

Recent research indicates that individuals who engage in infidelity within monogamous relationships may pose a greater level of risk than previously understood. This suggests that these participants are not solely risky due to their nonmonogamous nature, but rather, their lack of safer sex practices makes them even more dangerous than those involved in consensually negotiated nonmonogamy (Conley et al., 2012).

Below are a few guidelines to suggest to clients for maintaining good sexual health in ENM:

- Openly communicate with all sexual partners about STIs and discuss sexual histories.
- Openly and honestly communicate with their healthcare provider about their risk factors.
- Get tested often; every 3–6 months is sufficient.
- Use barriers: Condoms, dental dams, gloves, and medications.
- Create a To-Go Sex Kit; one should never depend on others for protection, so one must be prepared.

Pregnancy

When negotiating boundaries, agreements, and rules before opening up a relationship, many discuss the risks of STDs/STIs but rarely discuss the possibility of pregnancy. Pregnancy can occur when two fertile heterosexual individuals have penis-in-vagina (PIV) sex. Unless an individual who owns a uterus surgically removes said uterus or has any other medical procedure that eliminates the possibility of getting pregnant, pregnancy can occur when introduced to fertile testicles. For those in ENM relationships, an unexpected pregnancy can be very tricky to navigate. There are so many what-ifs and unknowns surrounding pregnancy, but when we add multiple partners to the equation, navigating through pregnancy can be overwhelming.

Fast Facts:

- According to the American Pregnancy Association, tubal ligation is one of the most effective ways to avoid an unwanted pregnancy for those who own fallopian tubes and having a vasectomy for those who own a vas deferens (Admin, APA, 2021).

  - The pregnancy rate after tubal ligation is around 1/1,000 after the first year and between 2 and 10/1,000 after five years.
  - While the risk is shallow, ectopic pregnancy after tubal ligation can occur.

- There is less than a 1% chance of pregnancy after a vasectomy.
- Due to a lack of research, the statistics for unplanned pregnancy within specific ENM relationship dynamics are scarce; however, there is limited data for polyamory relationships.

  - There was a qualitative study funded by the Association of Ontario Midwives that explores the lived experiences of polyamorous families with pregnancy and birth called POLYBABES. www.polybabes.ca

Exploring Pregnancy in ENM with the Client

There is no gentle way to have this conversation, but it is necessary when helping a couple navigate ENM.

Engaging in conversations about the potential of an unplanned pregnancy safeguards your relationship(s). The impact of an unexpected pregnancy can be complicated, causing significant strain. Even if having children was part of your plans or desires with your partner, the unpredictable nature of pregnancy can potentially jeopardize and even dismantle your relationship(s) (Burde, 2013).

Rip the band-aid off and ask the hard questions to create a contingency plan:

- "What happens if pregnancy occurs?"
- Client Response: "It won't happen; I am taking birth control."

- Explain the effectiveness of birth control to ensure they understand that when combined with a condom, pregnancy chances are significantly reduced but never null and void.
- Client Response: "I can't get pregnant because I have had a tubal ligation."
- Ensure that both partners have been surgically sterilized.

- What would the relationships between the biological parents, their other partners (consistent and secondary), and the children look like outside of the intimate connections among the parents?
- If the penis owner has **not** had a vasectomy, ask:

  - "What would happen if (the penis owner) were to get a secondary partner pregnant?"

    - Would the male partner want to be present in the child's life?
    - Would the primary couple request an abortion?

      - Requesting an abortion is not their choice, but it is always a question to explore.

    - What would happen if the biological mother refused to have an abortion?
    - How does the couple feel about co-parenting with another couple?
    - How would the consistent partner feel about the secondary partner moving in and raising the child?
    - If the vagina owner has **not** had a tubal ligation, ask:

      - "What would happen if (the vagina owner) were to get pregnant by a secondary partner?"

    - Would the primary partner have decision-making power if not the biological father?
    - What role would secondary relationships play in the child's life?
    - If the pregnancy is continued, what role would the biological father play in the child's life?

Regardless of how prepared a couple might feel to handle a pregnancy, there will be strong emotions if a pregnancy occurs, which is normal. Encourage the couple not to play the blame game. This was a journey they chose to take together, and they knew the risks involved. For more information about navigating an unplanned pregnancy within ENM, suggest the couples read Jessica Burde-Mahler's book *The Polyamory on Purpose Guide to Polyamory and Pregnancy* (Burde, 2013).

Social Risks and Stigma

If you don't fit nicely into society's mononormative mold, you will face social risks (persecution). Evaluate your practice. Do you perpetuate mononormativity while with clients without even thinking about it?

The ideologies and studies we encounter during our academic journeys, the applied experiences we gain through our internships and practice, the lexicon found in our intake forms, the content of our organization's websites, and even our continuous educational workshops are often permeated with the values and beliefs of mononormativity (Vaughan, 2022).

Those in ENM are not afforded any legal protections and policies, for example, multiple partner marriage, child custody, applying for housing, employment, etc., as those in monogamous relationships. Suppose we view ENM through a sexual orientation lens. In that case, it "is an exceptionally consistent predictor of public opinion ... [and] sexuality predicts attitudes at least as consistently, significantly, and substantially as gender, race, and education ..." (Schnabel, 2018).

Loss of Job, Social Standing, or Positions in Volunteer Organizations

Being in an ethical non-monogamous relationship can result in being fired from a place of employment, discriminated against in their neighborhood, and forced out of volunteer organizations with ZERO explanation.

Imagine you are standing around the "water cooler," AKA the Keurig, chatting about everyone's weekend plans. One co-worker excitedly announces:

- "My husband/wife and I have decided to have a baby, and we are going to start practicing trying this weekend!"
- Everyone expressed their happiness for the co-worker and provided well wishes.
- Another co-worker exclaims, "My partner and I are hosting an orgy at our house this weekend!"

Which statement will earn you a one-way ticket to HR and a boot out the door? It certainly isn't the co-worker who just announced they would be having sex with their partner all weekend to help procreate, but the co-worker who stated they would be having sex with their partner during the weekend for pleasure. They are dehumanized and viewed as deviant individuals (Rodrigues et al., 2021).

For those who embrace non-traditional relationships and lead fulfilling lives in non-monogamous dynamics, the relationship structure is not the primary concern (Sheff, 2017). Instead, the more significant issue is how others perceive and respond to these relationships. Planning for potential reactions and navigating them can be emotionally taxing for individuals in non-monogamous relationships when they choose to disclose their lifestyle to others. Additionally, non-monogamy can present challenges in work settings, as the need to conceal one's relationship may come with personal costs, and there is also a risk of encountering discriminatory practices based on their relationship choices (Sheff, 2017).

A client might have chaired a volunteer organization's board position for years, producing many happy constituents. Still, since coming out about their relationship dynamics, they have been released from their duties and banned from the organization. There have been ENM couples banned from coaching their children's sports teams, kids no longer allowed to spend the night with their children due to fear of being sexualized, and removed from being homeroom parents because other parents complained to administrators (Sheff, 2015). The research conducted by Conley and collaborators regarding the stigma attached to ENM posited that "participants assumed that people in monogamous relationships were happier in their relationships, sexually more satisfied, and simply better citizens than those in [ENM] relationships" (Conley et al., 2013, 25).

Loss of Friends and Family

I was fortunate enough to hide my podcast, website, and social media from my family for a while, but it happened. I got a call from my mother. She was frantic. One of my five brothers had finally found my podcast and sent a snippet to my other brothers, who then texted my mom with the following text message:

> "Mom, have you seen what YOUR daughter is doing? [Older brother's] sent me a link to a podcast where she is talking about sleeping with multiple people. SHE IS A SWINGER! And she has [my daughter, age 14 at the time] participating too. YOUR daughter is encouraging MY niece to masturbate! SHE BOUGHT HER A VIBRATOR!!!! Has she lost her freaking mind!"

As one can imagine, my Southern, religious momma couldn't "take the thought of her only daughter encouraging her perfect granddaughter to masturbate. Teaching her about *sex*, letting her know what I was doing in the bedroom, and buying her a vibrator!" I was floored by the phone call and even more confused when she told me I was encouraging my daughter to participate in BDSM. Yes, the message went on about several other aspects she "couldn't believe that I had the gall to do!"

The older brother who outed me to my family and then greatly exaggerated the truth went years without speaking to me. He can now tolerate me enough for holidays and important events, but I am not allowed to be alone with his children. My family understands that I am a certified sex therapist and educate people about healthy sex. Still, I was villainized for teaching my daughter about sex and providing a tool to help her discover pleasure for herself so she knows what to expect from future partners.

Unfortunately, my story is not uncommon. I work with clients dealing with the pain of rejection by their families and friends. I am confident that you will have an ENM couple or individual sitting across from you experiencing the same situation.

A New Orientation

One of the most startling revelations when opening up the relationship and exploring the many aspects of one's sexuality is when either or both partners declare they are gay, lesbian, or bisexual. On top of all the changes, challenges, and creativity a couple has experienced while on their ENM journey, a partner claiming their new sexual orientation can evoke contradicting feelings. There is exhilaration, possibly elements of comparison, and happiness, but negative emotions, such as uncertainty, rejection, and grief, will be mixed with excitement. A mixed-orientation couple, where one partner experiences a same-sex attraction while the other does not, will grieve the life they thought they had while celebrating their new life. Kays, Yarhouse, and Ripley (2014) found that most MOCs experience moderate levels of distress and are not highly satisfied with the overall quality of their relationship.

Various factors that influence the quality of relationships in marriages of convenience have been investigated through research (Kays, Yarhouse & Ripley, 2014). The study identified several important factors that predict the quality of relationships in mixed-orientation couples. Among these factors, commitment emerged as the most influential, accounting for a significant proportion of the observed variations. Partner-focused forgiveness also played a substantial role as the second strongest predictor, demonstrating a moderate effect size. Additionally, the distinction between contractual and covenantal marital values showed a relatively weaker association with the predictive relationship (Kays et al., 2014).

The results of Kays, Yarhouse, and Ripley's research study, *Relationship Factors and Quality Among Mixed-Orientation Couples,* provided clinicians insight into working with MOCs (2014):

- MOCs with higher levels of relationship commitment experience elevated relationship quality and overall satisfaction. Conversely, those with decreased levels of commitment experienced increased relationship distress.

- Impett, Beals, and Peplau characterized *relationship commitment* as "the degree to which an individual experiences long-term orientation toward a relationship, including the desire to maintain the relationship for better or for worse" (2001, 312).
- Partner-focused forgiveness is a substantial predictor of relationship quality.
  - Berry, Worthington, O'Conner, et al. defined *partner-focused forgiveness* as "the disposition to forgive [the] interpersonal transgressions [of an intimate partner] over time and across situations" (2005, p. 183)
- MOCs face many challenges and hurt feelings, chiefly during the disclosure process. A propensity for forgiveness toward a partner strongly indicates a couple's ability to work together during relationship distress.
- Encourage therapeutic strategies that strengthen a couple's relationship commitment and partner-focused forgiveness to enhance relationship quality, satisfaction, and longevity.

Designing Mixed-Orientation Relationships

When working with couples in marriages of convenience, it is crucial to recognize that each relationship is unique, leading to diverse outcomes. To facilitate a comprehensive exploration, several key areas can be addressed (Hawkins, Blanchard, Baldwin & Fawcett, 2008):

- **Exploration of Sexual and Emotional Desires**
  - The couple can be encouraged to create a living document that allows them to openly communicate and understand each other's romantic, sexual, and emotional needs and cravings. This process promotes transparency and supports the development of a more profound connection within the relationship.

- **Recreation of Intimacy**
  - Exploring and recreating intimacy across different dimensions is essential to reignite the passion. This includes emotional, sexual, spiritual, intellectual, and social aspects of their relationship. Couples can discover new ways to foster closeness and strengthen their bond by delving into these areas.

- **Support for New Sexual Orientation**
  - For couples navigating a shift in their sexual orientation due to their marriage of convenience, it is vital to provide resources, education, and information to assist both partners in understanding and embracing

their evolving identities. This support can empower the couple to navigate this relationship with confidence and knowledge.

- **Addressing Unknowns and Normalize Fears**

  - The couple should have open discussions to process and address their fears and hesitations regarding their marriage of convenience. By creating a safe space to discuss the unknowns and normalize their concerns, couples can better understand each other's perspectives and work toward building trust and a stronger foundation for their relationship.

These recommendations are based on the understanding that each marriage of convenience is unique and may require individualized approaches. As there is limited research specifically focused on marriages of convenience, it is essential to draw insights from related areas such as couples therapy, relationship satisfaction, and sexual orientation exploration.

Chapter Highlights

- Couples in the beginning stages of ENM exploration tend to immediately focus on the risks associated with the lifestyle. They worry about everything from contracting STIs to being disowned by their families.
- As a therapist, you must discuss their apprehensions and educate them on any associated risks.
- All relationships have emotional risks. However, in ENM relationships, chances are primarily increased due to multiple people being involved.

  - See mirror, mirror on the wall,
  - Self-soothing,
  - Pencil-in check-ins,
  - Expand comfort zone, and
  - Practice active listening to help clients be more vulnerable in ENM relationships.

- Fear of abandonment is also common in ENM relationships. Many individuals think their partner may leave them for someone else. Therapists need to guide clients through these thoughts and feelings.
- Ways to overcome fears of abandonment in ENM include:

  - Communicating these fears with their partner;
  - Scheduling specific moments to explore each partner's needs, wants, and thoughts, identifying where the fear is coming from and facing it; and
  - Taking responsibility for one's worries and realizing that fear of abandonment is a direct result of childhood.

- Resentment may present itself in ENM due to the many opportunities for insecurities.
- Partners may feel unimportant or burdened with unrealistic expectations.
- The key to avoiding resentment is to express one's feelings.
- Physical risks individuals in the lifestyle worry about include fear of STIs and pregnancy.
- Getting tested often and safe sex practices are ways to lessen the chances of contracting STIs and becoming pregnant or impregnating someone.
- Therapists should go over the protection guidelines, preventative measures, and the importance of maintaining sexual health with their clients.
- The social risks of ENM stem from a mononormative view of relationships. Individuals are often fearful that they'll lose their jobs, family members, and/or friends.
- Clinicians need to address these fears and provide guidance on navigating through them.
- Couples new to ENM may discover their sexual orientation has changed. This is not uncommon. This may bring about many challenges.
- Therapeutic resources and education that strengthen a couple's level of relationship commitment should be encouraged.
- Employ the Risks, Stigma, and Sexual Orientation treatment plan.

Treatment Plan: Risks, Stigma, and Sexual Orientation

Behavioral Manifestations

1 One or both partners have difficulty being vulnerable with other partners; one is struggling to know their primary partner is vulnerable with other partners.
2 One or both partners have difficulty being emotionally present with other partners; one partner is struggling with knowing their primary partner is emotionally present with other partners.
3 Inability to balance having a close relationship with someone while maintaining a separate one.
4 Does not practice safe sex with partners to decrease the chances of pregnancy and/or reduce the risk of getting Sexually Transmitted Infections.
5 Pregnancy resulting from a sexual encounter with an outside partner.
6 Violence occurs during a sexual experience with an outside partner or within the relationship due to a sexual experience during a group interaction.

7 Does not communicate about location when with other partners.

8 Hides ENM relationships from family and friends due to fear of judgment, rejection, and/or being ostracized.

9 Unable to agree on public spaces the primary partner can go to with other partners; disagreements on posting on social media about ENM; and arguments about events the couple would like to attend.

10 Disagreements about or concealing the amount of money invested in ENM happenings.

11 Suspicions regarding one partner spending money on another partner without their initial primary partner's consent.

12 One partner does not recognize the stigma associated with ENM.

13 One of the partners discloses that he/she/they are homosexual/bisexual/transgender.

Long-Term Client Goals

1 Able to choose and/or accept vulnerability and connection with outside partners.

2 Accept the differences in their partner's approach to being present with outside partners.

3 Sustain appropriate interpersonal boundaries within romantic relationships.

4 Engage in safe sex practices.

5 Terminate the relationship with any abusive partner and reclaim a healthy vision of self.

6 Agree upon a united decision about the completion or termination of the pregnancy.

7 Partners agree to share locations with other partners when going to new places.

8 Reduce the intensity of anxiety associated with fear of significant others (e.g., family, friends, and close community members) in their life finding out about their ENM relationship.

9 Reach an agreement on where their primary partners can go on dates with other partners, agree on social media content, and communicate effectively about events.

10 Open and honest communication about the amount of money spent on ENM happenings.

11 Reach a mutual agreement about how much money can be spent on others outside the initial primary relationship.

12 Partners acknowledge and respectfully accept the sexual orientation of the other and commit to overcoming irrational fears.

Short-Term Client Goals	Therapeutic Interventions
• Identify the emotional risks associated with being vulnerable and present with outside partners.	• Assist the couple in identifying emotional risks; falling in love, breakups, mismatched ENM interests, changes in the current relationship dynamic, etc.
• Identify and agree on what is present with outside partners would look like for each partner.	• Ask the partners to evaluate their ability to be vulnerable with others outside their primary relationship.
• Verbalize any fear of allowing themselves or their partners to be vulnerable to outside partners.	• Ask the partners to explore their emotions evoked by risky behaviors using "I" Messages.
• Identify the physical risks associated with having unprotected sexual activity and commit to practicing safe sex during future sexual encounters.	• Explore what safe sex means to each partner. Encourage them to clearly define boundaries surrounding safe-sex practices and have them commit to these agreements. • Assist each partner in identifying comfortable verbiage when requesting STI results from potential partners. • Identify the frequency each partner would feel comfortable getting STI testing. • Identify positive ways to ask potential partners for their STI test results.
• Detail the abusive or violent situation with the primary partner and/or with an outside partner.	• Explore the specific abusive situation and assess the immediate level of danger present. • Clarify the variety of feelings commonly associated with abusive or violent experiences; self-blame, embarrassment, shame, guilt, anxiety, etc. • Advise the couple or individual to seek legal assistance or protection from the offender.
• Identify and constructively discuss feelings associated with the unwanted/ unplanned pregnancy.	• Assist the couple in regulating their emotions via venting, bonding, exploring, and supporting solutions. • Assist the couple in recognizing the situation as a crisis and help them understand that their initial emotional response could cloud their sound judgment.
• List all available options and decide whether to continue or terminate the pregnancy.	• Inform the partners about the abortion laws in their state. • Conduct individual sessions with all involved parties to fully explore feelings, wants, and needs associated with the pregnancy.

(Continued)

Short-Term Client Goals	Therapeutic Interventions
	• Suggest that the pregnant partner seek individual therapy from an outside counselor to help process their feelings outside the group dynamic. • If the male partner of the primary couple is fathering a child with an outside sexual partner and she wants to complete the pregnancy, explore with the primary couple the options for co-parenting. • Advise the primary couple to seek legal counsel.
• Each partner explores potential social risks that could occur when practicing ENM.	• Assist the couple in identifying social risks; judgment from friends/family, loss of friends/family, family not allowing children around the couple, loss of a job, loss of community position, etc. • Help the couple identify how much social risk they are willing to accept in exchange for the benefits of ENM. • Identify a course of action for mitigating the determined social risks. Use the "*Risks and Stigmas*" activity in the resource section of this book.
• Openly describe and explore the situation resulting in a job loss and each partner's feelings about the situation.	• Examine the financial impact the loss of a job has created on the couple. • Refer the couple to legal counsel specializing in employment law to ensure the termination of employment was not discriminatory due to sexuality. • Identify the financial risks associated with ENM. • Facilitate money management skills that reflect careful planning, understanding, and thoughtful collaboration. • Settle on how decisions regarding financial control should be shared. • Assign the couple homework to create a budget for their new lifestyle. • Assist the couple in identifying financial risks: Job loss, dating site registrations, wardrobe expenses, travel and event expenses, and frequent health checkups at the doctor. • Ask partners to construct "I" Messages in the session to each other regarding their feelings and requests when risky financial behavior is observed.

(Continued)

Short-Term Client Goals	Therapeutic Interventions
• Discuss and process feelings resulting from the partner with the new orientation's revelation.	• Explore and verbalize irrational beliefs connected to sexual orientation that might trigger negative emotions. • Educate the partners about the origins of sexual orientation, explore faulty core beliefs, and replace them with healthy beliefs based on reality. Use the *"Mixed-Orientation Relationships"* activity in the resource section of this book.
• Provide a safe space for the couple to openly explore their anger, hurt, feelings of betrayal, etc., regarding the loss of their employment due to their lifestyle choices.	• Explore what feels emotionally safe and is too painful in the present situation regarding the primary partner bringing their same-sex partner around for visits at the primary house, spending overnights together, and being out in public spaces alone.

References

Admin, A. P. A. (2021). *Pregnancy after tubal ligation—Is it possible?* American Pregnancy Association. https://americanpregnancy.org/getting-pregnant/pregnancy-tubal-ligation/

American Psychiatric Association. (2013). *Diagnostic and statistical manual of mental disorders (5th ed.).* Arlington, VA: Author.

Anderson, S. (2020, September 7). *Fear of abandonment: A primal dilemma of insecurity and 10 ways to turn it around.* Medium. Retrieved September 11, 2022, from https://medium.com/abandonment-recovery/fear-of-abandonment-a-primal-dilemma-of-insecurity-and-10-ways-to-turn-it-around-4586a7dd10a8

Barker, M., & Langdridge, D. (2017). *Understanding non-monogamies.* Routledge.

Berry, J. W., Worthington, E. L., O'Connor, L. E., Parrott, L., & Wade, N. G. (2005). Forgivingness, vengeful rumination, and affective traits. *Journal of Personality, 73*(1), 183–226. 10.1111/j.1467-6494.2004.00308.x

Brown, B. (2012). *Daring greatly: How the courage to be vulnerable transforms the way we live, Love, parent, and lead.* Penguin Life.

Burde, J. (2013). *Polyamory and pregnancy.* CreateSpace Independent Publishing Platform.

Centers for Disease Control and Prevention. (2022, April 12). *Adolescents and STDs.* Centers for Disease Control and Prevention. Retrieved September 12, 2022, from https://www.cdc.gov/std/life-stages-populations/stdfact-teens.htm#:~:text=STDs%20are%20diseases%20that%20are,and%20passed%20on%20during%20sex

Conley, T. D., Moors, A. C., Matsick, J. L., & Ziegler, A. (2013). The fewer the merrier?: Assessing stigma surrounding consensually non-monogamous romantic relationships. *Analyses of Social Issues and Public Policy (ASAP), 13*(1), 1–30. 10.1111/j.1530-2415.2012.01286.x

Conley, T. D., Moors, A. C., Ziegler, A., & Karathanasis, C. (2012). Unfaithful individuals are less likely to practice safer sex than openly nonmonogamous individuals. *The Journal of Sexual Medicine, 9*(6), 1559–1565. 10.1111/j.1743-61 09.2012.02712.x

Davis, T. (2023). Retrieved from https://www.psychologytoday.com/us/blog/click-here-for-happiness/202302/5-self-soothing-techniques

Gottman, J. M., & Silver, N. (2015). *The seven principles for making marriage work: A practical guide from the country's foremost relationship expert.* Harmony.

Hardy, J. W., & Easton, D. (2017). *The Ethical Slut: A practical guide to polyamory, open relationships and other freedoms in sex and love.* Ten Speed Press.

Hawkins, A. J., Blanchard, V. L., Baldwin, S. A., & Fawcett, E. B. (2008). Does marriage and relationship education work? A meta-analytic study. *Journal of Consulting and Clinical Psychology, 76*(5), 723–734. 10.1037/a0012584

Impett, E. A., Beals, K. P., & Peplau, L. A. (2001). Testing the investment model of relationship commitment and stability in a longitudinal study of married couples. *Current Psychology, 20*(4), 312–326. 10.1007/s12144-001-1014-3

Jacobson, S. (2022, May 16). *Fear of abandonment—12 signs it is secretly sabotaging your relationships.* Harley Therapy™ Blog. Retrieved September 12, 2022, from https://www.harleytherapy.co.uk/counselling/fear-of-abandonment.htm

Johnson, S. (2008). *Hold me tight: Seven 7 conversations for a lifetime of love.* Little, Brown.

Johnson, S. (2019). *Attachment theory in practice: Emotionally Focused Therapy (EFT) with individuals, couples, and families.* Guilford Press.

Johnson, S. M., Makinen, J. A., & Millikin, J. W. (2001). Attachment injuries in couples' relationships: A new perspective on impasses in couples therapy. *Journal of Marital and Family Therapy, 27*(2), 145–155. 10.1111/j.1752-0606.2001. tb00342.x

Kays, J. L., Yarhouse, M. A., & Ripley, J. S. (2014). Relationship factors and quality among mixed-orientation couples. *Journal of Sex & Marital Therapy, 40*(6), 512–528. 10.1080/0092623x.2013.788107

Keelan, D. P. (2022, February 8). *Sentiment override: The bridge between the friendship and conflict management sides of a relationship.* Dr. Patrick Keelan, Calgary Psychologist. Retrieved September 11, 2022, from https://drpatrickkeelan. com/relationships/sentiment-override-the-bridge-between-the-friendship-and-conflict-management-sides-of-a-relationship/

Makinen, J. A., & Johnson, S. M. (2006). Resolving attachment injuries in couples using emotionally focused therapy: Steps toward forgiveness and reconciliation. *Journal of Consulting and Clinical Psychology, 74*(6), 1055–1064. 10.1037/0022-006X.74.6.1055

McGarey, M. R. (2018). "Your Relationship Toolkit: Strategies for Non-Monogamous Couples." (Source: ProQuest Dissertations Publishing.)

Mitchell, J. (2019). "Non-monogamy: A grounded theory study investigating the experiences and well-being of those involved in consensually non-monogamous relationships." (Source: ProQuest Dissertations Publishing.)

Orloff, J. (2020). *The Empath's survival guide: Life strategies for sensitive people.* Sounds True.

Powell, D. L. (2018). *Building open relationships: Your hands on guide to swinging, polyamory, and beyond!* Dr. Liz Powell.

Rajendrakumar, J. (2022, May 9). *Blame, resentment, and negative sentiment override.* The Gottman Institute. Retrieved September 11, 2022, from https:// www.gottman.com/blog/blame-resentment-and-negative-sentiment-override/

Rodrigues, D. L., Lopes, D., & Huic, A. (2021). What drives the dehumanization of consensual non-monogamous partners? *Archives of Sexual Behavior*, *50*(4), 1587–1597. 10.1007/s10508-020-01895-5

Schnabel, L. (2018). Sexual orientation and social attitudes. *Socius*. 10.1177/23 78023118769550

Sheff, E. (2015). *The polyamorists next door: Inside multiple-partner relationships and families*. Rowman & Littlefield.

Sheff, E. (2017, May 22). *Child custody issues for polyamorous families*. Psychology Today. Retrieved August 27, 2022, from https://www.psychologytoday.com/us/blog/the-polyamorists-next-door/201705/child-custody-issues-polyamorous-families

Sommerfeldt, S. (2019, March 26). How to reduce emotional barriers in your relationship [web log]. Retrieved September 10, 2022, from https://www.lovingrootsproject.com/allblogposts/emotionalbarriersinrelationships

Taormino, T. (2008). *Opening up: A guide to polyamory*. Cleis.

Vaughan, M. D. (2022). Introduction: Toward CNM-affirming, anti-oppressive clinical practice. In M. D. Vaughan & T. R. Burnes (Eds.), *The handbook of consensual non-monogamy (diverse sexualities, genders, and relationships)* (pp. 3–14). Rowman & Littlefield Publishers.

Veaux, F., Rickert, E., & Hardy, J. W. (2014). *More than two: A practical guide to ethical polyamory*. Thorntree Press.

Wenzel, S. (2019). *A happy life in an open relationship*. Chronicle Books.

Wiebe, S. A., Elliott, C., Johnson, S. M., Burgess Moser, M., Dalgleish, T. L., Lafontaine, M.-F., & Tasca, G. A. (2019). Attachment change in emotionally focused couple therapy and sexual satisfaction outcomes in a two-year follow-up study. *Journal of Couple & Relationship Therapy*, *18*(1), 1–21. 10.1080/15332691.2018.1481799

Wiebe, S. A., Johnson, S. M., & Lafontaine, M. F. (2020). Change in negative interaction and relationship satisfaction in couples in Emotion Focused Therapy: Examining process and outcome using the Ottawa Couple Therapy Process Measure. *Couple and Family Psychology: Research and Practice*, *9*(4), 248–262. 10.1037/cfp0000165

Step 5

Relationship Structure

Relationship Structure

Chapter 2 explored the many relationship structures available to your clients. We will examine how they connect and how the couple can uniquely design each ethical non-monogamy (ENM) relationship. The couple's preferred relationship dynamics will likely not look like any other relationship dynamic they encounter. Each partner brings their preferences, baggage, and comfort levels, allowing them to personalize their ENM journey.

In monogamy, expectations are defined, but in polyamory, they are not. There are no fixed models, only subtleties and complexities. This duality is both advantageous and challenging. Polyamory emphasizes that relationships are personal and customized to meet all individuals' unique needs. However, it also lacks a clear roadmap to achieve a successful relationship. Letting go of the norms of monogamy can be intimidating (Veaux, 2014).

Types of ENM: Each Definition Was Explained in Detail in Chapter 2

1 Monogamish
2 Polyamorous

   a Mono-poly
   b Solo Polyamory
   c Closed Vee
   d Triad
   e Hierarchical Polyamory
   f Non-Hierarchical Polyamory
   g Polyandry
   h Polygyny
   i Polyfidelity
   j Polyaffective

DOI: 10.4324/9781003464891-13

3 Open Relationships
4 Swinging
5 Casual Sex/Friends with Benefits (FWB)
6 Relationship Anarchy
7 Don't Ask, Don't Tell (DADT)
8 Deconstructing the "Relationship Elevator"

Maintaining Flexibility

ENM relationships come in various flavors; therefore, promoting flexibility with the couple is essential. They will go through many dynamics that do not work for them, find some elements of one relationship dynamic that benefit their relationship, and modify, redesign, and modify before they find precisely what works for them. The couple might have to battle mononormative thoughts from their past. All of this is very common and expected.

Developing a growth mindset is critical to maintaining flexibility during intense relationship change. In *Mindset: The New Psychology of Success*, Carol Dweck explains how individuals *think* about their partner and how their overall relationship matters. She further explains that a fixed mindset reflects the mentality of permanency. Things will not change and are set in stone, while a growth mindset communicates that with hard work and focus, we can develop and change over time.

Elizabeth Earnshaw, LMFT, Certified Gottman Therapist and contributing author for The Gottman Institute, in her article, *Change Your Thoughts, Change Your Relationship,* identified core beliefs about how partners treat each other throughout their relationship to facilitate a growth mindset, including

- We each can change and grow.
- I am not responsible for my partner's feelings (Romanelli, 2019).
- We recognize the importance of positive interactions.
- We each deserve integrity.
- We are entitled to empathy and compassion.
- We are willing and able to defend each other.
- We empower each other.

When people are single and have a fixed mindset, they believe their traits are fixed. ENM relationships exacerbate and multiply the contributing factors by the number of partners involved, the relationships, and the individuals.

People with a fixed mindset believe that different aspects of life, such as themselves, partners, and relationships, are unchangeable and will remain positive or negative. In contrast, the growth mindset emphasizes that these aspects can be developed and improved. According to this perspective, individuals and relationships have the potential to grow and change over time.

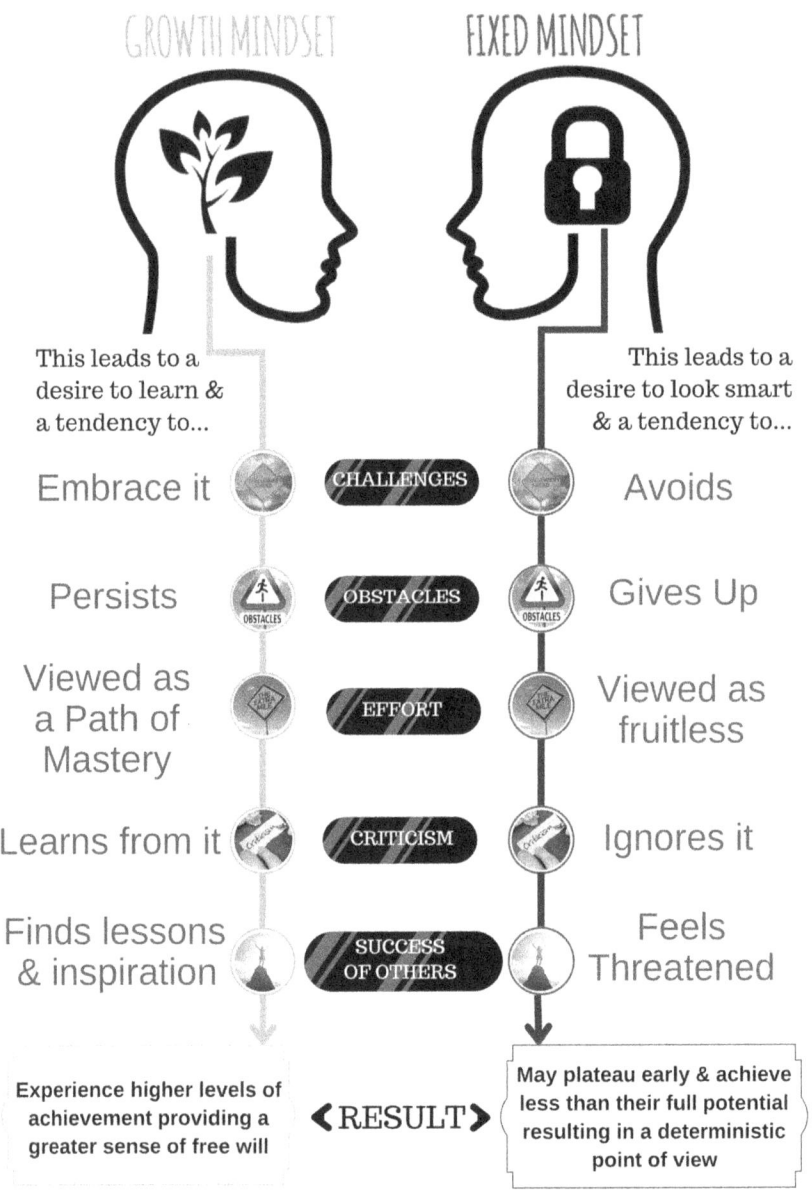

Figure S5.1 Growth vs. Fixed Mindset. Created by the Author.

Laying Out Your Lifestyle

Helping partners personalize their open relationship is essential to their journey because you are either setting them up for success or not. No pressure! The relationship structure will reflect the couple's values, needs, desires, and commitments. The clinician will help the couple outline their ideal open relationship, provide insight into elements the clients know about, and guide them in creating boundaries, agreements, and rules.

Guided Meditation Activity

* Have both partners close their eyes, take deep breaths, and relax.
* Have them imagine their ideal ENM relationship as you guide them through specific scenarios.
* Guiding questions:

  * Without censoring yourselves, imagine you can have anything you want. What does that look like?
  * Imagine your partner kissing another person in front of you. What do you feel in your body?
  * Envision yourself sitting to the side while your partner has penetrative sex with someone other than you. How does that make you feel?
  * How many romantic partners would you be comfortable having at one time?
  * Do you imagine having sex partners or relationships?

Forging the Framework

Research shows that successful ethical non-monogamy (ENM) relationships require exploration and open communication about various aspects, such as the individuals involved, the relationship dynamics, scheduling, and boundaries. While some individuals may initially claim not to have preferences or be open to anything, studies indicate this might not be entirely accurate.

A study by Moors et al. (2014) found that individuals in ENM relationships often experienced unexpected challenges and insecurities that had not been previously discussed or anticipated. These unanticipated issues could trigger emotional responses, even when jealousy was unexpected.

Therefore, individuals in ENM relationships must engage in thorough discussions and considerations of various details before embarking on this relationship style. While it may not be possible to plan for every potential obstacle or scenario, addressing as many details as possible can help establish a foundation for open communication and problem-solving when new issues arise (Taormino, 2008).

It is worth noting that every ENM relationship is unique, and what works for one couple may not work for another. Relationship agreements, regular check-ins, and ongoing communication have been identified as helpful strategies in ENM relationships (Barker & Langdridge, 2010).

The Who

When exploring who the clients are comfortable with and who they are not satisfied with, invite them to consider if gender preferences are required to help one or both partners feel safe.

- Are they comfortable with opposite-sex partners, or are they more comfortable with same-sex secondary partners?
- Does either partner have specific characteristic requirements, for example, "no tall blondes" or "no single men/women?"
- Discuss and process the roles the partners would like the secondary partners to fulfill, such as no dominant secondary partners.
- Last, have each partner delve into how familiar with secondary partners they are comfortable with. Would a partner want their primary partner to date a coworker? Do they only want to sleep with strangers?

The What

Establishing what each partner is comfortable with is a common area where partners feel they need to set limits for each other—whether it is setting sexual and BDSM limits, establishing requirements around safe sex practices, or "negotiat[ing] the nature of those relationships in terms of what [the author] loosely call[s] romantic/affectionate behavior" (Taormino, 2008, 127).

- Can they go on dates with regular sex partners?
- Are the partners comfortable with flirty emails, messages, or videos?
- How do they feel about their primary partners buying gifts for secondary partners?

If the couple is a practitioner of BDSM, have them explore what they are comfortable with their partner doing with others.

- What are their boundaries, agreements, or rules about power exchange with secondary partners?
- Do the partners have restrictions for scenes with other partners?
- Is it necessary to "create some form of role exclusivity within [their] non-monogamy" as a means of helping their partners better understand their

unique place in their primary partner's life to reduce feelings of jealousy (Taormino, 2008)?

The When

While those in ENM might have abundant love to share with others, and time is limited, when we are trying to raise kids, maintain employment, ensure intimacy with our primary partner, date multiple partners, flirt, and everything else, time is a precious resource.

- How often are the partners comfortable with sharing each other with others?
- How long would they prefer for dates to last?
- Would the partners reserve specific weeknights, days, and/or times for each other?

So many configurations can be implemented when they are comfortable sharing or seeing partners. Encourage the clients to explore each day of the week to ensure they are not missing anything important. Often, couples are excited to start or continue the new negotiations and forget established rituals for the primary family.

The Where

Determining where the couple is comfortable going depends on many factors. If they are not out to the general population, dating secondary partners could cause interesting rumors and other possible complications.

- Does the couple have hesitations about partners traveling to meet secondary partners?
- Would they prefer their primary partners to play with secondary partners only sexually when they go to adult clubs?
- Will they allow secondary partners to visit the family home for sexual experiences?
- Are any places in the house off-limits for secondary play?

The Art of Negotiation

As a certified sex therapist, I work with clients who saw *50 Shades of Grey* or "had a friend invite them to a house party," they slipped and fell into a chaotic ENM relationship without boundaries, agreements, or rules. They are now having significant relationship issues. For a relationship to succeed within ENM, the partners must discuss everything. Nothing should be implied or made up as they go along (Taormino, 2008).

When engaging in the negotiation process for ENM, it is vital to ensure that both partners are stable emotionally and that any unresolved issues are addressed beforehand (Barker & Langdridge, 2010). This sets the foundation for a favorable negotiation experience. It is crucial to approach the process openly, trust your partner, and genuinely believe they have your best interests at heart.

From the beginning, it is crucial to establish that the negotiation is not about outdoing each other or winning but rather about mutual respect and fairness. Each partner should feel that they have been treated respectfully and fairly throughout the process, with equitable rules that do not set anyone up for failure. The focus should be on accommodating the wants and needs of each individual and finding areas of compromise without anyone feeling pressured or coerced into agreeing to something that goes against their comfort levels or boundaries.

Maintaining a fair and consensual negotiation process is essential for the success of an ENM relationship. It ensures that both partners feel valued and heard and that their boundaries are respected.

Permission or Notification?

Those beginning to explore ENM will have mononormative habits that are very hard to break, and the idea of permission is one of the primary offenders. Veaux, in his book *More Than Two: A practical guide to ethical polyamory,* explained: "the idea that when we enter a relationship, we give up control over our actions to our partner" and seek permission before proceeding (2014, p. 247). To put it boldly, the primary partners become the gatekeepers of all new relationships.

If the couple's dynamics have one person being a gatekeeper, then the "permission model" would work well for them; however, the consensus prefers the notification model. The notification model represents well-defined boundaries, negotiated agreements, and rigid rules within a relationship, further solidifying security and equity by trusting each partner will do the right thing.

Veto Agreements

Veto agreements are the power to "say no" to potential secondary partners with no questions asked: "the agreed-upon ability for one person to tell another 'I want you to break up with your lover,' and have the breakup happen" (Veaux et al., 2014). As with anything today, there are optimists and naysayers regarding veto power. The overwhelming majority feel that veto agreements are fundamental for successful ENM relationships, but some agree they are necessary but rarely use them.

A veto in a relationship is an action taken by one person who holds the power to address an issue without the consent of others involved. It is binding, meaning the person using the veto expects their decision to be followed. Utilizing a veto shifts control from the individuals within the relationship to an external authority. This authority can resolve problems by eliminating a problematic partner or relationship. Much like nuclear weapons, vetoes can serve as a powerful tool for maintaining order, but their use can also significantly and permanently change the dynamics of the relationship.

While many feel the power to veto provides relationship security, they carry a very hefty price tag when used. The partner requesting the veto accepts they are breaking their primary partner's heart by removing a person from their life. When this occurs, damage to the primary relationship is unavoidable. Suppose feelings of love are beginning to develop or the primary partner is experiencing new relationship energy. Negative emotions will be attached to the veto request that must be processed so resentment does not manifest.

A common misconception about veto agreements is that the partner whose secondary relationship is being vetoed has no choice; however, the heartbroken partner can refuse to accept the veto request. The partner requesting the veto has to determine if they feel comfortable allowing the vetoed relationship to continue or walk away from the primary relationship.

A veto arrangement also makes the relationship more important than the people in it, because it requires that a relationship be ended without consideration for whether it is healthy or beneficial to the people in it. Nor does it consider the harm that may be done to them by the veto.

(Veaux et al., 2014)

Finding Common Grounds

Suppose a couple has had a negative experience with a veto request in a past relationship or feels uncomfortable with the power a veto implies. In that case, there are alternatives to veto agreements. John Gottman's extensive research on couples has proven that when couples are stuck in an argument that neither can win, facilitate a conversation that explores each partner's perspective to discover an acceptable compromise (Lisitsa, 2020).

While I present information about finding common ground to negotiate contested vetoes, teaching clients how to use this technique will benefit them when they are experiencing gridlock about any topic.

Finding Common Grounds

Yielding for the greater good:
Please engage in compromise with me, considering the love and respect we have for each other.

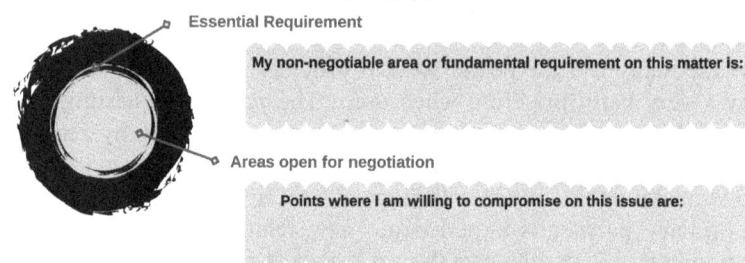

Essential Requirement

My non-negotiable area or fundamental requirement on this matter is:

Areas open for negotiation

Points where I am willing to compromise on this issue are:

Getting to 'YES' Guiding Questions

- Please clarify why this particular aspect is so important to you and why it cannot be compromised or negotiated?
- What are the underlying emotions and principles that shape your perspective on this matter?
- What are the shared objectives or aspirations that can be collectively pursued?
- What strategies or actions can be implemented to achieve these objectives together?
- What measures can be taken to establish a temporary agreement or middle ground between parties involved?
- In order to fulfill your fundamental requirements, what steps can be taken or assistance can be provided?

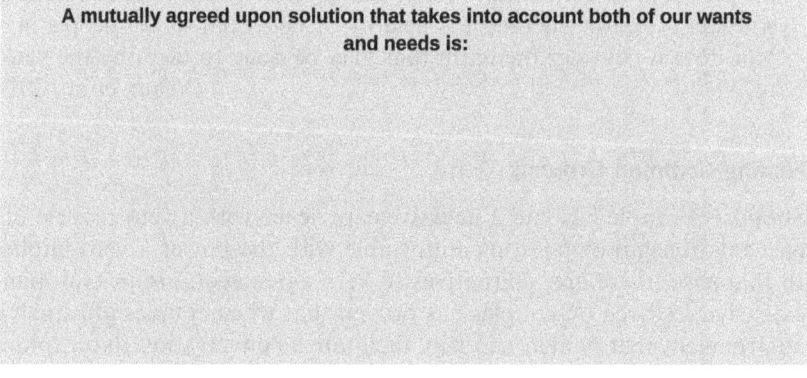

A mutually agreed upon solution that takes into account both of our wants and needs is:

Figure S5.2 Find Common Ground. Adapted from The Gottman Institute's Research.

Metamours Meeting

A metamour is a partner's partner. The relationship structure resembles a "V," with the point representing the shared, or hinge, partner and the legs representing each partner's partner (Chapman, 2010). The "leg" partners do not necessarily have a romantic relationship or even a friendship if that is how all involved partners choose to design their dynamics; however, metamours can be an essential resource for insight and support (Veaux et al., 2014).

Metamours can benefit a primary relationship, but no "rule" says that the primary and secondary partners must be best friends. It is recommended that the partners at least meet so everyone knows who the others are spending time with when away from each other. There are other helpful benefits metamours provide.

For example, Franklin Veaux recounted a time when he was the metamour and was able to provide support during a time of need (2014, p. 398):

The summer before we wrote [More Than Two: A practical guide to ethical polyamory], Eve [co-author and secondary partner] was in a serious bicycle accident that left her hospitalized for several days and disabled for weeks. At the time Peter [Eve's husband and primary partner] was living out of town, getting job experience in a new field while caring for his disabled mother. He happened to be in town when the accident happened, and he spent the weekend in the hospital with Eve, periodically stepping outside to call her other partners with updates. Two days after the accident, he had to head back to the town he was working in. Eve's girlfriend, Paloma, came to the hospital that evening and wheeled her in her wheelchair down the street for a sushi dinner, then

Simplified Metamour Explanation

Primary Partner   Secondary Partner

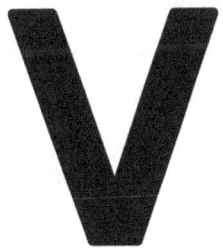

Shared (Hinge) Partner

Figure S5.3 Simplified Metamour Explanation. Created by the Author.

brought her back to the hospital room and stayed to cuddle. Later that night, Franklin arrived from Portland. He brought Eve home the next day and provided her with round-the-clock care for another week. In a crisis, everyone pitched in where they were needed as they were able.

Again, it is unrealistic to expect one person to provide for all of our needs, desires, and wants; therefore, metamours can help alleviate those expectations by incorporating more than one person to help fulfill their needs. Metamours can be intimidating in the beginning. As their therapist, it will be necessary to normalize those feelings and encourage them to push past those faulty beliefs as they mature.

Boundaries, Agreements, and Rules

Franklin Veaux and Eve Rickert comprehensively understand boundaries, agreements, and rules in their book, *More Than Two*. Much of the information in the following sections is based on their definitions.

Couples often use boundaries, agreements, and rules interchangeably; however, each term has a different meaning that must be explored with those in your office. While we will go into depth with each of these terms throughout this chapter, here is a brief explanation of each to help you better understand:

- A **boundary** concerns the self (me) and is established for the individual and their specific needs for obtaining emotional and physical safety within limits.
  - Individuals create conditions based on their needs, wants, and refusals.

- An **agreement** is a negotiation for all involved parties that discovers a common ground with other individuals to support their needs and desires; arrangements are equivalent to consent.
  - Mutual Accords support ALL individuals' needs, wants, and refusals.

- A **rule,** take it or leave it mentality is an irrevocable condition to solve problems and/or meet a need.
  - Decisions the couple agrees to are based on their needs, wants, and refusals that may impact others.

Boundaries

Boundaries are personal and solely concern the individual, and by understanding one's boundaries, agreements, and rules can be created to maximize overall satisfaction and empowerment (Veaux et al., 2014). Personal boundaries can be divided into two rugged categories: Physical boundaries and mental boundaries.

ENM clients have the right to establish and maintain their physical boundaries. They have the autonomy to decide how and when they want to be touched and who they want to be around or engage in intimate activities with. It is a common misconception that opening up a relationship means losing the ability to set these boundaries, but this is untrue.

In every aspect of life, individuals have the inherent right to choose what is best for them and to establish boundaries that align with their needs and comfort levels. This includes the physical aspects of relationships within ENM and other relationship styles. As Veaux expressed in his book *More Than Two*:

> "You may permanently set boundaries about your physical space and your body. If someone tells you it's not okay to assert a physical boundary—especially regarding who you will have sex with or who is allowed to touch you—look out! There's a problem."
>
> (Veaux, 2014)

As a clinician, supporting and validating clients' rights to assert their physical boundaries is essential, reminding them that their autonomy and agency remain intact even in ENM.

Setting mental boundaries is tricky because even the most mundane social interactions ignite possible mental and emotional boundaries (Veaux et al., 2014). Clients must understand that other members of their relationship dynamics are not responsible for their mental state and that they restrict their access, not a partner's behavior, when setting mental boundaries. Examples of boundaries that a couple could implement include:

- Not being involved with secondary partners who are not open and honest about everyone they are dating, having a sexual experience with, and/or spending a significant amount of time with. Everyone should know about everyone and consent to the relationships.
- They are choosing to refrain from having unprotected sex with partners who do not uphold adequate standards for their sexual health according to the primary couple's standards.

Agreements

These decisions affect more than one person, provide structure for managing expectations, and allow everyone to negotiate when necessary. Agreements are fluid, providing opportunities for growth and change within the individual and the partnerships. When agreeing to something one says they will do, acknowledge, or approve something someone else has proposed or desired.

That is a rule if an agreement does not allow for renegotiations by any involved parties. Also, a mandatory deal for others not permitted to negotiate is considered a rule. Here are some examples of ENM relationship agreements:

• The couple may agree for one of them to spend the night with a secondary partner if the desire is requested in advance and everyone has time to discuss it.
• If the couple is experiencing distress in the primary relationship, they agree to refrain from beginning new relationships with secondary partners.
• They agree to openly discuss sexual health information and safe sex practices with new partners.

Rules

Commonly, rules are established to preserve essential aspects of the relationship. It is up to the individual to follow the rules or break them with an understanding that a consequence could be enacted. Rules are non-negotiable declarations placed on another's behavior, fostering safety, security, and grit within the relationship; however, they are only as strong and valid as the person upholding them. Amelia Lichtenberg, Relationship Anarchist and artist, stated:

> The key trait that I sit with is that rules force the other party to take accountability for the wellness of the person setting the rule. Unlike boundaries, which serve a purpose of self-maintenance, rules can be set for any number of reasons – both healthy and unhealthy ones.
>
> (Lichtenberg, 2021)

Individuals may try to create rules that limit their partner's behavior but never fully clarify why that rule is necessary at this relationship stage. Rhea Orion stated that "rules can work if they can be followed and if partners are clear on how to carry them out in various situations" (2018, p. 45).

When a couple creates rules for their ENM relationship, discuss and process the following questions with them:

1   What is the purpose of the requested rule?
2   If implemented, would the rule serve its intended purpose? If so, how? If not, can it be redefined or clarified?

3   Is this rule the only foreseeable way to serve this purpose? If so, why? If not, explore other options and provide alternatives.

Creating a Relationship Contract

The relationship contract is not a legal document but a tool to help clients navigate ENM. Creating a relationship contract is a helpful exercise for couples to explore their desires, needs, hard limits, goals, and effective communication. The final step in the couple's activity is *Laying Out Your Lifestyle*. For many couples, creating a relationship and a contract solidifies their bond, limits miscommunication, and provides the framework for navigating issues when they arise.

Ground rules to establish with the clients before creating their relationship contract:

• The relationship contract will not make their relationship perfect.
• It does not provide a guarantee of any sort.
• It should not be weaponized.
• There will be issues that arise that were not covered in the contract.
• The contract is a living document that can be negotiated and modified anytime.
• The relationship contract cannot be used to justify bad behavior after the fact; for example, "Our relationship contract did not say anything about ... ."

Chapter Highlights

• The couple can uniquely design ENM relationships.
• Different ways relationships are structured are covered in Chapter 2.
• Maintaining flexibility often involves battling mononormative thoughts.
• Developing a growth mindset is essential to maintaining flexibility during times of extreme changes in a relationship. (See Guided Meditation activity.)
• Forging the framework of the relationship is of great importance.
• Therapists should help clients consider obstacles that may surface that the couple may not have previously thought of.
• Help them work through the "who, what, when, and where" of their ENM relationship.
• Teaching clients the art of negotiation is imperative.
• Clients should know that everything in an ENM relationship needs to be discussed.
• A model of permission may work for some. A model of notification after play has occurred may work for others. Educate clients in these

areas. Compromise should be practiced and understood. (See The Art of Compromise based on the Gottman Institute's Research.)

- Clinicians should familiarize couples with the differences between boundaries, agreements, and rules.
- Couples may also consider creating a relationship contract to lay out their lifestyle.
- Utilize the relationship structure, navigating jealousy and discovering compatibility, the common issues in ENM, managing relationships, and/or the established ENM & experiencing issues treatment plans.
- Also, see the Sexual History Interview. The interview should be held with each client individually.

Treatment Plan: Relationship Structure

Behavioral Manifestations

1   Personal distress resulting from a shift from monogamy to ENM.
2   Relationship distress due to disagreeing about the structure of the new ENM relationship.
3   One partner would rather stay monogamous, while the other wants ENM.
4   Unable to agree upon boundaries.
5   Personal distress regarding a primary partner's preferred characteristics for a potential romantic partner.
6   Unable to agree upon the familiarity of potential partners.
7   Individual distress after learning the primary partner's preferred orientation for a potential partner.
8   Lack of agreement regarding affection and sexual activities with romantic partners.
9   Unable to effectively negotiate desires and needs with a primary partner.

Long-Term Client Goals

1   Recognize many dynamics in ENM.
2   Open to exploring various relationship dynamics available in ENM.
3   Improve acceptance of non-monogamy mismatch.
4   Share ideas regarding boundaries, agreements, and rules.
5   Openly share concerns and insecurities with their partner about preferred characteristics, familiarity, and orientation for outside partners.
6   Agree or compromise on what each partner is comfortable with regarding affection and sexual activities with romantic partners.
7   Share ideas on how the primary partners can continue to meet each other's needs.

Short-Term Client Goals	Therapeutic Interventions
• Discuss the various relationship dynamics available in ENM.	• Educate the couple about the many types of relationship dynamics available in ENM. • Help partners identify the relationship dynamics that they are both comfortable with. • Encourage the couple to design their relationship the way they want to; encourage them not to censor their ideas; anything goes.
• Assist the couple in identifying their personal needs, desires, values, and goals for the relationship.	• Have each partner create an outline for what they want their ENM relationship to look like; use the *"Designing Your ENM Relationship"* activity found in the resource section of this book.

• Both partners read books and articles about non-monogamy mismatch and then report what they learned that helped them better understand ENM.	• Assign both partners to read books on ENM:
	  • *Opening Up* by Tristan Taormino
	  • *Building Open Relationships* by Dr. Liz Powell
	  • *Polysecure* by Jessica Fern
	  • *Rewriting The Rules* by Meg-John Barker

• Identify boundaries, agreements, and rules each partner is comfortable with regarding sexual play and intimate relationships.	• Educate the couple about boundaries and their purpose for ENM relationships; they can set boundaries for anything they can control having to do with themselves. • Educate the couple about agreements and their purpose for ENM relationships, making decisions for the couple as a whole, and each partner can renegotiate agreements at any time. • Assist the couple with individually creating agreements that will help them feel emotionally, mentally, and physically safe. Assign the *"Boundaries, Agreements, & Rules, Oh My!"* assignment in this book's resource section. • Educate the couple about rules and their purpose for ENM relationships; rules are a "take it or leave it" mentality.
• Each partner identifies their preferred characteristics, familiarity, and orientation for outside partners.	• Assist the couple in identifying: Who all their potential romantic partners might be; what types of activities they do as well as the nature of their romantic relationship; the frequency and duration of their time together, where they are comfortable with each other taking romantic partners too. Use the *"Designing*

(Continued)

Short-Term Client Goals	Therapeutic Interventions
	Your ENM Relationship" activity found in the resource section of this book.
• Both partners agree on how they would like to approach each other when they want to negotiate elements of their ENM relationship.	• Have the couple establish how they would like to approach the negotiation process. • Assist the couple in identifying what approaching the negotiating process from a place of stability would look like in their relationship.
• The couple signs a relationship contract for the boundaries, agreements, and rules for their ENM relationship.	• Have the couple create a relationship contract based on the information from "Designing Your ENM Relationship" activity. • Have the couple agree upon the relationship contract and sign the contract. Use the "Relationship Contract" activity in the resource section of this book.

References

Barker, M., & Langdridge, D. (2010). *Understanding non-monogamies*. Routledge.

Chapman, M. (2010). *What does polyamory look like?: Polydiverse patterns of loving and living in modern polyamorous relationships*. iUniverse Inc.

Lichtenberg, A. (2021). *Relationship anarchy—Love is the action—Amelia Lichtenberg*. Amelia Lichtenberg. Retrieved October 13, 2022, from https://www.amelialichtenberg.com/loveistheaction/tag/relationship+anarchy

Lisitsa, E. (2020, December 28). *Manage conflict: The art of compromise*. The Gottman Institute. Retrieved September 15, 2022, from https://www.gottman.com/blog/manage-conflict-the-art-of-compromise/

Moors, A. C., Conley, T. D., & Chopik, W. J. (2014). Attached to monogamy? Avoidance predicts willingness to engage (but not actual engagement) in consensual non-monogamy. *SAGE Journals, 32*(2). https://journals.sagepub.com/doi/full/10.1177/0265407514529065

Orion, R. (2018). *A therapist's guide to consensual nonmonogamy: Polyamory, swinging, and open marriage*. Routledge.

Romanelli, A. (2019). *You are not responsible for your partner's feelings*. Psychology Today. Retrieved September 14, 2022, from https://www.psychologytoday.com/us/blog/the-other-side-relationships/201908/you-are-not-responsible-your-partners-feelings

Taormino, T. (2008). *Opening up: A guide to polyamory*. Cleis.

Veaux, F., Rickert, E., & Hardy, J. W. (2014). *More than two: A practical guide to ethical polyamory*. Thorntree Press.

Navigating Jealousy, Rejection Sensitivity and Discovering Compersion

Navigating Jealousy, Rejection Sensitivity, and Discovering Compersion

This week, I had a client express concern about the growth in their ethical non-monogamy (ENM) relationship because they were experiencing jealousy, and their partner told them that ENM might not be for them because "there is no jealousy in ENM." Personally and professionally, I can adamantly proclaim that jealousy is a natural part of all relationship dynamics, monogamous and/or non-monogamous. Still, how one manages those feelings makes the difference in relationships.

According to Mogilski et al., jealousy is triggered when individuals perceive a threat to their romantic relationship, whether real or imagined (2019). This threat can arise from factors such as the presence and quality of potential rivals, discrepancies in attractiveness or satisfaction within the relationship, thoughts or stories of a partner's involvement with someone else, and signs of emotional or sexual withdrawal from the partner. These cues can lead individuals to believe their relationship is unstable or at risk of ending. Jealousy is a natural reaction in response to these perceived threats.

Jealousy wears many faces and is constructed on layers of emotions, including but not limited to insecurity, fear of loss, fear of abandonment, inadequacy, and helplessness. Jealous feelings are beyond the control of the person experiencing the emotion; however, jealous actions in response to the feelings can be controlled. Jealous actions attempt to regain control over a situation by creating a false sense of safety and security. Trying to maintain a partner's behavior "undermine[s] intimacy by telling [the] partner that [they are not trusted] ... [and they] don't believe [their] affection is genuine" (Veaux et al., 2014, 125).

ENM relationships are diverse and contingent on individual preferences; therefore, independent relationships are negotiated and refined continuously throughout the relationship, allowing for constant growth

DOI: 10.4324/9781003464891-14

and change (Musson, 2019). When jealousy is experienced, the brain's reptilian parts try to communicate without words. The jealousy could be trying to articulate significant issues within the relationship, or the jealous feelings could be the angry inner child stomping their foot because they didn't get what they wanted. It is up to the individual to decide what the jealousy is attempting to represent. Humans are quick to associate jealousy with the behaviors of others instead of owning the feelings that might be a direct result of insecurities. Ideally, those in ENM relationships have or are learning mature communication skills; however, jealousy can be triggered unexpectedly, resulting in a communication breakdown.

Navigating Jealousy

When helping clients navigate their jealousy, please encourage them to explore how they experience jealousy and find healthier, more manageable, less overwhelming patterns. A large-scale research project, *Agreements, rules and agentic fidelity in polyamorous relationships,* conducted by Kassia Wosick-Correa, found that:

> Agentic fidelity involves remaining loyal to the process of establishing agreements and rules, respecting oneself and one's partners through following the rules and being self-aware on a very individual level.
>
> (Wosick-Correa, 2009: 58)

By placing focus on the importance of preserving uniqueness through agentic fidelity, disruptions, fractures, or breaches in the stipulations of a relationship are approached as boundary, agreement, or rule violations instead of disrupting the core of a relationship, similar to what jealousy creates in monogamous relationships (Musson, 2019). Furthermore, creating situations that promote specialness within the relationship by sharing specific interactions or locations with certain partners can reduce jealousy.

Regardless of agentic fidelity or being aware of extradyadic relationships allowing for secondary romantic or sexual relationships, jealousy is one of the primary factors when couples come to therapy. As a society, we are not taught how to navigate jealousy, providing an increased opportunity for strong emotional or physical reactions.

Jealousy is a complex emotional response that can be categorized into different types based on the underlying motivations and triggers. Buunk (1997) categorizes jealousy into three main types: reactive, preventive, and anxious.

Reactive jealousy is a response to the actual engagement of one's partner in intimate behaviors with someone else (Barelds & Barelds-Dijkstra, 2007). It arises when there is clear evidence or confirmation of a partner's infidelity or betrayal. This type of jealousy is often characterized by strong emotional reactions such as anger, hurt, and a sense of betrayal.

As the name suggests, preventive jealousy involves efforts to limit contact between one's partner and individuals of the opposite sex (Barelds & Barelds-Dijkstra, 2007). Individuals experiencing preventive jealousy may try to control or restrict their partner's interactions with others, often out of fear of potential infidelity. In extreme cases, preventive jealousy can lead to acts of violence or possessive behavior.

Anxious jealousy is a cognitive process where the individual imagines their partner becoming emotionally or sexually involved with someone else (Barelds & Barelds-Dijkstra, 2007). Feelings of anxiety, suspicion, worry, distrust, and upset characterize it. Anxiously jealous individuals often have

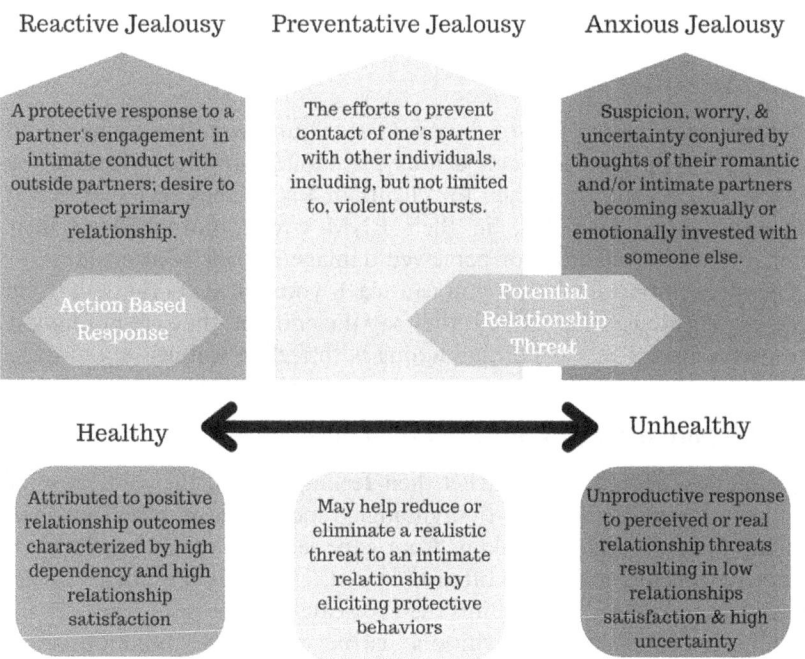

Three Types of Jealousy

Reactive Jealousy

A protective response to a partner's engagement in intimate conduct with outside partners; desire to protect primary relationship.

Action Based Response

Preventative Jealousy

The efforts to prevent contact of one's partner with other individuals, including, but not limited to, violent outbursts.

Potential Relationship Threat

Anxious Jealousy

Suspicion, worry, & uncertainty conjured by thoughts of their romantic and/or intimate partners becoming sexually or emotionally invested with someone else.

Healthy ←——————→ Unhealthy

Attributed to positive relationship outcomes characterized by high dependency and high relationship satisfaction

May help reduce or eliminate a realistic threat to an intimate relationship by eliciting protective behaviors

Unproductive response to perceived or real relationship threats resulting in low relationships satisfaction & high uncertainty

Adapted from *Personality, birth order and attachment styles as related to various types of jealousy* by B.P. Buunk, 1997

Figure S6.1 Types of Jealousy. Adapted from Research Conducted by Abraham P. Buunk (1997).

intrusive thoughts and engage in excessive monitoring or checking behaviors in an attempt to alleviate their fears.

While reactive jealousy is triggered by actual evidence of infidelity, both preventive and anxious jealousy can be fueled by real extradyadic involvement or the perception of potential relationship threats. In preventive and anxious jealousy, the triggers can range from harmless interactions to imagined scenarios, highlighting the cognitive and emotional nature of these types of jealousy.

Understanding the different types of jealousy can provide insights into the complex dynamics of romantic relationships and help individuals navigate and manage their feelings of jealousy.

In the research study, *Three Types of Jealousy and Their Relation to Dependency, Uncertainty, and Satisfaction,* Buunk and Dijkstra found that distinguishing between the different categories of jealousy could aid in the understanding of the various effects jealousy has on the overall quality of romantic and intimate relationships allowing clinicians to tailor their therapeutic strategies to help clients with coping with their negative expressions of jealousy (2021).

Step 1: Accept the Feelings

It will be standard for you to discover that your clients have never been taught how to navigate through jealousy, let alone know how to accept the feelings. When jealousy occurs for clients in ENM, they feel shame and guilt confounded by others in their ENM circles, not allowing their jealousy to cause reactions or perceived damage in their relationships.

The most important lesson you can teach your clients is that everyone experiences jealousy <period>. If they say they do not, they are not honest with themselves. There is nothing wrong with feeling jealous.

Step 2: Separate the Triggers from the Causation

Encouraging clients to deconstruct their feelings to find the root cause of their jealousy and addressing that entangled mess is more beneficial than focusing on the trigger. Speaking from experience, managing jealousy is extremely difficult, and more often than not, I immediately focus on the trigger before looking deeper into the root cause.

Suppose a couple presents with one partner reporting a situation where they were overwhelmed by jealousy when they saw their partner kissing another person and acting irrationally. The kiss triggered the jealousy; however, a root cause must be uncovered and processed. The root cause could have been a fear of being replaced, feeling left out, or feeling territorial.

Step 3: Try to Understand the Feelings

More times than not, jealousy stems from fear, fear of being alone, fear of abandonment, fear of losing your partner, fear of rejection, and fear of being left out. The jealousy isn't about the person igniting those feelings for the client. It is what the feelings represent to them: fear. The fear is real, but the message it sends them is not valid. Understanding the root cause of jealousy takes time and practice. Jealousy can make clients want to react uncharacteristically but encourage them to take a breath and explore the root cause.

Step 4: Talk about the Feelings

Talking about feelings is an excellent opportunity to practice "I" Messages with clients. Taking ownership of the jealous feeling and talking to their partner is not easy, but being assertive is helpful.

Example of "I" Message:

I felt insecure when I saw you passionately kiss them because it had been a while since you kissed me passionately. You did not do anything wrong by kissing them. I need your love and support as I process my fear of her getting something I am not.

Step 5: Choose Security

Insecurity is unpleasant, unwelcomed, and, most of the time, unfounded, but trying to tell a client experiencing a meltdown that their feelings of insecurity are false could cause damage in the therapeutic process. Remind them that relationships become what they practice. If they tell themselves that their partner does not love them, that their partner is going to leave them, or that they are not good enough for the relationship, those things will become true. If they believe they are valuable to their partner and worthy of their lives, their actions and behaviors will match those beliefs. Please encourage them to choose security over insecurity.

New Relationship Energy (NRE)

Nothing can trigger jealousy quicker than NRE. This energy is addicting, overwhelming, perfect, and traumatic all at the same time! The energy source for your current cocktail of neurotransmitters can make the worst day perfect with a straightforward text! We have all been there: twitterpated, giddy, bubbly, everything-is-absolutely-perfect, you-are-my-missing-puzzle-piece feeling that occurs when you start something with someone new.

I proudly proclaim that NRE is the most intoxicating, obsessive-compulsive experience sprinkled with the potential for the most gut-wrenching, crying-on-the-bathroom-floor pain one will ever experience and topped with sheer euphoria.

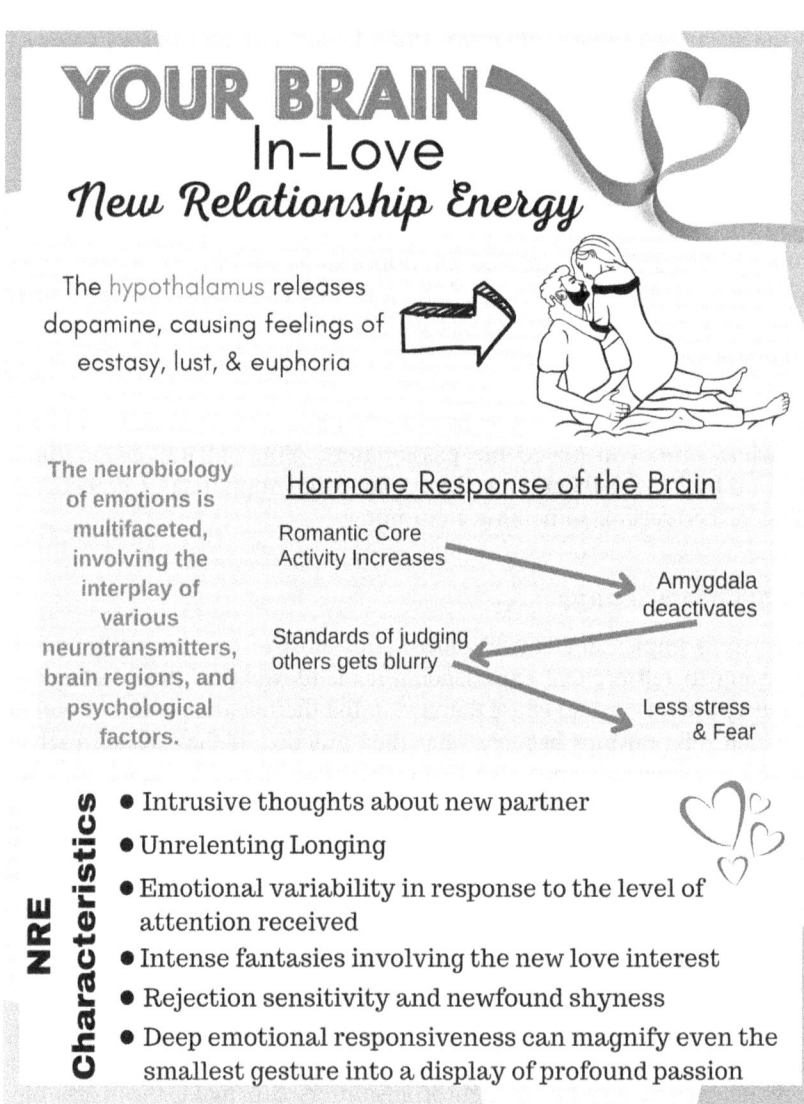

YOUR BRAIN
In-Love
New Relationship Energy

The hypothalamus releases dopamine, causing feelings of ecstasy, lust, & euphoria

The neurobiology of emotions is multifaceted, involving the interplay of various neurotransmitters, brain regions, and psychological factors.

Hormone Response of the Brain

Romantic Core Activity Increases

Amygdala deactivates

Standards of judging others gets blurry

Less stress & Fear

NRE Characteristics

- Intrusive thoughts about new partner
- Unrelenting Longing
- Emotional variability in response to the level of attention received
- Intense fantasies involving the new love interest
- Rejection sensitivity and newfound shyness
- Deep emotional responsiveness can magnify even the smallest gesture into a display of profound passion

Figure S6.2 Your Brain in Love. Adapted from *Love and Limerence: The Experience of Being in Love*, by Dorothy Tennov (1998).

From a biological perspective, our attraction toward someone triggers a complex set of chemical reactions in our brain and body. The release of neurotransmitters such as dopamine, serotonin, and norepinephrine creates a sense of euphoria and excitement, along with a range of emotional responses such as infatuation and devotion (Veaux et al., 2014). These chemicals can also lead to obsessive-compulsive behaviors and a heightened sense of physical lust.

Research has shown that the brain regions involved in romantic love include the reward center, responsible for feelings of pleasure, and the amygdala, which processes emotions such as fear and arousal (Fisher et al., 2016). These changes in brain activity can also lead to a sense of mysticism and a desire to pursue a deeper connection with the object of one's affection.

From an evolutionary perspective, our attraction to others is driven by the desire to reproduce and ensure the survival of our species. This biological drive can manifest as intense physical and emotional attraction that encourages us to seek out the most desirable partners (Fisher et al., 2016). Our bodies are designed to respond to cues indicating strong genetic compatibility and reproductive fitness, such as physical appearance and scent (Ferreira et al., 2020). While these biological factors may drive us, it's important to remember that a successful and fulfilling relationship requires more than just physical attraction.

Dorothy Tennov, psychologist and author of *Love and Limerence: The Experience of Being in Love,* interviewed 500 volunteers about what falling in love was like and identified common characteristics (1998):

- Intrusive thoughts about their newest energy source of biochemical cocktail
- Incessant yearning
- Emotional variability in response to the level of attention received
- Rejection sensitivity and shyness
- Striking fantasies involving the love interest
- Intense sensitivity to actions and behaviors often turns the smallest gesture into profound passion being displayed.

Helping Clients Survive Relationship Energy

Congratulations! One of the partners is experiencing NRE, and their life is perfect! Nevertheless, their partner feels slighted, jealous, ignored, unimportant, and other negative emotions. Due to the rush of neurotransmitters, their new relationship is more fulfilling than their existing relationship. The love-struck partner might begin to idolize their new partner and unknowingly create chaos in their other relationships.

NRE is not harmful but can be destructive if not handled properly.

Theoretically, NRE can last for years, resulting in other relationships crumbling. The key to maintaining sanity for the sidelined partner is to be patient and communicate their feelings frequently. Please encourage them to allow the NRE partner to ride the high within limits. While in session, establish NRE ground rules and build checkpoints for the primary couple to ensure they consider everyone's needs.

While NRE affects each person differently, some foundational principles can help sail their ship to calmer waters, including

- The person in the grips of NRE is not in their typical mindset; they are flooded with feel-good chemicals, so they should not make significant decisions during this time.
- Communication is critical; if the NRE partner's actions and behaviors make their existing partner feel insecure, neglected, and/or unimportant, they must speak up.
  - Caveat: "Patience in communication is also key because a partner in the throes of NRE may not hear [them] the first time" (Veaux et al., 2014, 260).
- Ensure that the NRE client understands that their judgments and perceptions are biased, further impairing their judgment.
- Support the logical partner as they try to offer an objective view of the situation or express concern about the budding relationship; however, amid the NRE haze, their partner could accuse them of being jealous or unsupportive, and those feelings must be addressed.
- Encourage the NRE partner to use their newfound sexual energy and inspiration in all their relationships instead of focusing solely on the new relationship.
- Cautiously observe the client's patterns with NRE to ensure they are not jumping from one relationship to another when the NRE dissipates. Some individuals are addicted to the feelings they experience because of NRE and constantly seek new relationships to fill their needs. Frequently requiring NRE can be exceedingly hurtful for consistent partners in their lives.

When working with a couple wanting to open their relationship for the first time, have them complete the NRE activity in this book's resource section. This activity is excellent for those who have allowed NRE to impact their relationships in the past and want to explore healthier ways to manage those feelings in future relationships so they are not damaging their other relationships.

Rejection Sensitivity Dysphoria (RSD)

As of the writing of this book, RSD is not a mental health condition listed in the Diagnostic and Statistical Manual of Mental Disorders, Fifth Edition, Text Revision (DSM-5-TR, 2017); therefore, RSD has no set of empirical, quantifiable criteria for an official diagnosis. While there is no formal diagnosis for RSD, it is a brain-based symptom and likely an innate characteristic of ADHD (Dodson, 2022).

For most people, rejection makes them feel undesired and unwelcome, but rejection, perceived or actual, can feel traumatic for someone with RSD. Those with RSD feel an extreme emotional response to any feelings of rejection, including feeling left out, criticism, or negative opinions. They feel like failures, lash out in anger, or their self-esteem drops almost instantly.

RSD can have a crucial impact on seeking and/or keeping relationships. Dating is complicated for those with RSD due to the hyperfocus placed on any feeling of rejection. The rapid mood changes can imitate the individual's perception of the trigger, ranging from an emotional breakdown with suicidal ideations to full-blown rage at the situation or person. Mood dysregulation can fluctuate quickly, resulting in multiple episodes daily (Dodson, 2022).

These individuals require constant reassurance from their partner(s) and will routinely second-guess their actions and behaviors. The fear of not being "good enough" contributes to them withholding their true feelings from their partner(s) at times of escalating conflict with exaggerated anger that feels harsher than the situation called for at the moment.

> Dysphoria is the Greek word meaning unbearable; it's use emphasizes the severe physical and emotional pain suffered by people with RSD when they encounter real or perceived rejection, criticism, or teasing.
> ~ William Dodson, M.D., LF-APA

Figure S6.3 Definition of Dysphoria. Created by the Author.

How Does RSD Manifest in ENM

It's understandable to have a love/hate relationship with the ENM lifestyle when experiencing Rejection Sensitivity Dysphoria (RSD). RSD refers to the intense emotional reactivity and sensitivity to perceived rejection or criticism (Surman et al., 2019). While the lifestyle can offer affirmations and positive experiences, it can also trigger feelings of rejection in individuals with RSD.

Even if someone with RSD is not being rejected, their brain and emotions may interpret situations as such. This can lead to a rollercoaster of emotions and difficulties controlling these intense reactions. The rapid and intense emotional shifts can create awkward situations and affect the overall participation experience in ENM.

Discovering the concept of RSD and understanding its impact can be transformative for individuals who have experienced these emotional challenges. It allows them to recognize and process their intense emotions quickly, preventing them from ruining or overshadowing their experiences. This knowledge empowers individuals to navigate the ENM lifestyle with greater awareness and emotional resilience.

Sharing personal experiences with others is valuable, as it raises awareness of RSD and can help individuals who may be going through similar experiences but are unaware of the condition. For example, a couple's silence or lack of communication after a positive playdate may trigger individuals with RSD to ruminate on perceived faults or flaws in their behavior, even when nothing was actually wrong. This fixation on self-criticism can lead to unnecessary tension with partners and hours or days wasted on unfounded self-analysis.

By openly discussing RSD, individuals can raise awareness, promote understanding, and foster a more supportive and empathetic environment in the ENM community.

Common Characteristics of RSD

According to William Dodson, M.D., LF-APA, the following are common behaviors exhibited by those with RSD (Dodson, 2022):

- Emotional outbursts in response to perceived or actual criticism or rejection
  - Anger, rage, or burst into tears
- Disengagement during social situations
- Negative inner dialogue accompanied by thoughts of self-harm
- Habitual people-pleasers who avoid social settings where they might be criticized or fail at a task
- Constantly feeling attacked in relationships leads those with RSD to be very defensive during confrontations.
- Strive for perfectionism and avoid starting projects or functions if there is a chance of failure.
- Perseveration or the inability to move past a topic after the conversation has moved on
- Ruminations or obsessive thoughts that interfere with cognitive activity

Discovering Compersion

The word COMPERSION was invented by the Kerista Commune based in the Haight-Ashbury of San Francisco from 1971 to 1991 and defined as "the opposite of jealousy, positive feelings about your partner's other intimacies" (Kerista Commune, n.d.).

Throughout the years, others have expanded on their original definition of compersion; for example,

> Compersion is our wholehearted participation in the happiness of others. It is the sympathetic joy we feel for somebody else, even when their positive experience does not involve or benefit us directly. Thus, compersion can be thought of as the opposite of jealousy and possessiveness.
>
> (Dr. Marie Thouin, n. d., Love InSight)

> Compersion, sometimes referred to as the opposite of jealousy, is a well-known term among those who practice consensual non-monogamy, which refers to any romantic relationship where people consensually form non-exclusive romantic partnerships.
>
> (Eric W. Dolan, 2021, PsyPost)

> Compersion is an important concept for non-monogamous people. Often described as jealousy's opposite, compersion labels positive feelings toward the intimacy of a beloved with other people. Since many people think jealousy is ordinary, intransigent, and even appropriate, compersion can seem psychologically and ethically dubious.
>
> (Luke Brunning, 2020, Journal of the American
> Philosophical Association)

While there is no unified definition of compersion, the majority agree that it is the opposite of jealousy and the happiness experienced when your partner is happy with or receiving pleasure from other partners. Research is limited at the time of this writing. Flicker and colleagues created a quantitative scale, The COMPERSe (Classifying Our Metamour/Partner Emotional Response Scale), explaining that it is "grounded in a qualitative understanding of consensually non-monogamous (CNM) individuals' lived experience of compersion" (Flicker et al., 2021, p. 1569).

Through their research, Flicker and colleagues found a three-factor scale for determining compersion:

1 Happiness about Partner/Metamour Relationship (HPMR),
2 Excitement for New Connections (ENC), and
3 Sexual Arousal.

If clients are struggling with the concept of compersion or frustrated that they have not experienced it, yes, explore the components of compersion with them. Farrell (2022) strengthens the importance of open and honest communication when building compersion by suggesting that clinicians help reinforce healthy communication skills through mindfulness and acceptance.

Chapter Highlights

- Jealousy is a natural part of all relationship dynamics, monogamous and/or non-monogamous. How one manages those feelings makes the difference in relationships.
- Jealousy happens in response to a genuine or perceived threat to a relationship, which includes various features of the physical and social environment that produce the opinion that one's current romantic relationship may be unstable or at risk of ending.
- ENM relationships vary and depend upon individual preferences; independent relationships are discussed and refined incessantly throughout the relationship, allowing for constant growth and shifts.
- When clinicians assist clients in navigating their jealousy, clients should be encouraged to explore how they experience jealousy and find healthy patterns that are more practicable and less consuming.
- Regardless of agentic fidelity or being aware of extradyadic relationships allowing for secondary romantic or sexual relationships, jealousy is one of the primary factors when couples come to therapy.
- Based on the research of Abraham P. Buunk, there are three types of jealousy (1997).

  - Reactive jealousy refers to the response to one's partner's engagement in intimate behaviors.
  - Preventive jealousy refers to efforts to prevent contact of one's partner with individuals of the opposite sex, which may even include acts of violence to limit their mate's autonomy.
  - Anxious jealousy refers to an active cognitive process in which the individual generates images of their mate becoming sexually or emotionally involved with someone else and experiences feelings of anxiety, suspicion, worry, distrust, and upset.

- Restorative steps to help clients cope with their negative expressions of jealousy include:

    Step 1: Accepting the Feelings
    Step 2: Separating the Triggers from the Causation
    Step 3: Trying to Understand the Feelings
    Step 4: Talking about the Feelings
    Step 5: Choosing Security

- There are two ways to participate in non-monogamy. This is either consensually or unknowingly.
- As with infidelity in monogamous relationships, infidelity in ENM relationships is just as, if not more, devastating and negatively impactful because the hurt partner was willing to share.
- Cheating will be defined differently with each couple, and their therapist must understand their individualized definition of infidelity so assumptions can be eliminated.
- New Relationship Energy (NRE)

  - Intrusive thoughts about their newest energy source of biochemical cocktail
  - Incessant yearning
  - Mood fluctuations according to the amount of attention given
  - Rejection sensitivity and shyness
  - Striking fantasies involving the love interest
  - Intense sensitivity to actions and behaviors often turns the smallest gesture into profound passion being displayed.
  - See NRE activity.

- Common behaviors exhibited by those with RSD can include:

  - Emotional outbursts in response to perceived or actual criticism or rejection (anger, rage, or bursting into tears)
  - Disengagement during social situations
  - Negative inner dialogue accompanied by thoughts of self-harm
  - Habitual people-pleasers who avoid social settings where they might be criticized or fail at a task
  - Constantly feeling attacked when in relationships leads them to be very defensive during times of confrontation
  - Strive for perfectionism and avoid starting projects or functions if there is a chance of failure
  - Perseveration or the inability to move past a topic after the conversation has moved on
  - Ruminations or obsessive thoughts that interfere with cognitive activity

- While there is no unified definition of compersion, the majority agree that it is the opposite of jealousy and the happiness experienced when your partner is happy with or receiving pleasure from other partners. Research is limited at the time of this writing.
- Three-factor scale for determining compersion:

  1 Happiness about Partner/Metamour Relationship (HPMR),
  2 Excitement for New Connections (ENC), and
  3 Sexual Arousal

Treatment Plan: Navigating Jealousy, Rejection Sensitivity, and Discovering Compersion

Behavioral Manifestations

1   Concerns about losing their primary partner's love, awareness, and intimacy to another romantic partner
2   One partner is envious of another
3   Verbally undervalues oneself; constantly compares self to others; never feels good enough within the relationship
4   Inability to share their primary partner
5   When caught up in the NRE, the primary partner feels ignored or unimportant
6   Fear of being excluded from a partner's activities
7   Avoidance of expressing feelings associated with anything negative about the relationship due to fear of their partner rejecting them
8   Refuses to discuss their partner's jealous feelings in a positive way that promotes emotional safety within the relationship
9   Unable to manage time effectively
10   Notably sensitive to perceived or actual rejection from others
11   Debilitating fear that their primary partner will leave them for another romantic partner
12   The resentment felt from feeling pressured to do something they were not ready for or did not want to do

Long-Term Client Goals

1   Develop open and honest communication about fears of loss within the relationship
2   Recognize and replace envious thoughts with healthy, realistic inner dialogue
3   Demonstrate an understanding that their primary partner loves them and is not looking to replace them with a romantic interest
4   Acknowledge that their primary partner is not a possession to be had and that they can share their partner without fear of losing them
5   Find a balance between NRE experienced with a new romantic interest and saving time and energy for the original partner
6   Validate and own their jealous feelings
7   Practice self-care when jealous feelings arise
8   Listen to your partner's concerns and feelings without judgment
9   Ensure that time and energy are managed effectively
10   Effectively manages feelings of rejection sensitivity

11 Rationally evaluate the relationship dynamics creating the fear of abandonment and increasing trust within the relationship
12 Learn to express your feelings even when they are challenging to talk about; resentment, betrayal, or fear
13 Ability to have intermittent feelings of compersion toward primary partner

Short-Term Client Goals	Therapeutic Interventions
• Recognize and clarify feelings of jealousy in the relationship.	• Have the partners identify jealous behaviors and label the type of jealousy they have experienced. Use the "Types of Jealousy" activity in the resource section.
• Deconstruct faulty mononormative beliefs about jealousy.	• Challenge flawed beliefs about jealousy created by society. Use the "Mononormative No More!" activity in the resource section.
• Verbalize an understanding that overcoming jealousy is a process and not a quick fix.	• Ask both partners to share their understanding of jealousy as a process. • Advise the partners about jealousy being a learned behavior that can be unlearned with practice and communication. • Help the jealous or both partners discover the source of their jealousy and process those experiences. • Have each partner discuss previous times in their relationship when they felt jealousy and identify healthy ways to resolve the issue(s) causing those feelings.
• Strategize as a team healthy ways to practice self-care when feelings of jealousy arise.	• Help each partner identify self-care activities that can help them process their feelings when their partners are with metamours.
• Verbalize an understanding of how envy can create competitiveness within the relationship. Identify areas of concern.	• Assess for any envious feelings within the relationship, including comparing oneself to their metamours, wanting something the metamour has that they do not (smaller waist, larger breast, larger penis), and encourage the partner to create a list of positive characteristics about themselves.
• Identify any sources of insecurity and explore how insecurities can manifest within their relationship.	• Encourage the insecure partner to separate themselves from their primary partner's desires and secondary relationships that do not immediately involve them. • Assist the insecure partner in identifying if the source of their insecurities stems from their overactive imagination and encourage them to evaluate the reality of the situation.

(Continued)

Short-Term Client Goals	Therapeutic Interventions
	• Discuss ways to provide reassurance during their partner's distress with the non-insecure partner.
• Verbalize a willingness to explore feelings of resentment, betrayal, or fear, perceived or real, and identify associated behaviors.	• Assist the partner in identifying coping strategies and mindfulness activities to utilize during emotional dysregulation.
• Verbalize a willingness to explore feelings of abandonment, perceived or actual, and identify behaviors associated with fear of abandonment.	• Assist the partner in identifying coping strategies and mindfulness activities to utilize during emotional dysregulation.
• Verbalize a willingness to explore feelings of rejection, perceived or actual.	• Reassure the couple that feelings of rejection are not uncommon in any relationship but can be intensified by ENM. • Educate the partners about Rejection Sensitivity Dysphoria (RSD), hypersensitivity, and acute susceptibility to rejection. Use the "The Pain is Real" handout in the resource section of this book. • Have the rejection-sensitive partner complete the "Rejection Sensitivity Quiz" in the resource section of this book to identify how sensitive they are to rejection. Have the rejection-sensitive partner share the results with their partner. • Utilize Cognitive Behavioral Therapy (CBT) to create an understanding of faulty thoughts and patterns that contribute to negative behavior.
• Recognize, confront, and change rejection-induced inner dialogue with self-talk that promotes aggressive behavior.	• Explore the client's negative thoughts of rejection triggering the aggressive behavior and replace them with positive self-talk that evokes the desired behavior. Use the "The Pain is Real" handout in the resource section of this book.
• Verbalize feelings of compersion when they are experienced.	• Discuss the difference between comparison and jealousy with the couple and how compersion is not a natural emotional response and takes practice to develop. Assign each partner the "Compersion" activity found in the resource section of this book.

(Continued)

Short-Term Client Goals	Therapeutic Interventions
	• Provide the couple with the role-play scenarios, *"What-If"* from the resource section of this book and have them explore how they would handle each situation.
• Recognize how NRE affects your primary relationship.	• Discuss and process how NRE can positively and negatively impact existing relationships. • Have the couple complete the *"Managing NRE"* activity.

References

Barelds, D. P., & Barelds-Dijkstra, P. (2007). Relations between different types of jealousy and self and partner perceptions of Relationship Quality. *Clinical Psychology & Psychotherapy, 14*(3), 176–188. 10.1002/cpp.532

Brunning, L. (2020). Compersion: An alternative to jealousy? *Journal of the American Philosophical Association, 6*(2), 225–245. 10.1017/apa.2019.35

Buunk, B.P. (1997). Personality, birth order and attachment styles as related to various types of jealousy. *Personality and Individual Differences, 23,* 997–1006.

Diagnostic and statistical manual of mental disorders: DSM-5. (2017). CBS Publishers & Distributors, Pvt. Ltd.

Dodson, W. (2022, July 11). *New insights into rejection sensitive dysphoria.* ADDitude.

Dolan, E. W. (2021, September 5). *Psychologists have created a new tool to measure the phenomenon called compersion.* PsyPost. Retrieved September 27, 2022, from https://www.psypost.org/2021/09/psychologists-have-created-a-new-tool-to-measure-the-phenomenon-called-compersion-61822

Farrell, R. M. (2022). Polyam Affect, working with emotions in CNM. In M. D. Vaughan & T. R. Burnes (Eds.), *The handbook of consensual non-monogamy: Affirming mental health practice* (pp. 74–96). Essay, Rowman & Littlefield.

Ferreira, L., Fink, B., Grammer, K., & Neave, N. (2020). Human body odor and sexual attraction: An updated review. *Archives of Sexual Behavior, 49*(5), 1631–1657.

Fisher, H., Xu, X., Aron, A., & Brown, L. L. (2016). Intense, passionate, romantic love: A natural addiction? How the fields that investigate romance and substance abuse can inform each other. *Frontiers in Psychology, 7,* 687.

Flicker, S. M., Vaughan, M. D., & Meyers, L. S. (2021). Feeling good about your partners' relationships: Compersion in consensually non-monogamous relationships. *Archives of Sexual Behavior, 50*(4), 1569–1586. 10.1007/s10508-021-01985-y

Kerista Commune. Kerista.commune—the historical record. (n.d.). Retrieved September 27, 2022, from https://www.kerista.com/kerista.html

Mogilski, J. K., Reeve, S. D., Nicolas, S. C., Donaldson, S. H., Mitchell, V. E., & Welling, L. L. (2019). Jealousy, consent, and compersion within monogamous and consensually non-monogamous romantic relationships. *Archives of Sexual Behavior, 48*(6), 1811–1828. 10.1007/s10508-018-1286-4

Musson, C. (2019). Polyamorous jealousy: Group differences in jealousy and mate retention behaviors between polyamorous and monogamous relationships. *Honors Capstones, 904.*

Surman, C. B. H., Asherson, P., & Shah, H. J. (2019). Rejection sensitive dysphoria in ADHD diagnosed individuals. *Current Psychiatry Reports, 21*(12), 128.

Tennov, D. (1998). *Love and limerence: The experience of being in Love.* Scarborough House.

Thouin, M. (n.d.). *Compersion: A radical love phenomenon.* What is compersion? Retrieved September 27, 2022, from https://www.whatiscompersion.com/home

Veaux, F., Rickert, E., & Hardy, J. W. (2014). *More than two: A practical guide to ethical polyamory.* Thorntree Press.

Wosick-Correa, K. (2009). Agreements, rules and agentic fidelity in polyamorous relationships. *Psychology and Sexuality, 1*(1), 44–61. 10.1080/19419891003634471

Step 7

Common Issues in ENM

Common Issues in ENM

Speaking from experience, there is no secret how-to template that gets passed down when you decide to open your relationship that provides us with the winning formula for relationship success. We are all out here trying to figure this out, just like everyone else. We make big mistakes. We make little mistakes and every other mistake in between. The difference for those in ENM relationships is the way they view the rupture or fracture within the relationship. We are all love-struck idiots fumbling awkwardly, trying to catch our crush's attention.

ENM individuals will face the same challenges as monogamous folks, but some added complexities are unique to open relationships, such as breakups and broken boundaries. Creating a plan of action with your clients for when things go wrong sets them up for success. There will be complications and tears, but there will also be growth, love, and acceptance for your clients.

Breakups

In her book, *The Polyamory Breakup Book*, Kathy Labriola, a prominent voice in discussing ENM relationships, provides valuable insights into the complex dynamics and challenges that can arise within non-monogamous (ENM) relationships (Labriola, 2019). Labriola acknowledges that not all polyamorous relationships end happily ever after and that many individuals experience ups and downs, often resulting in painful breakups (Labriola, 2019). However, over time, they develop essential relationship skills, learn to choose compatible partners, and identify the open relationship model that suits them best. It should be noted that some individuals struggle to learn from their experiences and continue to repeat the same mistakes indefinitely.

When a breakup occurs within the ENM community, former partners might still attend the same events, parties, or social gatherings (Labriola, 2019).

DOI: 10.4324/9781003464891-15

As a result, amicable separations are preferred to avoid awkward interactions. It is vital to recognize that, regardless of the nature of the breakup, it still hurts. Having other partners does not reduce the pain of losing a partner that an individual cared about, spent time with, grew with, and possibly loved.

Last, it is essential to dispel the misconception that individuals in ENM relationships possess a heightened relationship awareness that monogamous individuals do not have. In reality, many ENM breakups occur for the same reasons that end monogamous relationships. Despite this, Labriola's work emphasizes the importance of personal growth and self-awareness in navigating these unique relationship structures (Labriola, 2019). Labriola's contribution provides valuable guidance for anyone seeking to navigate the complexities of ENM relationships (Labriola, 2019).

Kathy Labriola (2019) established a list of reasons that usually end relationships, monogamous and ENM that she calls The Big Seven:

1 Sexual issues
2 Money discordance
3 Cohabitating controversy
4 Contention regarding autonomy and intimacy
5 Substance abuse
6 Untreated/undiagnosed mental health conditions
7 Abuse: Mental, emotional, physical

According to Kathy Labriola, one of the most common reasons for these relationships to end is when one partner discovers they are inherently monogamous (Labriola, 2019). Labriola emphasizes that this situation is something that many individuals in ENM have encountered at least once, particularly when entering into secondary relationships or those with no long-term expectations (Labriola, 2019). This realization presents a significant challenge as it cannot be quickly resolved or compromised. Labriola's insights underscore the importance of transparent and sincere communication within ENM relationships. It is vital to recognize that, despite the best intentions, not everyone is suited for this relationship structure. Consequently, it becomes crucial to consider compatibility carefully when engaging in ENM dynamics.

Another misconception, even held by novice participants of ENM, is that breaking up with a secondary partner will not hurt as much as breaking up with a consistent partner or as much as breaking up in a monogamous relationship. THAT IS A LIE! They hurt <period>!

When I experienced a breakup for the first time in ENM, I was bedridden with depression and physically hurt. I truly loved my secondary partner and wanted to share much more with him before the breakup. My partner would find me crying on the floor in my closet, holding and reassuring me. We broke up over a year ago, and I still feel a pull in my heart when someone mentions his name.

My healing journey aligned with Kathy's recommendations for surviving an ENM breakup, and hopefully, teaching your clients these skills will help them heal when they experience a separation (Labriola, 2019).

1 Self-care: I took time to do things I needed or wanted. I did it without guilt if I wanted to eat a gallon of ice cream. If I wanted to lay in bed and cry all day, I cried all damn day. Self-care will look different for everyone, but they must allow themselves the opportunity to take care of themselves. The timeframes will vary as well. I only allowed myself to wallow for a week. Then, I found healthier ways to grieve and return to seeing my clients.

2 Grieve what was lost and learn from the experience: I allowed myself to grieve the adventures we never took, the sex we would never have again, the time we spent talking to each other, and the loss of my friend. As I began to heal, I found the nuggets of knowledge I learned along the way and explored how to incorporate what I enjoyed most about that relationship into other relationships. My partner and I had deep conversations about how we could improve our relationship due to our positive experiences. Encourage your clients to explore the good, the bad, and the ugly together. They will grow closer because of it.

3 After the initial shock was gone and I could breathe again, I focused on maintaining and strengthening my remaining relationships. Thankfully, they all rallied around and supported me, but I must continue investing in those relationships. Remind your clients that just because one relationship ended does not mean that the other relationships get to take a back seat. They are responsible for maintaining those as well.

4 When I was ready, I faced public scrutiny. My ENM friends and family held me up while my monogamous friends and family tore me down. They would say things like, "We knew that would never work," "What did you expect to happen," or the one that hit the hardest for me, "I told you this would happen, now just suck it up and deal with it." Encourage your clients to lean on those who support them and take the snide comments with a grain of salt. It is easier said than done, but it will help.

As with any loss, encourage the client to take time to grieve the relationship, and if they have a primary partner, ensure they are being supported as well. Educate the client about the stages of grief and guide their consistent partner so they can help them as well.

Broken Boundaries, Agreements, and Rules

Previously, we discussed creating boundaries, agreements, and rules, but what happens when those are not followed or broken? Due to the amount of time spent discussing needs, desires, their hard limits, the negotiation process that can take days if not weeks, tears shed, and the overall emotional toll it takes to create boundaries, agreements, and rules when there is a violation, it is devastating.

When a couple presents in relationship distress due to a violation of a boundary, agreement, or rule, it is essential that the clinician fully understand the weight of the breach. Forgetting to call their partner each day when they are out of town is less heavy than having sex with someone when they agreed not to. The pain for both is real, but helping a couple navigate the violation might be easier if the response to the fracture is appropriate.

Managing the Chaos

As the expert in the room, the couple will look to you for guidance to untangle the mess the violation has created. The first step is to have everyone acknowledge what happened and share their story. Explore all possible circumstances: Is there a gray area in a boundary or agreement, was there a miscommunication of some sort, was it unfortunate timing, or was the boundary, agreement, or rule blatantly broken? Examine the offender's intentions and motivations and probe for more profound issues that could have contributed to the violation, for example, anger, jealousy, resentment, or revenge.

After determining the why and all details in between, delve into the couple's boundaries, agreements, and rules, allowing each partner to share their thoughts and feelings about them. Did they agree to something they did not want to agree to? Was the offender pushing boundaries to see how far they could go? Allow each client to speak candidly about their thoughts to evaluate if modifications are needed to their existing agreement.

After the emotions have been expressed, tears have been shed, and a decision has been made to repair the relationship and guide the couple in exploring ways to reestablish trust. As we all know, reestablishing trust in relationships is never easy, but it is mandatory if they want a healthy relationship again. Reassure them that boundaries, agreements, and rules can be negotiated and updated as needed, but they have to discuss the possible changes BEFORE jumping off a cliff into more chaos.

Mismatched Libidos

A prevalent complaint that brings a couple, monogamous or ENM, to therapy is a difference in libido. One partner is upset that the other doesn't want sex as much as they once did, and now the high libido partner is conjuring up nonsensical ideas regarding infidelity, loss of attraction, and anything else that have read in the latest issue of their favorite magazine about why their partner no longer wants to have sex with them. It is unrealistic to believe that partners will be sexually in sync throughout their relationship.

In their book *Building Open Relationships*, Liz Powell presents a compelling analogy to shed light on the challenges of having mismatched libidos (Powell, 2018). They use the example of one partner wanting to eat three times a day while the other prefers to eat only once. This analogy effectively demonstrates the struggle to find a compromise that satisfies both individuals. It leads to one person eating when they do not want to or the other goes hungry. As a result, the partner with a higher libido may feel resentful or deprived, while the partner with a lower libido may feel overwhelmed and constantly pressured. Powell's analogy effectively captures the complexities and potential frustrations of dealing with mismatched libidos in a relationship.

There are infinite possibilities for a decreased libido, and then top that with the ever-changing appetite for frequency. I have experienced this in my former relationship. My libido was higher than my partner's for a duration, and a separate partner met my sexual needs. I allowed my partner the space to work through his issues without the added stress of being frustrated that my sexual needs were going unmet.

Normalize, Normalize, Normalize, Don't Pathologize

Mismatched libidos can be very frustrating; however, it does not mean the end of a relationship. But it does mean more communication and compromise. It is natural for sex drives to ebb and flow throughout the relationship, and a lifetime for that matter, but that does not mean something is *wrong* with an individual. Experiencing a low libido can occur for anyone: Monogamous, ENM, or with solo sex. The more clients understand themselves, the quicker they can create better sexual experiences for themselves and their partners.

Let us explore some of the major players when exploring a decreased libido with couples:

- Hormones/Biology
  - On average, a cis-gendered female has a 28-day menstrual cycle where hormone levels rise and fall as quickly as a two-year-old child's interest in anything. These rapid hormone changes make the lucky person feel physically and emotionally out of control.

- The female hormonal cycle:
  - Menstrual phase
  - Follicular phase
  - Ovulation phase
  - Luteal phase

- On average, a cis-gendered male has a 24-hour cycle where their testosterone levels are highest in the morning and lowest in the evening.

- Stress disrupts the body's natural hormone balance
- Specific medication can suppress libido
- Traumatic events, past and present, can negatively affect one's libido
- Body image: If you do not feel sexy, then more than likely, you do not want to be sexual
- Relationship distress
- Not having the kind of sex they desire, so why have it at all mentality?

Therapeutic Interventions for Mismatched Libidos

Are There Medical Factors Contributing to Their Lack of Desire?

Rule out any external factors contributing to their lack of desire. I have clients schedule a visit with their general practitioner to discuss their symptoms and complete blood work to ensure they produce the necessary hormones for their bodies to function correctly. Often, clients return to therapy reporting that their hormone levels were alarmingly low and their doctor started them on hormone replacement therapy.

Hormone imbalances are different for men and women. If you are not a practicing medical doctor, please do not use the following information to diagnose your clients. This list is strictly informational.

Women who may be experiencing hormonal imbalances might report the following:

- Vaginal dryness or general discomfort
- Pain during penetration
- Skin tags
- Shifts in menstrual cycles
- Abnormal breakouts on the face, chest, or back
- Hair loss
- Night sweats
- Darkening of the skin, notably around the groin, neck, and breasts

Men who may be experiencing an imbalance in testosterone levels may report the following:

• Tender breast
• Increase in breast tissue
• Decreased libido
• Inability to concentrate
• Decrease in bone mass
• Hair thinning or loss
• A decline in muscle mass
• Erectile disappointment

While the client is in the office with their doctor, have them discuss their current medications and any possible sexual side effects that could stem from specific medicines.

Explore the Current Stressors in Their Lives

Stress and sex have a fascinating relationship. Is the lack of sexual desire caused by stress, or does sex reduce the effects of stress on the body? Some will use sex for stress relief, while others will experience more stress because they don't want sex.

Emily Nagoski, a renowned educator, researcher, activist, and author of *Come As You Are*, has expanded upon the dual control model of sexual response originally formulated by Erick Janssen and John Bancroft at the Kinsey Institute (Nagoski, 2015). Nagoski provides a simplified explanation of this model, making it more accessible for readers to understand its workings. Within the central nervous system, which comprises the brain and spinal cord, Nagoski describes a collaboration between "accelerators" and "brakes" (Nagoski, 2015). Drawing an analogy, she explains that the sympathetic nervous system functions as the "accelerator," while the parasympathetic nervous system serves as the "brakes," specifically in the realm of sexual response. The central insight of the dual control model is the recognition that the principles governing other parts of the nervous system also hold for the brain's involvement in sexual activity, involving both sexual accelerators and sexual brakes (Nagoski, 2015).

The dual control model of sexual response has two components: The Sexual Excitation System (SES) and the Sexual Inhibition System (SIS) (Janssen & Bancroft, 2006). The SES accelerates the sexual reaction (Janssen & Bancroft, 2006). It receives sexually relevant information—the thought of sweat running down Jason Momoa's body, the smell of one's favorite fragrance, or any other sexually stimulating sense—sending the sexy message from the brain to the genitals, encouraging them to turn on. The SES never sleeps and continuously scans the environment for sexy stimuli, so people get turned on unexpectedly (Janssen & Bancroft, 2006).

The SIS, or the brakes of sexual response, scans the environment for potential threats and explores reasons not to get turned on, for example, during a business meeting. The SIS also provides a rational pause to ensure the individual is not taking unnecessary sexual risks. Like the SES, our SIS never sleeps and constantly scans for potential environmental threats.

> Here's how sexual desire really works. First, *arousal* begins when you activate the accelerator and take pressure off the brake—turn on the ons and turn off the offs. And then *desire* comes along when arousal meets a great context.
>
> (Nagoski, 2015: 226)

During stress, our sympathetic nervous system accelerates, causing physical responses such as increased heart rate, tense muscles, and/or headaches. None of those signals are sexy, but they signal the flight or fight. When the stress has been eliminated, our parasympathetic nervous system applies the brakes, allowing us to relax. Still, when we are exposed to chronic stress, our accelerator feels stuck on high, causing our bodies to work overtime, never allowing the brakes to kick in, allowing for relaxation.

The Gottman Institute recommends that couples have daily stress-reducing conversations where each partner can talk about their day without fear of judgment and encourage the couple to tackle the stressful situation as a team (Lisitsa, 2020).

Also, Emily Nagoski offers worksheets and guides in her book *Come As You Are, which* I often provide for clients when exploring low libido (Nagoski, 2015).

Are They Having the Sex They Want to Have?

Many people have never been allowed to explore their sexual desires due to stigma, shame, embarrassment, or other reasons. When I ask couples what type of sex they would like, many have the most perplexed look because they only know one way. At this time, I give each of them a copy of the Sexual Preferences Questionnaire, have them complete it while in session, and then exchange it with their partners. I like to have the couple do this in the office in case there is a sexual preference discovered that causes a partner distress or negative feelings. Ensure you are normalizing the choices and reminding them there are ways to work around the request if they are uncomfortable providing that for their partner.

I will also have them create a *Sex Menu* based on their discoveries and request that they try to complete three items on the menu before their next session with me. You must remind them that if they are overwhelmed by demand or unsure how to fulfill a desire, they can ask for help or tell their partner no. The beauty of ENM is that if one partner does not feel comfortable providing a desire, they can explore that desire with another partner.

Risk-Aware Sex Protocols and Fluid Bonding

In previous sections of this book, we discussed the risks associated with ENM. We will now explore how to encourage clients to incorporate risk-reducing protocols into their relationships. We have already established that sex is risky with multiple partners, but there are many ways of reducing the risk of transmitting an STI/STD by practicing safer sex.

Each individual will create their protocols for themselves, and then the primary couple can explore those with each other and decide if they want to add them to their lists. Theoretically, a couple's risk-aware sex protocols should match, but there are times they do not, and this is where they need to negotiate how they would like to proceed for them to both feel heard.

Fluid bonding with a partner or partners is a very personal and weighted decision that affects everyone within the relationship and their partners. Fluid bonding is having sex unbarriered with a partner or partners. When a client or couple is exploring fluid bonding with others, we have several discussions in our session together before the fluid bond with another. I want to ensure that they think about everything before deciding.

Here are the things we explore in session before they fluid bond:

- Why are you considering fluid bonding, and what benefits are you expecting?
- What STD/STI risks are you opening yourself up to, and how can you manage those risks to keep your other partners safe?
- Do you want to have a fluid bond for all sexual acts you participate in, or are there hard limits for you? For example, unbarriered sex for vaginal and oral pleasure but protection for anal? Dental dams? Gloves for digital penetration?
- Who are the partners that will need to agree to this choice you are making to fluid bond with another person?
- How often would you like to request STI/STD test results from partners you have fluid bonded with?
- Do you want to fluid bond with a partner to strengthen the relationship or enhance intimacy?

When clients want to fluid bond with another partner, they must clarify and set boundaries BEFORE it. I have had many clients do the work on their end and go into a situation where they think that everyone is on the same page, only to find out that the person they have fluid bonded with doesn't see the relationship dynamics the same way or didn't have a clear understanding, so boundaries are broken.

Harm Reduction Sexual Practices

Harm reduction sexual practices prioritize the physical and emotional safety of individuals who are sexually active by using intentional methods to mitigate potential risks such as sexually transmitted infections (STIs), unwanted pregnancies, and sexual assault. Dr. Evelin Dacker, a sex-positive integrative primary care physician from Salem, Oregon, emphasizes that harm-reduction sexual practices involve communication, education, and consent and do not shame individuals for their sexual choices (Dacker, 2022).

Dacker developed the STARS method to help individuals navigate safer sex practices through the exploration of sexuality and the promotion of healthy relationships with oneself and others.

• Sexual Health/STI Status
• Turn-ons
• Avoid
• Relationship Intentions/Expectations
• Safety

Harm reduction sexual practices recognize that individuals have different levels of comfort and risk tolerance and seek to provide a non-judgmental approach to sexual wellness while empowering individuals to make informed decisions that respect their boundaries and the boundaries of their partner(s) (Dacker, 2022).

Talking about Sexual Health and STI Status

The topic of STIs and sexual health can sometimes be uncomfortable to discuss due to the societal stigma surrounding it. However, having a conversation about it is crucial to ensure a safe and pleasurable sexual experience. Dr. Dacker recommends the following tips to help guide the discussion (Dacker, 2022):

• Start by sharing your information, including when you were last tested for STIs, what specific infections you were tested for, and your test results
• Educate your partner on the difference between a "basic" panel and a "full" panel of tests. An introductory panel typically checks for HIV,

Syphilis, Gonorrhea, and Chlamydia. In contrast, a full panel includes those infections and Hepatitis B and C, Herpes Simplex Virus I and II
• Use the phrases "positive" or "negative" instead of "clean" or "dirty" to reduce the stigma associated with STIs
• Discuss how frequently you get tested. Generally, it's good practice to get tested every three months if you have multiple sexual partners
• Ask your partner about their own sexual health and testing history

Remember, having an open and honest conversation about sexual health is an integral part of ensuring a safe and enjoyable sexual experience for everyone involved. And while it may seem uncomfortable at first, normalizing discussions around sexual health can ultimately benefit everyone's overall health and well-being.

Unveiling Turn-Ons for Connection and Intimacy

Clients are guided to explore and articulate their turn-ons using the following strategies:

1 Self-exploration:

   • Clients are encouraged to delve into their desires and pinpoint what arouses them.
   • They are then prompted to practice expressing these turn-ons as if talking to a potential partner.

2 Effective Communication:

   • Examples of practical expressions include:

     • "I become aroused by ..."
     • "I find pleasure in being touched on my ..."
     • "My erogenous zones include ..."

   • Clients are encouraged to discuss and explore their erogenous zones with their partners.
   • Expressions such as:

     • "I derive pleasure from receiving ..."
     • "I derive pleasure from giving ..."
     • "I appreciate both kinky and vanilla sexual play."

Understanding and effectively communicating turn-ons and preferences are essential components of a satisfying and consensual sexual experience. By encouraging clients to explore their desires, communicate openly, and establish clear boundaries, we aim to promote healthier and more fulfilling connections. Let us prioritize conversations about turn-ons and preferences, creating a safe space to express individual needs and desires for the benefit and satisfaction of all individuals and their partners.

Navigating Aversions, Boundaries, and Triggers

When working with clients, the counselor must encourage them to focus on the importance of recognizing and respecting boundaries, aversions, and triggers within sexual relationships. Building upon previously established relationship boundaries, couples are guided in exploring areas that may be off-limits during their sexual encounters.

Example questions provided to facilitate open and honest conversations are

- "I get turned off when someone does ..."
- "At this time, I am not interested in ..." and
- "Due to past trauma, I am easily triggered by ..."

By acknowledging and addressing these aversions and triggers, couples can create a safe and consensual sexual environment, fostering emotional well-being and mutual satisfaction.

Understanding Relationship Intentions and Communicating Expectations

The therapist emphasizes the importance of discussing intentions and expectations in relationships, acknowledging that it may be challenging. Clients are encouraged to explore and adapt their desires and preferences based on individual encounters and partners. Despite the potential fear of rejection, it is crucial to have upfront conversations to manage expectations effectively.

Example conversation prompts are aimed at fostering open and honest communication, such as

- "My sexual orientation is ..." and
- "I am looking for—with you."
    - options including FWB, long-term relationship, ENM dating, and a D/s dynamic,
- "This is what sex means to me ..." and
- "After a sexual experience, I like to ... ."

Encouraging clients to have these conversations helps reduce unrealistic expectations and fosters healthier, more fulfilling relationships.

Prioritizing Safety beyond Physical Protection

This element emphasizes that sexual safety extends beyond the use of barriers and birth control. Partners are encouraged to explore emotional, spiritual, and psychological safety before, during, and after sexual experiences. This requires an open and honest conversation between partners to establish boundaries and preferences.

Clients are asked to consider various scenarios, such as their stance on drug and alcohol use during sexual encounters, how their body responds when they don't feel safe, whether mental health or emotional factors need disclosure to potential partners, and whether spiritual or religious values influence their preferred style of sexual play. Physical limits are also highlighted, and partners should know what the body can and cannot handle. By prioritizing safety, clients can promote a healthier and more respectful sexual environment, building trust and intimacy with their partners.

Revealing/Accepting Partner Kinks and Fetishes

Normalize, Normalize, Normalize, Don't Pathologize!

In his 2018 book, *Tell Me What You Want,* Justin J. Lehmiller conducted the largest survey of sexual fantasies, finding that 98% of Americans have a variety of sexual fantasies, identifying seven significant themes representing sexual desire (Lehmiller, 2018):

- Multipartner sex
- Power, control, and rough sex
- Novelty, adventure, and variety
- Taboo and forbidden sex
- Partner sharing and ENM relationships
- Passion and romance
- Erotic flexibility, most notably, homoeroticism and gender-bending

Your client is neither unique nor alone in kinks and fetishes, making clinicians need to normalize their feelings. If the client opens up to you individually, allow them the space and time to choose how and when they discuss this with their consistent partner. They have been holding on to this secret for a long time, and there is no need to push them to discuss it before they are ready.

Encourage Them to Embrace Their Kink

Remind them that it is their right to enjoy and explore what feels good. If they aren't already doing so, have them masturbate to images or videos of their kink, being mindful of how it makes them feel to experience and embrace it finally. If unsure where to begin, provide the client with a list of ethical porn sites. Also, please encourage them to connect with other kinky individuals and educate themselves. They don't have to share the same kinks, but building a community of like-minded individuals helps remove the stigma.

Self-Disclose to a Consistent Partner

When the kinky client is ready to share their secret with their partner(s), help them frame it as an exciting discovery instead of *having* to tell them. Ready yourself with facts and statistics about the kink or fetish so that you can help further normalize it to their partners and answer any questions they may have. The self-disclosure is about supporting each of them individually and as a couple by combating shame via the increasing connection.

Assist the Non-Kinky Client in Finding Ways to Participate

The non-kinky client may be overwhelmed by the disclosure and unsure how to incorporate the kink or fetish into their sex life, which is expected. Reassure the non-kinky client that they do not *have* to do anything uncomfortable and help them explore suitable alternatives to help feel the kinky partner's desire.

I have found that when one partner opens up about their kink and fetishes to their consistent partner, the once non-kinky partner feels comfortable opening up about their kinks or fetishes. This revelation tends to be a massive relief for both partners.

However, there are times when non-kinky clients are shocked and feel as if they have been lied to for the entire duration of their relationship. Again, arm yourself with the facts to help normalize the kinky client holding on to their secret for so long.

I encourage clinicians who have the potential to work with kinky clients to read *The Leather Couch, Clinical Practice with Kinky Client* by Stefani Goerlich.

> *The Leather Couch* provides a comprehensive overview of the BDSM and kink community and guides clinicians on how to meet the unique relational and mental health needs of its members.
>
> (Goerlich, 2021: 1)

Mononormative Mindset

Monogamy has been the accepted relationship model for centuries, and societal privileges are afforded to monogamous couples that are not provided for ENM relationships. Due to the mononormative mindset of society, even ENM relationships tend to have a monogamous hangover mindset at times, which can negatively impact ENM relationships. There is a "fair amount of energy and effort unlearning problematic monogamy mindset lessons about how love and dating are supposed to go" for those practicing ENM (Powell, 2018, p. 125).

Vaughan (2022) provided insight into a related concept called *amatonormativity,* where the societal message of long-term monogamous romantic relationships is intrinsically relevant and the most beneficial relationship model for adults, reducing ENM relationships to a second-class, criticized status. Furthermore, the negativity portrays ENM individuals as selfish, immoral, and characterized as being less human. A recent study in the journal *Archives of Sexual Behavior* found that the general public tends to dehumanize—seen as having less love to provide to partners, less compassion, and lascivious behavior—those in ENM relationships (Rodrigues et al., 2021).

"The polyamorous continuum" acknowledges that each person's life consists of various relationships, including long-term and short-lived, romantic and platonic, and those that defy conventional labels (Rothschild, 2018). The polyamorous lifestyle affirms that individuals have the autonomy to shape their relationships through open communication, expressing their needs, negotiating boundaries, and obtaining consent rather than conforming to prescribed norms. Embracing the idea of the polyamorous continuum and existence opens possibilities to question and deconstruct monogamy as a social institution (Rothschild, 2018).

This process of deconstruction could potentially be integrated into the existing monogamous framework, as practical changes are needed alongside theoretical concepts. While this thought experiment makes radical polyamorous ideas more accessible to individuals who may not pursue polyamory themselves, it also validates the legitimacy of embracing diverse forms of sexual and romantic expressions (Rothschild, 2018). It encourages reflection on the prioritization of romantic relationships over platonic ones, embracing the fluidity and adaptability of relationships, and challenging societal expectations dictated by monogamy. Ultimately, this mindset empowers individuals to consider and pursue the relationships that align with their desires rather than trying to fit into predefined societal molds.

Clients will have a monogamy hangover and cling to mononormative beliefs. There might be clients stuck on the idea of the fairy tale model where they believe in one true love and want to hold on to their consistent partner at all costs. You could have clients who practice coercion instead of consent due to the normalization of control and coercion in our society. Providing your clients with a broader viewpoint can assist them in shedding the mononormative hangover they might experience when transitioning to ENM.

Time Management

Nothing can knock the breath out of a relationship faster than over-scheduling, forgetting about important events, or the inability to manage time in multiple relationships properly. While your clients might have limitless love to give, they only have 24 hours within a day to give to those they are close to, their professions, their children, other family members, and possibly multiple partners. The inability to manage time correctly can cause opportunities for jealousy to brew if not adequately handled.

Those most successful in ENM have strong time management skills or are at least willing to learn time management skills rather quickly. Great tools can be utilized to ensure everyone is on the same page, partners don't begin to feel like they are not receiving equal attention, and time is not lost due to miscommunication. If they want to use a shared calendar with secondary partners, have them negotiate expectations and boundaries.

Veaux et al. provided suggestions to explore with your clients, including (2014):

- What are you willing to share with others?
- How do you want your partners to interact with your calendar?
- Do you want partners to see the full details of your calendar or only see that they are busy with no explanation listed?
- Will they grant permission for partners to add events directly to their calendars, or would they prefer invitations be sent so they can accept or deny the possibility?

Suggestions for clients who have difficulties tracking time include (Powell, 2018):

1 Always refer to their calendar before committing to a date or event to reduce double booking, inadvertently causing a partner to feel unimportant
2 Could you immediately put it on their calendar when making plans with others? Life is busy, and things are quickly forgotten
3 Build check-in times weekly to review upcoming events

4 Set notifications for events to help reduce losing track of time and possibly forgetting events

In their book, *Building Open Relationships,* Liz Powell provided that learning to balance and prioritize time clients should (Powell, 2018):

- Pay themselves first by setting aside time for their own needs
- Create a "gray space" in the calendar for unexpected happenings

Ensure an equal balance between personal needs, partner dates, self-care activities, and time with children.

Chapter Highlights

- Breaking up in ENM is painful, and clinicians should facilitate the grief and loss with the hurt partner
- A good resource is *The Polyamory Breakup Book* by Kathy Labriola
- Boundaries, agreements, and rules are essential to ensure emotional and physical safety in ENM; when those are broken, the repercussions are sometimes devastating
- When a couple presents with mismatched libidos, normalize their feelings and foster healthy communication to find an equitable solution
- Encourage the couple to explore risk-aware sex protocols and fluid bonding negotiations before they play with outside partners
- Teach the STARS acronym for risk-aware sex protocols

  - Sexual Health/STI Status
  - Turn-ons
  - Avoid
  - Relationship Intentions/Expectations
  - Safety

- When partners reveal kinks and fetishes to the other, normalize their desires and help the non-kinky partner understand that they are not required to provide these requests for their partner if they are uncomfortable. Help find suitable ways for the non-kinky partner to participate within their comfort level
- Normalize the mononormative hangover, help the clients identify where they might be stuck in their old thought patterns, and help them grow through those hangups
- Time management can be a common issue when beginning ENM. Encourage the couple to have an honest conversation about improving their time management skills so they are not unintentionally hurting their consistent partner

Treatment Plan: Common Issues in ENM

Behavioral Manifestations

1 Depression, grief, and withdrawal resulting from a breakup with a partner
2 Confusion surrounding how to best support a primary partner as they experience depression, grief, and withdrawal resulting from a breakup with a secondary partner
3 Unable to uphold boundaries and agreements previously determined in the primary relationship
4 One partner engages in sexual behavior (penetration and/or oral sexual activity) and/or nonsexual behavior (sharing intimate details, being secretive, hiding communication) that disregards previously negotiated boundaries, agreements, and/or rules
5 There are differences within the relationship that contribute to distress between the primary couple and/or outside partners
6 Unable to communicate sexual kinks, desires, and needs with a partner due to fear of adverse reactions from a partner
7 Having an extreme emotional reaction to a miscommunication within the relationship
8 Misrepresenting needs and desires and then experiencing emotional dysregulation when needs and desires are not met by their partner
9 Conflict resulting from the inability to deconstruct mononormative ideologies
10 Insecurities and anxiety originate from a metamour, new or existing, within the ENM dynamic

Long-Term Client Goals

1 Properly communicate grief and depressed feelings with the primary partner without withdrawing from the relationship
2 Support the grieving partner by encouraging self-care and insightful reflection, reassuring them that the primary relationship is positive, and helping with any public relations surrounding the breakup
3 Negotiate boundaries, adapt agreements to reflect cohesiveness in the relationships, and commit to discussing boundaries and agreements that need to be negotiated before breaking them
4 Rebuild trust within the relationship
5 Partners recommit to maintaining appropriate boundaries, upholding agreements, and following rules with other partners
6 Renegotiate the relationship agreement to ensure compliance with identified differences contributing to relationship distress

7 Openly explore where the miscommunication occurred, and each partner accepts personal responsibility for their contribution

8 Unapologetically discuss sexual kinks, desires, and needs with their partner

9 Using healthy communication skills, openly explore realistic desires and needs with their partner

10 Recognize how mononormative beliefs imposed by society have negatively affected the primary relationship

11 Communicate feelings of insecurity and anxiety resulting from a metamour with the primary partner and provide insight into how the primary partner can provide reassurance

Short-Term Client Goals	Therapeutic Interventions
• The grieving partner verbalizes feelings resulting from the recent breakup with a secondary partner.	• Encourage the non-grieving partner to provide emotional support, compassion, and empathy. • Educate the non-grieving partner about experiencing vicarious grief while supporting their grieving partner. • Educate the couple about the stages of grief and help the grieving partner identify their grieving stage.
• Non-grieving partner supports the grieving partner in reclaiming serenity and joy gradually.	• Facilitate the healing process by encouraging the grieving partner to practice self-care, provide a supportive place to grieve the lost relationship openly, remind them of their commitment to their other relationships, including yours, and assist them with handling the public relations required for an ENM breakup. Provide *"Breaking up in ENM"* in this book's resource section.
• Identify boundaries, agreements, and rules that need further clarification, adjustments, or revisions.	• Educate the couple about boundaries and their purpose for ENM relationships; they can set boundaries for anything they can control having to do with themselves. • Have each partner provide clarity about their boundaries, agreements, and rules to reduce or avoid future disagreements. • Normalize both partners' feelings of betrayal, mistrust, and uncertainty as they navigate feelings associated with the broken boundary and/or disagreement. • Have the partners create "I" messages in the session to express how the fracture in the

(Continued)

Short-Term Client Goals	Therapeutic Interventions
	relationship has made them feel and how they would prefer to move forward. Use the *"I" Messages* handout provided in the resource section of this book.
	• Encourage the offending partner to apologize and commit to actively upholding the negotiated boundaries and agreements.
	• Suppose the offending partner feels as if they are unable to uphold the negotiated boundaries successfully. In that case, agreements and rules encourage them to explore why they are unable to complete this request and offer possible solutions.
	• Normalize both partners' feelings of betrayal, mistrust, and uncertainty as they navigate feelings associated with the broken boundary and/or disagreement.
	• Assist the couple with individually creating boundaries that will help them feel emotionally, mentally, and physically safe. Assign *"Boundaries, Agreements, & Rules, Oh My!"* assignment found in the resource section of this book.
	• Verbalize a healthy understanding of forgiveness as a process, not a one-time event.
	• The therapist creates a "No Secrets Policy" with the couple, outlining that the therapist will not keep secrets from another partner, ensuring the couple understands the therapist's role is for the collective well-being of the couple as a unit.
	• Have the couple update their existing relationship contract and sign the new version of the contract. Use the *"Relationship Contract"* activity in the resource section of this book.
	• Have each partner write a letter to the other expressing their emotions evoked by the broken boundary, agreement, and/or rule.
• Discuss emotions evoked by the broken boundary, agreement, and/or rule in a clear and considerate manner.	• Have the partners discuss their feelings about the broken boundary, agreement, and/or rule and ask them to rate themselves using a 1–10 (one equaling not being very clear and ten being very clear) scale on how **clear** they felt they were.

(Continued)

Short-Term Client Goals	Therapeutic Interventions
	• Have the partners discuss their feelings about the broken boundary, agreement, and/or rule and ask them to rate themselves using a scale of 1–10 (one equaling not being very clear and ten being very clear) on how **considerate** they felt they were. • Educate the clients on creating and utilizing a Behavior Change POA effectively. Use the *"Behavior Change POA"* activity in the resource section of this book.
• Verbalize a healthy understanding of forgiveness as a process, not a one-time event.	• Explore each partner's definition of forgiveness and create a common understanding for processing emotions moving forward. • Explore any hesitations or fears regarding extending forgiveness.
• Determine the level of trust between the partners regarding various aspects of the relationship.	• Have each partner answer the following questions (Baucom et at., p. 321): 1 "I trust you to _____." 2 "I trust you with _____." 3 (Right now) "I don't trust you to _____." 4 (Right now) "I don't trust you with _____." 5 "I have some but not full trust regarding _____." • Assign trust-building activities to assist the couple with rebuilding trust within the relationship.
• Verbalize sexual kinks, fetishes, preferences, desires, and needs without fear of judgment or embarrassment.	• Teach the partners to openly communicate about their sexual kinks, fetishes, preferences, desires, and needs without fear of judgment or embarrassment. • Teach the couple active listening skills by having Partner 1 discuss their desires and needs while Partner 2 listens. Partner 2 summarizes what they heard and asks Partner 1 if what they heard was correct. If Partner 2 reflects back incorrect information, then Partner 1 clarifies, ensuring they feet listened to before moving on in the discussion. • Normalize the sexual kinks, fetishes, preferences, desires, and needs and encourage the couple to find support groups, online or in person and/or suggest educational

(Continued)

Short-Term Client Goals	Therapeutic Interventions
	reading material to help clients "develop positive models of others with similar predilections" (Goerlich, 2021).
	• Recognize that disclosing a kink or fetish can be distressing for a non-kinky partner resulting in feelings of catastrophe; contextualize the new revelation while normalizing the information of the disclosure (Goerlich, 2021).
	• Help the non-kinky partner to realize that sexuality is a journey and their partner's disclosed kink or fetish does not have to be fulfilled immediately; encourage the couple to explore ways to begin incorporating elements of the identified kink and/or fetish into the relationship in a less intimidating manner.
	• Help the couple identify secondary partners that might be more suited to fulfill the kinky partner's need for a specific request.
• Understand the origin of traditional mononormative beliefs and how those beliefs affect the current relationship.	• Have the couple create a list of mononormative beliefs currently affecting their decision-making skills. Use the *"Mononormative No More!"* activity in this book's resource sections to help the couple identify the mononormative ideas they are struggling with as they move into ENM.
	• Assist the couple in creating antidotes to their mononormative beliefs that result in issues for the primary relationship.
• Recognize and clarify feelings of jealousy and/or anxiety in the relationship toward a metamour.	• Help the jealous/anxious partner, or both partners, to discover the source of their jealousy/insecurities about the metamour and process those feelings.
	• Encourage the jealous/anxious partner to spend time with the metamour and develop a relationship to combat negative feelings.
	• Reassure the couple that it is not required for all partners to want to spend time together or always to get along; suggest ways for all involved partners to brainstorm solutions to help alleviate jealous or anxious feelings that will benefit everyone.
	• Suggest using John Gottman's Rituals of Connection to help establish meaningful

(Continued)

Short-Term Client Goals	Therapeutic Interventions
	activities unique to the primary relationship and encourage feelings of emotional safety.
• Verbalize the type of sex you would like to have without fear of judgment, shame, or guilt.	• Provide each partner a copy of the *"My Sexual Preferences Questionnaire"* for them to complete individually. After completing the activity, have them discuss and process their discoveries with each other. • Based on what they have learned, have them create a *"Sex Menu"* encouraging them to try a few of the new discoveries over the next few weeks.

References

Dacker, E. M. (2022). *The relationship talk workbook.* Maketimeforthetalk.com.

Goerlich, S. (2021). *The leather couch: Clinical practice with kinky clients.* Routledge.

Janssen, E., & Bancroft, J. (2006). The dual control model: The role of sexual inhibition & excitation in sexual arousal and behavior. In E. Janssen (Ed.), *The psychophysiology of sex.* Bloomington, IN: Indiana University press.

Labriola, K. (2019). *Polyamory breakup book: Causes, prevention, and survival.* Thorntree Press, LLC.

Lehmiller, J. J. (2018). *Tell me what you want: The science of sexual desire and how it can help you improve your sex life.* Da Capo Lifelong Books.

Lisitsa, E. (2020, December 28). *Manage conflict: The art of compromise.* The Gottman Institute. Retrieved September 15, 2022, from https://www.gottman.com/blog/manage-conflict-the-art-of-compromise/

Nagoski, E. (2015). *Come as you are: The surprising new science that will transform your sex life.* Simon & Schuster.

Powell, D. L. (2018). *Building open relationships: Your hands on guide to swinging, polyamory, and beyond!* Dr. Liz Powell.

Rodrigues, D. L., Lopes, D., & Huic, A. (2021). What drives the dehumanization of consensual non-monogamous partners? *Archives of Sexual Behavior, 50*(4), 1587–1597. 10.1007/s10508-020-01895-5

Rothschild, L. (2018, February 12). *Compulsory monogamy and polyamorous Existence.* Feminist and Queer Legal Theory. Retrieved October 2, 2022, from https://www.academia.edu/35902793/Compulsory_Monogamy_and_Polyamorous_Existence_pdf

Vaughan, M. D. (2022). Introduction: Toward CNM-affirming, anti-oppressive clinical practice. In M. D. Vaughan & T. R. Burnes (Eds.), *The Handbook of consensual non-monogamy (diverse sexualities, genders, and relationships)* (pp. 3–14). Rowman & Littlefield Publishers.

Veaux, F., Rickert, E., & Hardy, J. W. (2014). *More than two: A practical guide to ethical polyamory.* Thorntree Press.

Step 8

Managing Relationships

Managing Relationships

One of the most challenging aspects of ENM is managing relationships. The clients are adding multiple relationships that will require attention, love, and more communication than they have ever had in previous relationships. For clinicians, there is the possibility that couples therapy could turn into working with multiple adults in one relationship. Throughout this chapter, we will evaluate how therapists can assist their clients with managing various relationships and how the clinician can effectively manage a network of relationships with multiple people in a poly community.

Living Authentically

Psychologist and author of *Building Open Relationship,* Dr. Liz Powell, expressed, "The biggest misconception about coming out is that it's a one-time decision ... [because] in reality, coming out is a daily, minute-by-minute decision about how much information we share about ourselves with others" (2018, p. 261). There are many benefits of coming out as ENM. Everyone deserves to live their lives "genuinely, completely and honestly." Still, it can be too dangerous for some, and the risks are not worth the rewards (Human Rights Campaign Foundation, 2020). I encourage you to refer to Step 4: Risks, Stigma, and Sexual Orientation, to review the discussed risks associated with being part of the ENM community.

Being Outed vs. Being Out

Being allowed to share the news of their chosen lifestyle is always best for ENM relationships. Unfortunately, some participants of ENM are deprived of the choice to properly come out to their friends, family, and

DOI: 10.4324/9781003464891-16

general community due to other selfish individuals assuming they know what is best for the ENM individual/couple. According to the contributing author Steven Nelson from LGBTQ and ALL, a mental health blog and directory for the LGBTQ+ community, "'outing' is when someone discloses the sexual orientation or gender identity of an LGBTQ+ person without their consent ... [and] creates issues of privacy, choice, and harm" (Nelson, 2022).

The couple and/or individual who was "outed" will need to go through the grieving process for the choice of determining their coming-out narrative being taken from them. They will need to grieve their former lives and be provided coping strategies for grief. As a mental health provider, regardless of the main population you work with, I can imagine that you have helped clients process and work through times in their lives when secrets were shared or others created damage, and I trust your toolbox has strategies for those situations. Those will all come in handy with this population as well.

Most importantly, remind the client that their choice to be ENM is not wrong, sinful, or any other negative term that has been personally associated with them when being outed. Please encourage them to hold their heads high and address the situation logically instead of emotionally by providing education and acknowledging presented concerns. (You may also want to review the common misconceptions from Chapter 4: Clinical Misconceptions about ENM.)

Clinicians play a crucial role in assisting couples in creating a narrative that suits their needs and preferences. Drawing from Tristan Taormino's book *Opening Up*, it is emphasized that coming out about one's lifestyle does not have to be done with everyone in their life (2008). Selectivity is often necessary, and it is essential to consider specific individuals: Immediate or extended family members, children, ex-partners or spouses, friends, acquaintances, neighbors, employers, co-workers, employees, landlords, lawyers, and doctors. Each person in this network may have a different level of involvement or observation of the relationship, making it essential to discern whom to disclose to. By carefully navigating the process of sharing their lifestyle choices, couples can create a supportive environment tailored to their unique circumstances.

Setting up the client for a successful coming-out experience will require therapists to assist the client(s) in determining the following:

- Who do they want to know about their ENM relationship status?

  - What are the benefits of telling those they have selected?
  - What are the negative possibilities for telling those they have chosen?

- How do they want to tell those they have selected?
- When do they feel would be the best time to talk to them?
- How will they address their selected population's concerns?

  - Assist them in creating a response for the following concerns:

    - ENM is not God's intention, and they are sinning.
    - The dangers of STI/STDs with having multiple partners.
    - Others think they need therapy for a mental health disorder because they have chosen ENM.
    - Responses for those concerned about the individual not finding the *right person* yet, but when they do, they will be monogamous.
    - Destroying their primary relationship/marriage or questions about their dissatisfaction with their current relationship/partner.

Couple Privilege

Couple privilege is a real issue in modern relationships, where some couples may prioritize their relationship over others, leading to a power imbalance in a non-monogamous or polyamorous setup. The idea of couple privilege has been discussed in sociology and psychology, and several studies have been conducted to understand its prevalence and impact.

One study found that individuals who identify as monogamous typically view monogamous relationships as superior to other relationship practices, leading to the marginalization of non-monogamous individuals (Barker, 2015). It was also found that individuals who identify as non-monogamous often experience feelings of stigmatization and social exclusion due to the privilege given to couple-centric relationships.

If a couple is seeking to establish a non-monogamous relationship, it is crucial to acknowledge and address the privilege that comes with being in a primary relationship (Conley, 2013). Couples must recognize that all relationships are unique, and hierarchical structures or unequal power dynamics can hinder the success of an open relationship.

To combat couple privilege, communication, honesty, and transparency are essential. Couples must be willing to listen and understand others' perspectives and prioritize respect and consent in all relationships they establish (Barker & Langdridge, 2011). Educating oneself and seeking professional guidance can also aid in navigating the complexities of non-monogamous relationships.

Benefits and Risks of Coming Out to the Children

The therapist explores the significant and personal decision of discussing non-monogamous relationships with children. Clients are provided with guidance on considering various factors in this decision-making process. Insights from Elisabeth Sheff, an esteemed authority on polyamorous families, shed light on the crucial elements to ponder (Sheff, 2021). Age plays a pivotal role in assessing the extent of children's exposure to their parents' partners. Additionally, evaluating the potential impact on the family's well-being is vital. By thoughtfully considering these aspects, parents can make a well-informed decision that aligns with their family's unique dynamics and fosters an environment of understanding and support for their children's emotional well-being.

Age of Child

Children's understanding of complex relationship dynamics evolves as they grow older, and their questions about their parents' relationship choices may vary depending on their age. Research in developmental psychology has shed light on how children's understanding of non-traditional family structures develops over time (Golding, 2018).

In the early years, children, particularly preschool-aged and younger, have limited knowledge and understanding of relationship complexities (Kennedy, 2019). They tend to accept their parents' relationships with other adults as usual without questioning or having significant curiosity about them. This is because young children's cognitive abilities are still developing, and their focus is primarily on basic needs and immediate family interactions.

However, as children enter elementary school, their cognitive abilities and social awareness progress, and they may start comparing their family structure with their peers. At this stage, questions about non-traditional relationship dynamics may arise. Children may notice that their family structure differs from what they observe in their classmates' families and may seek clarification or further information from their parents (Golding, 2018).

Parents need to be prepared to address these questions in an age-appropriate manner. Honest and open communication is vital, allowing children to feel heard and understood. Providing simple explanations that reflect the child's developmental level can help them understand the complexities of their parents' relationships (Kennedy, 2019). This can be done by emphasizing concepts like love, trust, and open communication among all involved parties.

It is worth noting that each child is unique, and their understanding of relationships may develop at different rates. Some children may have more advanced cognitive abilities and may ask more detailed questions at an earlier age. In contrast, others may take longer to express curiosity about their parents' relationship choices.

Between the ages of 5 and 10, children have a basic understanding of kissing relationships with their parents. Still, upon reaching adolescence, they begin to develop a more complex understanding of relationships, sexuality, and adult interactions. During adolescence, kids will require more information from their support team (parents and extended parents, if applicable) about many things, especially the dynamics of the significant relationships in their lives. Children in middle school and high school are developing the ability to understand complex relationships and how they strategically fit into the larger society; therefore, it will be essential to help the clients determine what information they want to be disclosed about their family to others, and what information they prefer to keep private (Sheff, 2021).

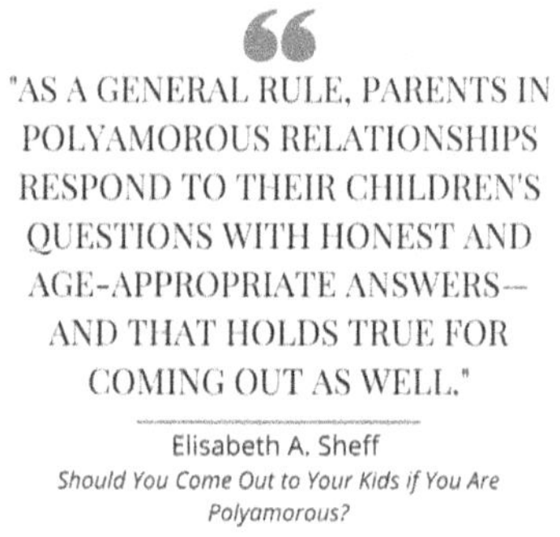

> 66
> "AS A GENERAL RULE, PARENTS IN POLYAMOROUS RELATIONSHIPS RESPOND TO THEIR CHILDREN'S QUESTIONS WITH HONEST AND AGE-APPROPRIATE ANSWERS— AND THAT HOLDS TRUE FOR COMING OUT AS WELL."
>
> Elisabeth A. Sheff
> *Should You Come Out to Your Kids if You Are Polyamorous?*

Figure S8.1 Quote by Elisabeth A. Sheff. Created by the Author.

Exposure to Significant Others

The decision of whether to introduce a new partner to children in the context of non-monogamous or polyamorous relationships is a complex and individual one. Clients need to consider various factors, including the nature of the relationship and the level of involvement the partner has with the children (Sheff, 2013). The age and maturity of the children also play a role in determining how much information should be disclosed.

If the relationship with a new partner primarily revolves around a sexual connection and the partner is not expected to have much interaction with the children, it may not be advisable to introduce them (Sheff, 2013). Introducing a new person to a child's life can create confusion and potential disruption if the relationship does not develop into a long-term commitment. It is essential to prioritize stability and consistency for children, especially daily.

On the other hand, if the partner(s) in the non-monogamous relationship are around frequently and have a significant role in the children's lives, it becomes more essential to disclose information about the relationship in an age-appropriate manner. Children can be resilient and accepting of diverse family structures if they receive open and honest communication from their parents (Bauermeister & Gee, 2016). This may involve explaining the nature of the relationship, the roles and responsibilities of everyone, and reassurance that the child's needs and well-being are a priority for all involved.

Parents must consider their children's emotional well-being throughout the process of introducing new partners. Regular and open dialogues should be encouraged, allowing children to express their concerns and ask questions (Haritaworn et al., 2006). Parents should be prepared to offer support and reassurance, ensuring that the child feels secure and loved.

It is worth noting that there is limited research specifically addressing the introduction of multiple partners to children in non-monogamous or polyamorous relationships. Therefore, individuals need to seek professional guidance and consider their unique family dynamics when making decisions regarding the involvement of partners in their children's lives.

Level of Risk

Clients who are considering whether their children should keep their non-monogamous relationships a secret should carefully examine the potential risks and considerations involved. Here are some questions to help guide this exploration:

1 Is there a risk if children disclose their parent's relationship status to certain family members, ex-spouses, or others? It is crucial to assess the potential consequences, such as strained family relationships or legal implications, particularly in custody agreements.
2 Do the clients identify with marginalized identities, especially those related to sexual orientation and gender? Marginalized communities may already face discrimination and stigma, and adding the disclosure of non-traditional family dynamics could potentially compound these challenges. It is essential to consider whether the clients and their children can sustain another disadvantage and if it is worth exposing themselves to potential harm (Sheff, 2021; Powell, 2018).
3 Are the children frequently around the clients' co-workers? If so, disclosing the family dynamics may lead to employment discrimination or prejudice, affecting the clients' professional lives. This consideration becomes particularly important if the clients live in areas without legal protections for individuals in non-traditional relationships.

It is essential to approach these questions from a place of understanding that children may unintentionally share information without fully grasping the potential consequences. Adult family members must be prepared to face any retribution or adverse reactions that may arise if their child discloses non-monogamous relationship dynamics to others in the community.

Whether children should keep their parent's ENM relationships a secret depends on various factors, including the potential risks involved and the client's readiness to address and navigate any challenges that may arise from disclosure.

Chosen Family

Chosen families have become a significant aspect of non-monogamous relationships, providing emotional support, understanding, and acceptance that may not always be found within a person's family of origin or traditional societal structures (Taormino, 2008). These relationships go beyond mere friendships, as they often involve deep emotional connections and a sense of kinship with individuals who share similar relationship values and lifestyles.

Encouraging clients to build a chosen family, or "tribe," can offer numerous benefits. These connections can provide unwavering support during challenging times and celebrations of milestones within their non-monogamous relationships. Chosen families can also provide valuable education and guidance as members share their experiences, wisdom, and knowledge about navigating non-traditional relationship dynamics.

One of the essential aspects of chosen families is creating a judgment-free space for individuals in non-monogamous relationships. By surrounding themselves with like-minded individuals, clients can find acceptance, understanding, and validation for their relationship choices. This sense of belonging can help clients build resilience, self-confidence, and emotional well-being.

Chosen families can vary, ranging from small intimate groups to more extensive networks of individuals. Some individuals may create closed, exclusive networks, while others may opt for more open and fluid connections that allow new members to join over time (Taormino, 2008). The structure and dynamics of chosen families are highly personal and depend on the preferences and needs of the individuals involved.

In conclusion, chosen families play a vital role in enhancing the lives of individuals in non-monogamous relationships. These relationships offer a sense of belonging, support, and understanding that may not always be found within traditional family structures. By cultivating these connections, clients can create a supportive community that aligns with their values and provides a safe space for their non-monogamous relationships to thrive.

Managing Multiple Relationships with ENM Clients

Multiple relationships can be complex for therapists working with clients in non-monogamous relationships. These relationships occur when a therapist is in a professional role with a person while having another role or relationship with the same person or someone closely associated with them (American Psychological Association [APA], 2002).

Therapists who work with non-monogamous clients often encounter situations where multiple relationships are unavoidable. Elizabeth Duke, a clinical psychologist and member of the APA's Divisions 32 and 44, highlights the challenges clinicians face in ENM communities, stating that avoiding multiple relationships can be impossible in these contexts. Moreover, the additional complexities of romantic and sexual webs within polycules can amplify emotional distress for both ENM clinicians and clinicians working with ENM clients (Duke, 2022).

In response to these challenges, Dr. Duke, as a polyamorous clinician and Clinical Director at LifeWorks Psychotherapy Center, has developed guidelines based on her understanding and synthesis of ethical codes. These guidelines focus on three main categories:

1 **Scope of competence/cultural humility:** Therapists must assess their competence and cultural humility in working with non-monogamous clients. This includes exploring their knowledge, training, and understanding of ENM dynamics and acknowledging and addressing any biases they may have.
2 **Navigating multiple relationships:** Therapists must understand the unique ethical considerations and challenges when working with clients in ENM relationships. This involves setting clear boundaries, managing potential conflicts of interest, and maintaining objectivity in therapeutic relationships.
3 **Confidentiality:** Therapists must maintain the confidentiality of all individuals involved in non-monogamous relationships. This may require discussing and establishing agreements regarding confidentiality with clients and being aware of any potential breaches that may occur within the multiple relationship dynamics (Duke, 2022).

By following these guidelines, therapists can navigate the complexities of multiple relationships in ENM contexts while upholding ethical standards and providing effective client support.

Scope of Competence/Cultural Humility

When considering whether to work with clients in non-monogamous relationships, therapists need to assess their ethical ability. Elizabeth Duke, in her guidelines for therapists working with ENM clients, identifies certain statements that clinicians should reflect upon to determine if they can ethically work with ENM couples/individuals (Duke, 2022):

1 Therapists who have not openly announced their participation in ENM, limiting their ability to secure supervision/consultation, may face challenges in effectively supporting ENM clients. Openly acknowledging their involvement in ENM can help therapists connect with other professionals knowledgeable about non-monogamy and access appropriate supervision or consultation.
2 Therapists who currently pathologize ENM may not be suitable for working with ENM clients. Therapists must approach non-monogamous relationships without bias or judgment and recognize that ENM is a valid and legitimate relationship style.
3 Therapists who struggle with overcoming preconceived notions about mononormativity may find it challenging to provide non-judgmental and affirmative support to ENM clients. Mononormativity refers to the societal assumption that monogamy is the only valid and accepted form of romantic relationship. Clinicians need to examine their biases and work toward understanding, validating, and respecting the diverse relationship styles of their ENM clients.

Additionally, it is essential for therapists working with ENM clients to regularly engage in consultation/supervision with other therapists who are knowledgeable about ENM. Consultation/supervision provides a safe space for therapists to discuss challenges, seek guidance, and gain insights from peers who have experience in working with ENM populations.

Therapists can also benefit from conversing with other clinicians working with ENM populations to learn how they manage entangled relationships. These conversations can provide valuable insights, strategies, and perspectives on maintaining boundaries, managing conflicts of interest, and addressing the unique dynamics of non-monogamous relationships.

Furthermore, therapists actively involved in the happenings within the ENM community can deepen their understanding of ENM dynamics, challenges, and experiences. This involvement can include attending ENM community events, workshops, or conferences, engaging with online forums or support groups, and keeping up-to-date with relevant research and resources.

By considering these aspects and actively engaging with the ENM community and knowledgeable clinicians, therapists can enhance their competence and provide ethical and practical support to clients in non-monogamous relationships.

Navigating Multiple Relationships

In working with clients in non-monogamous relationships, therapists should openly discuss with clients the hazards associated with having intersecting social circles. Elizabeth Duke emphasizes the importance of addressing this potential challenge in her guidelines for therapists working with ENM clients (Duke, 2022).

To ensure informed consent and client autonomy, therapists should allow clients to choose whether they want to continue therapy, considering the potential risks associated with intersecting social circles. This discussion enables clients to assess their comfort level and make decisions that align with their needs and preferences.

Suppose the client decides that they are uncomfortable continuing the therapeutic relationship due to overlapping social circles. In that case, the therapist should ethically provide referrals for ENM clinicians if such professionals are available. However, in some cases, there may be a limited number of ENM clinicians in a particular area. In such situations, the therapist can explore the possibility of providing consultation about ENM to a therapist who can offer services to the client, ensuring that the client's needs are still met.

Maintaining confidentiality is a crucial aspect of therapy. However, when intersecting social circles are present, therapists may need to use their clinical judgment to determine the appropriate level of self-disclosure for the clients. This self-disclosure should be done to protect the confidentiality of all individuals involved while addressing the potential impact of multiple relationships.

If an ENM therapist discovers that an established client has entered a relationship with an individual within their relationship circle, seeking consultation or supervision is essential. The therapist should handle this situation with sensitivity and ensure that the shared partner of the therapist–client relationship remains unaware of the therapeutic relationship. The therapist must communicate with the client about the dual relationship and encourage them to disclose the revelation to the shared partner if clinically appropriate.

By openly discussing intersecting social circles, providing options for continued therapy, offering appropriate referrals, using clinical judgment for self-disclosure, and ensuring ethical management of dual relationships, therapists can navigate the hazards associated with multiple relationships in ENM contexts.

Confidentiality

In working with clients in non-monogamous relationships, therapists can implement strategies to support the unique dynamics and relationships within these contexts. Elizabeth Duke suggests two approaches in her guidelines for therapists working with ENM clients: Creating and implementing a "HIPAA+" office policy and actively notating polycules and/or relationship trains (Duke, 2022).

Creating and implementing a "HIPAA+" office policy involves extending the Health Insurance Portability and Accountability Act (HIPAA) principles to protect individuals' privacy and confidentiality within polycules or relationship trains. This entails taking extra measures to ensure that all individuals involved in the ENM relationships, including metamours (partners' partners), know the therapist's commitment to confidentiality.

Therapists can discuss and obtain consent from all parties involved regarding information-sharing and the involvement of multiple relationships within therapy sessions. Clear boundaries and communication protocols can help maintain confidentiality and respect everyone's autonomy and privacy within the polycule or relationship train.

Active notation of polycules and/or relationship trains refers to the therapist's deliberate documentation of the interconnected relationships within ENM contexts. This practice can help therapists understand and remember the complex dynamics and connections between individuals involved in the client's life.

By actively notating polycules and/or relationship training during the therapy process, therapists can gain insights into the support systems, dependencies, and potential conflicts within the client's relationships. This documentation can assist therapists in effectively addressing the needs of the client and their network of relationships during the therapeutic journey.

These two strategies, creating a "HIPAA+" office policy and actively notating polycules and/or relationship trains, emphasize respecting confidentiality and managing the complex dynamics in ENM relationships. By implementing these approaches, therapists can create a safe and inclusive therapeutic environment that acknowledges and supports the diverse relationships within the client's life.

Chapter Highlights

- Living an authentic lifestyle can be challenging for those new to living out in the open with their lifestyle. Therapists should normalize their fears and help them find comfortable ways to introduce themselves to being out.
- When a couple is outed before they are ready, this can be devastating and have serious repercussions. Help the couple grieve their former life and embrace the new elements that will follow.
- Couple privilege is consistent with the monogamy hangover and places more value on pair bonding than other relationship dynamics.
- Explore the positives and negatives about coming out to the client's children and help them form age-appropriate language to talk to their children if they choose to self-disclose.
- Due to the close-knit community of ENM, therapists might find themselves in a situation where they are managing multiple relationships with ENM clients; therefore, creating a safe space for the therapist and the clients is vital. Ensuring confidentiality is the most critical element when managing multiple relationships within ENM.

Treatment Plan: Managing Relationships

Behavioral Manifestations

1 Concealing open relationship dynamics from significant others, such as family, friends, and community members, due to fear of rejection and/or retaliation.
2 Relationship dynamics were shared with others without the permission of the primary couple.
3 Having limited or no social support network outside of the monogamous networks previously created.
4 The choice of who to openly talk about relationship dynamics was removed by an outside party "outing" the couple or partner.
5 The children discover parents' open relationship dynamics.
6 Cut off or removed from social, family, and/or religious networks due to open relationship dynamics.

Long-Term Client Goals

1 Disclose relationship dynamics to significant others, such as family, friends, and community members, when/if both partners feel they are ready to do so.

2 Reduce anxiety and fear associated with relationship dynamics being shared with others without permission.
3 Create a community or join a community of like-minded individuals who can provide support and guidance using ENM narratives.
4 Determine who needs to know about chosen relationship dynamics and how they are informed.
5 Openly discuss relationship dynamics with children using age-appropriate terminology.
6 Create a supportive community of like-minded individuals or a chosen family that will supplement the family and communal support that was removed after beginning ENM.
7 The couple decides to maintain privacy regarding their ENM relationship status.

Short-Term Client Goals	Therapeutic Interventions
• List the benefits and reservations of being open about the relationship dynamics with family, friends, and community.	• Have the couple explore the benefits and negatives of sharing their open relationship dynamics with others. • If the partners are not in agreement about openly proclaiming their new relationship dynamics, have each partner list their reasonings and preferences, ensure the listener shows respect for the other partner's point of view, and withhold further criticism while they explore their feelings.
• Verbalize feelings regarding not being afforded the choice to tell others about the ENM relationship dynamics.	• Assist the couple in exploring their feelings, and normalize feelings of loss, anger, betrayal, and shame associated with being "outed." • If only one partner is hurt or angry, encourage the other partner to support the hurt/angry partner and listen to their concerns in a way that fosters support and understanding. • Help the couple understand that coming out is not a one-time choice, and they will have to determine daily what information they will share with others in their daily lives. • Educating the couple about "couple privilege" and how those couples tend to blend in and are afforded more benefits than those who stand out.
• Identify the amount of information each partner is comfortable sharing with the children.	• Provide the couple with research regarding how non-monogamy affects kids. Suggest they research Dr. Elizabeth Sheff. • Suggest to the couple age-appropriate conversations that can help broach the topic of ENM with their children.

(Continued)

Short-Term Client Goals	Therapeutic Interventions
	• Educate the couple about issues resulting from their children telling friends and teachers about their ENM relationship.
• Verbalize an understanding of the importance of finding a supportive community.	• Common issues include other parents not allowing their children to spend time at the family house, teachers passing judgment, CPS notified, grandparents causing problems, the social community rejecting children, etc.
• Express the importance of keeping the ENM relationship status a secret.	• Assist the couple by providing information for local ENM communities and online resources.
	• Explore the importance of creating a community, or chosen family, as a means of support.
	• Create a list of positives and negatives regarding being "out" about being ENM.
	• Explore any safety concerns that might arise from making the ENM relationship status public knowledge; children's school, employment concerns, hostile family members, child custody considerations, etc.
	• Create an agreement between the partners regarding how they will handle specific situations as they arise due to being ENM; social media, dating secondary partners in public, questions about trips or events from others, responses for nosey neighbors, etc. Use the "Risks and Stigmas" activity in the resource section of this book.

References

American Psychological Association. (2002). Ethical Principles of Psychologists and Code of Conduct. Retrieved from https://www.apa.org/ethics/code/index

Barker, M. (2015). A critique of the monogamy hangover: An argument for ethical polyamory. *Policy and Politics*, *43*(2), 171–185.

Barker, M., & Langdridge, D. (2011). Whatever happened to non-monogamies? Critical reflections on recent research and theory. *Sexualities*, *14*(5), 618–635.

Bauermeister, J. A., & Gee, G. C. (2016). Heteronormativity and sexual partnering among bisexually-active Latino young men. *Archives of Sexual Behavior*, *45*(3), 519–538.

Conley, T. D. (2013). Monogamish: The new rules of marriage. *Psychology Today*. Retrieved from https://www.psychologytoday.com/us/blog/the-long-reach-childhood/201306/monogamish-the-new-rules-marriage.

Duke, E. A. (2022). Ethical clinical practice with consensual non-monogamous clients. In M. D. Vaughan & T. R. Burnes (Eds.), *The handbook of consensual non-monogamy: Affirming mental health practice* (pp. 266–282). Rowman & Littlefield.

Duke, E. D. (2022). Multiple relationships in psychology of diverse-sexual-orientation and relationship-style communities. In Z. Britton (Ed.), *Handbook of cultural practices: Considerations for psychological practice* (pp. 271–280). Oxford University Press.

Golding, J. M., & Wilt, J. (2018). Children's understanding of non-traditional family structures: A review and commentary on current research. *Journal of Divorce & Remarriage, 59*(3), 224–241.

Haritaworn, J., Lin, C., Klesse, C., & Brown, G. (2006). Queering paradigms. *Qualitative Sociology Review, 2*(3), 345–366.

Human Rights Campaign Foundation. (2020). Coming out: Living authentically as lesbian, gay and bisexual+. *Human Rights Campaign.* https://issuu.com/humanrightscampaign/docs/comingout-lgb_-resource-2020

Kennedy, J. L. (2019). Children's understanding of non-traditional families. *The Oxford Research Encyclopedia of Communication.* Retrieved from 10.1093/acrefore/9780190228613.013.730

Nelson, S. (2022, January 7). *What is outing and why is it harmful?* LGBTQ and ALL. Retrieved October 10, 2022, from https://www.lgbtqandall.com/what-is-outing-and-why-is-it-harmful/

Powell, D. L. (2018). *Building open relationships: Your hands on guide to swinging, polyamory, and beyond!* Dr. Liz Powell.

Powell, R. L. (2018). Mental health disparities in polyamorous individuals. *Journal of Feminist Family Therapy, 30*(3), 126–149.

Sheff, E. (2013). Polyamorous families, same-sex marriage, and the slippery slope. *Journal of Contemporary Ethnography, 42*(2), 124–155.

Sheff, E. (2021). *The polyamorists next door: Inside multiple-partner relationships and families.* Rowman & Littlefield.

Sheff, E. A. (2021, November 15). *Should you come out to your kids if you are polyamorous?* Psychology Today. Retrieved October 10, 2022, from https://www.psychologytoday.com/us/blog/the-polyamorists-next-door/202111/should-you-come-out-your-kids-if-you-are-polyamorous

Taormino, T. (2008). *Opening up: A guide to polyamory.* Cleis.

Established ENM Clients Experiencing Issues

Established ENM Clients Experiencing Issues

As with any relationship, the question is never IF things go wrong, but rather WHEN they have hiccups. The most experienced practitioners of ethical non-monog (ENM) have hiccups, and if a couple denies that fact, they are not being honest with themselves. Anecdotally, ENM challenges every aspect of one's life because of the overwhelming support for monogamous relationships.

There are many couples that I have had the pleasure of therapeutically working with that have been involved in ENM for decades; however, they experienced a setback and needed guidance to get back on track. I firmly believe that a relationship check-up is always beneficial regardless of how long a couple has been ENM. In this chapter, we will explore common issues experienced ENM couples face and how you, as their therapist, can help them navigate their predicament.

Changes in Relationship Status with Secondary Partners

Using the term *secondary partner* contributes to the impression that the individual is not as important as the primary partner and alludes to a hierarchical relationship; however, I am using this term to differentiate between partners throughout this chapter. Everyone is important and deserves equal treatment unless previously arranged through conversations and agreements.

In their book *Building Open Relationships,* Dr. Liz Powell uses the terms "upleveling" and "downleveling" to describe the modifications in the seriousness of these relationships (2018). They explain that these terms are based on mainstream dating understandings, where more sincerity, entwinement, and commitment are considered "moving up." At the same time, fewer elements are seen as "moving down" (Powell, 2018, p. 220).

Similarly, in her book *Stepping Off the Relationship Escalator: Uncommon Love and Life,* Amy Gahran refers to the conventional template of relationships as the "relationship escalator" (Gahran, 2017). This template follows a linear progression from initial attraction and

DOI: 10.4324/9781003464891-17

dating to being sexually and romantically involved, becoming exclusive, adopting a shared couple identity, merging lives, and ultimately leading to marriage and having children, with the commitment lasting until death.

Dr. Powell also provides the following disclaimer (that is perfectly stated, so I could not bring myself to try and find a *better* way to say it), "thinking about relationships as having 'levels' often encourages us to try and fit the people in our lives into boxes rather than just allowing what happens between the two of us to find its shape" (Powell, 2018, p. 220).

Primary to Primary: Upleveling

Regardless of the terminology, when a primary partner begins to get closer to a secondary partner, A.K.A., a metamour, the opportunity for jealousy appears out of nowhere. Change throughout life is inevitable, but growth is an individual choice that everyone can experience if they are open to it.

Primary to primary upleveling is when a primary partner approaches the other primary partner, revealing their desire to uplevel with a secondary partner. Unfortunately, a primary partner could have an unpleasant reaction to the request for their significant other to uplevel with their secondary relationship, resulting in hurt feelings, misunderstandings, jealousy, and resentment.

Clinical Considerations

Areas of exploration with a couple experiencing difficulties with primary to primary upleveling:

- *Distressed Partner*
  - Do they feel pressured or coerced into accepting the uplevel?
    - Did the primary partner present the proposal as "if you love me, then you will let me have this" or "if you don't accept this, then we will break up"?
  - How do they feel a level change of seriousness will affect their ERE with their primary partner?
  - Has their primary partner experienced new relationship energy (NRE), and if so, how did that affect their overall relationship?
  - In their opinion, how does the metamour positively contribute to the primary relationship?
  - In their opinion, how does the metamour negatively contribute to the primary relationship?
  - Assess their attachment style.
    - Explain that attachment styles can change from one relationship to another and even within a specific relationship, in this situation, their primary relationship (Fern, 2020).

- Explore their understanding of and ability to experience compersion.
- Educate the client about primal panic compared to jealousy, encouraging them to label their feelings appropriately.

  - According to Jessica Fern, primal panic occurs when attachment-related threats, perceived or actual, are present:

    - Potential loss of attachment figure (in this case, their primary partner)
    - Separation from our attachment figure
    - Loss of access to primary partner for extended periods or more prolonged than previously experienced

  - Identify how the distressed client self-soothes when experiencing primal panic and suggest modifications for self-destructive behaviors.
  - "When primal attachment panic gets mislabeled as jealousy, the partner experiencing it can be left thinking that there is something wrong with them, that this is their issue to figure out on their own, and that they should be better at doing [ENM]" (Fern, 2020, p. 144).

- *Upleveling Partner*
  - How do they feel a level change of seriousness will affect their established relationship energy (ERE) with their primary partner?
  - Have them examine how they presented the information to their primary partner.

    - How did they begin the conversation, and what was their emotional tone for the proposal?

  - Have they experienced NRE with previous secondary partners, and if so, what were their behaviors in response to those intense feelings?

    - If they disclose that their behavior left their primary partner feeling distressed, identify actions that can be implemented to ensure their primary partner doesn't feel the way they previously did.

  - In their opinion, how does the metamour positively contribute to the primary relationship?
  - In their opinion, how does the metamour negatively contribute to the primary relationship?
  - Remind the upleveling partner that they have had time to sit with their feelings for some time; therefore, they may feel their primary partner overreached when proposed initially.
  - If the distressed partner identifies with primal panic, how can the upleveling partner assist them in creating healthy coping mechanisms?

Secondary to Primary: Upleveling

When a secondary partner has approached a primary partner requesting that the current relationship move toward higher levels of commitment or entanglement, the primary partner can experience negative feelings about the request, further triggering insecurities. Commonly, most therapists respond with some form of, "If it is going to cause these negative feelings for your partner, why would you entertain that option?" but an ENM-aware therapist should explore the emotions, get to the root of the emotional distress, and encourage compromise. For many couples, this conversation was not originally negotiated when opening their relationship, thus the basis for the current conflict.

Clinical Considerations

Areas of exploration with a couple experiencing difficulties with metamour to primary upleveling:

- *Distressed Partner*

  - How do they feel a level change of seriousness will affect their ERE with their primary partner?
  - Has their primary partner experienced NRE, and if so, how did that affect their overall relationship?
  - Explore the relationship dynamics between the distressed partner and their metamour.

    - Does the distressed partner feel disrespected by their metamour?
    - Discuss and process perceived expectations, identifying whether they were realistic or unrealistic.

  - In their opinion, how does the metamour positively contribute to the primary relationship?
  - In their opinion, how does the metamour negatively contribute to the primary relationship?
  - Differentiate between primal panic and jealousy, allowing the distressed partner to identify where the negative emotions stem from.
  - Do they feel the metamour is using coercion with the primary partner?
  - How would the distressed partner like to be approached in the future by their primary partner when upleveling with a metamour?

- *Upleveling Partner*

  - Do they feel pressured or coerced into accepting the uplevel?

    - Did the secondary partner present the request as "If you love me" or "We do this or break up?"

- Have them examine how they presented the information to their primary partner.

  - How did they begin the conversation, and what was their emotional tone for the proposal?

- Did they explore what they wanted to achieve by upleveling before presenting it to their primary partner?

  - How much time would they like to spend together moving forward?
  - How would they like to label each other if labels are a thing for them?
  - Do they want to share holidays with their secondary partner?
  - Are they requesting this relationship be public knowledge?

- How do they feel a level change of seriousness will affect their ERE with their primary partner?
- Remind the upleveling partner that they have had time to sit with their feelings before presenting this to their primary partner; therefore, significant emotional reactions are not uncharacteristic.
- Are they trying to be the go-between for their primary and secondary partners?
- Do they unknowingly (or knowingly) employ coercion to sway their primary partner's decision?

Primary to Primary: Downleveling

Primary to primary dowleveling is when a primary partner tells the other primary partner they are downleveling with a secondary partner. This realization can evoke positive and negative emotions for both partners that must be discussed and processed. When metamours are close friends, downleveling can damage their relationship, resulting in emotional distress all the way around. This rendered both primary partners grieving and confused about how to move forward concerning relationships with the third person.

There are many reasons that downleveling occurs in secondary relationships, with a few being listed below (Powell, 2018):

- Circumstances in one's life change
- Each partner undergoes changes that are not compatible with each other
- NRE has run its course
- Conflict within the relationship

Clinical Considerations

Areas of exploration with a couple experiencing difficulties with primary-to-primary downleveling:

- *Distressed Partner*

  - While both primary partners might be distressed, for this demonstration, I am referring to the pivot partner, the shared partner of the primary and secondary partners, as the distressed partner.
  - Assist the distressed partner in determining why they feel/felt the need to request a downlevel within the relationship dynamics.
  - Explore what they enjoyed most about their connection with the secondary partner.
  - Identify the relationship dynamics they would like to maintain with the secondary partner.

    - Do they want to break up with the secondary partner completely?
    - Do they want to maintain a sexual relationship with the secondary partner?
    - Are they able to maintain emotional support for the secondary partner? If so, have them detail their limitations for emotional support.

  - How do they expect them to respond without discussing their need for downleveling with their secondary partner?
  - Create talking points for the distressed client to have prepared before they downlevel with their secondary partner.

    - Do they have the capacity to process the change in relationship dynamics with their secondary partner?
    - Are there any limitations to holding their secondary partner's feelings while they process the change?
    - How do they want to greet each other when/if they see each other at a community event?
    - How would they like to share their downleveling with others, if at all?

  - If they have already discussed their need for downleveling with their secondary partner, was there anything surprising they felt during the conversation?
  - Discuss and process how their primary partner can support them during emotional distress.
  - Remind the distressed partner that they have had time to sit with their feelings before presenting this to their primary partner; therefore, significant emotional reactions are not uncharacteristic.
  - Explore the grieving process with the distressed client, helping them identify their current stage of grief.

- Encourage the client to create a self-care plan of action to help them with the grieving process.

- *Supportive Primary Partner*

  - Inquire about the relationship dynamics between metamours.
  - Provide them the opportunity to express their feelings regarding the downleveling.

    - Ensure they are presenting their feelings non-judgmentally, providing redirection when necessary.
    - Assess for feelings of guilt or responsibility and normalize as needed, if needed.

  - How does the supportive primary partner feel about continuing the friendship if the metamours were close?

    - As a couple, please encourage them to identify realistic and unrealistic expectations for the metamours relationship after the downleveling.

  - Explore the grieving process with the distressed client, helping them identify their current stage of grief.

Secondary to Primary: Downleveling

This occurs when the secondary partner approaches the primary partner, requesting they downlevel their relationship. The primary partner could be caught off guard, resulting in uncharacteristic emotional distress.

Clinical Considerations

Areas of exploration with a couple experiencing difficulties with primary to primary downleveling:

- *Distressed Partner*

  - While both primary partners might be distressed, for this demonstration, I am referring to the pivot partner, the shared partner of the primary and secondary partners, as the distressed partner.
  - Remind them that there is no right or wrong way to downlevel with partners and that their feelings are valid.

- Discuss and process how the secondary partner presented their request for downleveling to them.

  - Identify the positive and negative takeaways from the overall conversation.
  - What are the relationship dynamics moving forward?

- Discuss and process the distressed partner's reaction to the request.

  - Was this request a surprise, or did they feel things were changing within the secondary relationship?

- Encourage the client to create a self-care plan of action to help them with the grieving process.

- *Supportive Primary Partner*

  - Remind them that there is no right or wrong way to downlevel with partners and that their feelings are valid.
  - Inquire about the relationship dynamics between metamours.
  - Provide them the opportunity to express their feelings regarding the downleveling.

    - Ensure they are presenting their feelings non-judgmentally, providing redirection when necessary.
    - Assess for feelings of guilt or responsibility and normalize as needed, if needed.

  - How does the supportive primary partner feel about continuing the friendship if the metamours were close?

    - As a couple, please encourage them to identify realistic and unrealistic expectations for the metamours relationship after the downleveling.

  - Explore the grieving process with the distressed client, helping them identify their current stage of grief.
  - If the supportive primary partner harbors negative feelings, encourage them to explore those feelings in an individual session if necessary.

    - Negative feelings toward someone who has hurt a loved one are common, but voicing those negative feelings when the primary partner is grieving will not foster emotional healing.

Table S9.1 Creative Space

Take advantage of this space and unleash your creativity by creating a mind map or flowchart that will help you grasp and consolidate "Downleveling" and "Upleveling" to your clients.

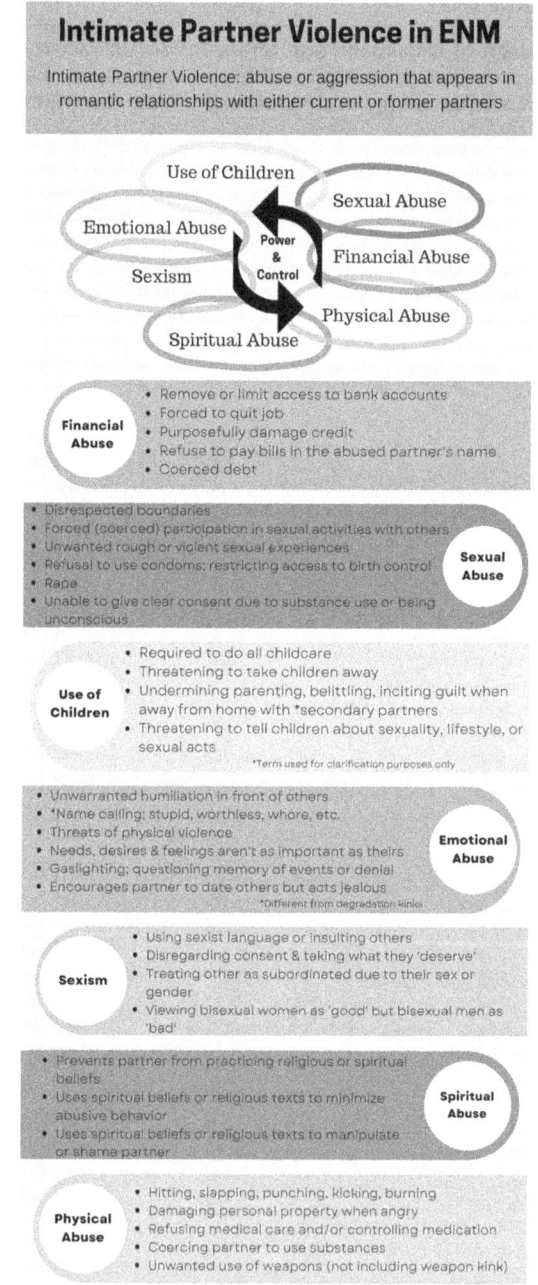

Figure S9.1 Intimate Partner Violence in ENM. Created by the Author.

Identifying Abuse in the Lifestyle

Intimate Partner Violence (IPV) can be present in ENM relationships, just like in any other relationship dynamic. According to Sandra Knispel, the Communications Officer at the University of Rochester, approximately one in four women and almost one in ten men in America have experienced IPV. In an article discussing intimate partner violence titled *What is intimate partner violence? It's not just physical abuse*; Knispel interviewed Catherine Cerulli, the director of the University of Rochester's Susan B. Anthony Center and the Laboratory of Interpersonal Violence and Victimization (Knispel, 2022).

Intimate partner violence can occur between individuals in an intimate relationship, regardless of marital status, current or former dating status, or the presence of a romantic relationship. It can take various forms, including emotional abuse, psychological abuse (such as coercive control), economic abuse, physical abuse, sexual abuse, and even the use of children to obtain the abuser's desired outcomes.

While IPV and domestic violence are often used interchangeably, IPV is a subcategory of domestic violence. According to Cerulli, domestic violence includes but is not limited to elder abuse, sibling abuse, and IPV and can occur by an individual who does not reside at the exact location (Knispel, 2022). Women Against Abuse, a 501(c)(3) nonprofit agency in Philadelphia, provided "the abusive partner may use oppression systems already set in our society to assert his or her privileges against the other person" (Types of Abuse, n.d.).

Overwhelmed by Multiple Relationships Demanding Attention

Managing multiple romantic relationships can indeed be overwhelming, leading to feelings of stress and complexity. It is important for therapists to assist clients in exploring various strategies to address these challenges and provide support.

The following approaches can be explored with clients who are feeling overwhelmed by multiple relationships:

- **Discuss and process contributing factors**
  - Encourage clients to identify and list the broad themes that contribute to their feelings of overwhelm. By narrowing down these themes, clients can gain insight into specific areas that may be causing stress within their work, family, and romantic relationships.

- **Time management**

  - Help clients examine how they are balancing their time between different areas of their lives. This could involve exploring techniques for effectively managing work tasks, spending quality time with family, and allocating sufficient time and energy to each romantic partner.

- **Identify unrealistic expectations**

  - Address any unrealistic expectations placed on clients by themselves or others. This could involve exploring whether clients are trying to meet unattainable standards in various aspects of their relationships.

- **Establish areas of control**

  - Work with clients to identify aspects within their control that can be changed to alleviate overwhelm. This may involve restructuring work schedules, delegating tasks, setting boundaries, or creating shared calendars to communicate availability.

- **Scarcity mindset vs. abundance mindset**

  - Educate clients about the distinction between viewing relationships through a scarcity mindset (feeling limited in options) and an abundance mindset (recognizing the availability of love and potential partners). Encourage clients to shift their mindset to one of abundance, which can alleviate the fear of abandonment and reduce the inclination to overcommit or sacrifice self-care.

- **Practice mindfulness and self-acceptance**

  - Help clients cultivate mindfulness by focusing on the present moment and observing their thoughts and emotions without judgment. Encourage acceptance of negative thoughts or emotions and guide clients in developing a plan of action to address concerns or self-care needs.

- **Explore self-care practices**

  - Support clients in incorporating small moments of self-care into their daily routine. This could include activities such as stretching breaks, brief walks, guided meditation, journaling, dancing, or engaging in art.

- **Avoid reliance on substances**

  - Ensure that clients are not turning to drugs or alcohol as coping mechanisms for stress. Facilitate discussions and exploration of healthier stress management strategies.

By guiding clients through these strategies, therapists can assist them in navigating the challenges of managing multiple relationships while prioritizing self-care and reducing overwhelm.

Mismatched Evolvement in ENM

Change is a perpetual aspect of our lives, and it can come suddenly, like an inescapable wrecking ball. However, one must deliberately strive toward growth when faced with change. Couples may encounter challenges in their relationship growth, particularly if one partner is progressing faster than the other, owing to the societal norm of monogamy. In this article, we will delve into two different perspectives: Hierarchical and non-hierarchical.

Using the hierarchical framework, the couple can only grow as fast as the slowest member of their dyad; therefore, resentment and jealousy can occur when one partner is growing fast. Explore areas where the slow-growing partner might be stuck while normalizing individual growth and acceptance.

While a person can be stuck where they are emotionally for absolutely ANY reason, and that is perfectly acceptable, there are some common reasons therapists can explore with their clients if they are having a hard time identifying where they are stuck:

- **Monogamy hangover**
  - Believing there is only "one" person for them
  - Feeling as if they have to do everything together
  - Uncomfortable being alone
  - Ownership/codependency
  - Attaching personal value to the quality of the relationship
  - Connecting the overall health of the relationship to the amount of sex they are having

- **Jealousy, insecurity, and fear of abandonment**
  - Partner dating someone more attractive than their partner

    - The subjective view of self
    - Increase self-esteem

  - Age differences
  - Different socio-economic status
  - Outward expression or NRE
  - Using unique names, "pet" names, with other partners

- **Weak boundaries, agreements, and/or rules**

  - Clarity might be needed for the stuck partner.

- **Poor communication**
- **Mismatched libido**
- **Unable, or not comfortable with, communicating their needs**
- **Feeling like they are easily replaceable**

Individuals in non-hierarchical ENM relationships encounter similar challenges as those in hierarchical ENM relationships, with the distinction that all partners are given equal consideration in decision-making processes. It is important to debunk the misconception that non-hierarchical relationships are free-for-all or endless orgies, as that portrayal is unrealistic. Here are some common stuck points for clients practicing non-hierarchical ENM:

- **Inability to effectively communicate**

  - ENM (especially polyamory) is complicated
  - Multiple personalities, several points of view, and more egos to consider

- **Afraid of heartbreak**

  - ENM requires vulnerability, and vulnerability can be painful
  - Unable to control the direction of relationships

    - Explore their boundaries, agreements, and rules, identifying unrealistic requests.

- **Sharing your partner is hard**

  - Having a hard time letting go of the "mine, mine, mine" mindset
  - Uncomfortable with equality of some sort

- **Confrontation**

  - Unable to get along with a metamour(s)

Providing support to ENM individuals can be intricate, especially when their partners are on different journey stages. Sometimes, one partner may struggle to recognize the exact point they are stuck at. In such cases, comprehending common reasons why individuals hit stuck points can aid in identifying the problem swiftly. During some sessions, clients may struggle to recall the underlying issues hindering their progress. Assigning them tasks to help them evaluate their thoughts and feelings can be invaluable.

Chapter Highlights

- Changes in relationship status with secondary partners can be challenging to accept for consistent partners who may not understand why this is occurring. Normalizing being able to love multiple partners and ensuring the clients see this as emotional growth instead of regression.

- In their book *Building Open Relationships,* Dr. Liz Powell refers to these relationship modifications as "changes in levels of seriousness," further explaining that they are utilizing terms such as "Upleveling" and "Downleveling" due to "mainstream dating understandings, more seriousness/entwinement/commitment is considered 'moving up,' and less of those are considered 'moving down'" (Powell, 2018, p. 220).

- Identifying abuse in ENM is a critical task for clinicians. For some couples, intimate partner violence can be disguised as ENM, but it has no place in ENM.
- Individuals can become overwhelmed when multiple partners require their attention, making consistent partners feel unimportant, unheard, and left out. Encourage the couple to find equitable ways to share their time with each partner so negative feelings do not develop.
- There might be times when one partner is more involved than the other or receives more attention from potential partners, which can lead to resentment and jealousy. Normalize these feelings and encourage the couple to find equitable ways to participate in ENM.

Treatment Plan: Established ENM and Experiencing Issues

Behavioral Manifestations

1 Relationship distress resulting from a requested change in the relationship dynamics with a secondary partner.
2 Relationship distress is caused by increased emotional feelings toward a secondary partner, i.e., falling in love.
3 Personal distress resulting from one partner ending a relationship with a secondary partner.
4 Relationship distress is caused by frequent arguments or strong disagreements stemming from one partner having emotional distress (decreased sex).
5 Deliberately causing psychological and/or physical pain or injury to a partner; preventing communication with others, gaslighting, destructive behaviors, threats of violence, denial of basic needs, deliberate unsafe play, inappropriate boundaries, anger in kink, and/or any physical violence resulting in unwanted injuries.
6 Inability to stay equally invested in multiple relationships demanding attention.
7 Relationship distress due to one partner evolving and growing in ENM faster than the other.

Long-Term Client Goals

1   Allow for growth within secondary relationships without fear of losing the primary partner/relationship.
2   Communicate underlying feelings about the change in feelings for a secondary partner instead of lashing out and/or being defensive.
3   Hold space and support the grieving partner as they process the loss.
4   Eradicate all psychological and physical abuse identified within the relationship.
5   Adequately balance the demands of having multiple romantic and/or intimate relationships simultaneously.
6   Support each other's growth and development within ENM without shaming or making one partner feel guilty.

Short-Term Client Goals	Therapeutic Interventions
• Describe the initial emotions experienced resulting from the partner requesting a change in dynamics with a secondary partner.	• Recognize that changes to the original relationship agreement can devastate a consistent partner. • Normalize feelings of jealousy, anxiety, fear, etc., and identify mononormative beliefs contributing to emotional dysregulation. • Tension or hesitancy when discussing elements of the relationship dynamics due to fear of upsetting the other person. • Encourage the emotionally dysregulated partner to reframe their negative mindset about the situation by evaluating why they chose to be ENM. • Conduct a session with the emotionally dysregulated client to explore where the negative emotions stem from and address the issue's root. • Explore with the couple how changing the relationship dynamics with a secondary partner would affect the primary relationship.
• Identify and share negative self-talk resulting from the primary partner having deeper feelings for a secondary partner than initially agreed upon.	• Educate the distressed partner on how a significant change in the primary relationship dynamics can elicit grief and assist them in identifying their stage of grief. • Normalize any feelings of betrayal experienced by the consistent partner changing the agreed-upon relationship dynamics.

(Continued)

Short-Term Client Goals	Therapeutic Interventions
• Demonstrate an understanding of how the attachment style affects emotional safety, regulation of stress, ability to adapt, and resilience.	• Have the partners practice "I" messages while in the session. Use the *"I" Messages* handout provided in the resource section of this book. • Help the partners identify how their attachment style contributes to their ability, or lack thereof, to trust their primary partner, offer forgiveness, and respond with constructive behavior instead of impulsive behavior. • Learn and apply skills that facilitate trust in significant others and find peace when not in their immediate presence.
• Tension or hesitancy when discussing elements of the relationship dynamics due to fear of upsetting the other person.	• Ask open-ended questions that help facilitate the process of evaluating reactions to specific situations, styles of play, coercion, or other behaviors that might come across as abuse.
• Identify and discuss times when consent was violated and/or recognize a power imbalance within the primary relationship.	• If the violated partner is in imminent danger in an individual session, create a plan of action to help remove them from the abusive environment. • Educate the clients about equality of expectations as the difference between domestic violence and consensual kink (Goerlich, 2021). • Explore the four characteristics of the components of safe, sane, and consensual: (1) Consensuality, (2) use of a "safe word," (3) flexibility of roles, and (4) reciprocity of satisfaction (Goerlich, 2021). • Assist the couple in negotiating boundaries, agreements, and rules when participating in kinky behavior. • Assist the couple in creating a standard definition of abuse outside their negotiated kink agreement.
• The violating partner acknowledges and accepts responsibility for non-consensual behaviors and verbally commits to The Wheel of Nonviolence and Equality.	• Educate the couple about The Wheel of Power and Control compared to The Wheel of Nonviolence and Equality. • Provide copies of the handout and have the couple assess whether abuse, control, and/or coercion is present in the relationship.

(Continued)

Short-Term Client Goals	Therapeutic Interventions
• Verbalize feelings stemming from the primary partner's inability to manage multiple relationships at one time equally.	• The hurt partner verbalizes their feelings surrounding the consistent partner's inability to manage multiple relationships at one time effectively. • Have the couple revisit the other partner who is not upholding their relationship contract and highlight agreements they feel. • Encourage the inattentive partner to evaluate their contribution to the state of the relationship. • Encourage the inconsistent partner to honestly evaluate their ability to provide adequate attention and support in multiple relationships. • Assist the hurt partner in identifying realistic expectations vs. unrealistic expectations. • Have each partner create a list of compromises they will employ to find satisfaction within their relationship.
• Each partner identifies how they feel they have grown since beginning their ENM journey.	• Normalizing ENM as a process and growth is a personal journey for each partner. • Assist the couple in understanding that ENM is a process and encourage them to move comfortably for the slowest member of the relationship.
• Identify self-talk assumptions that are aimed at problem-solving, directly pertain to the circumstances, and are reality-based.	• Ensure that self-talk and/or inner dialogue meet the following criteria: Beneficial, valid, and connected to the situation. If not, have the struggling partner modify their inner dialogue to include the above criteria. For example: "My partner doesn't love me anymore because they aren't giving me the attention I need" can become "My partner can't read my mind, so if I want more time with them, I need to request that directly from them."
• Select preferred outcomes that are satisfying and achievable for both partners.	• Have the partner express if they can successfully achieve the desired outcome. For example: "My partner doesn't want to make time for me" can become "I will invite them to dinner and talk about how we can make more time for each other."

References

Fern, J. (2020). *Polysecure: Attachment, trauma and consensual nonmonogamy.* Thorntree Press, LLC.

Gahran, A. (2017). *Stepping off the relationship escalator: Uncommon Love and life.* Off the Escalator Enterprises, LLC.

Goerlich, S. (2021). *The leather couch: Clinical practice with kinky clients.* Routledge.

Knispel, S. (2022, April 19). *What is intimate partner violence? It's not just physical abuse.* News Center. Retrieved October 12, 2022, from https://www.rochester.edu/newscenter/what-is-intimate-partner-violence-domestic-violence-516342/

Powell, D. L. (2018). *Building open relationships: Your hands on guide to swinging, polyamory, and beyond!* Dr. Liz Powell.

Types of abuse. Women Against Abuse. (n.d.). Retrieved October 12, 2022, from https://www.womenagainstabuse.org/education-resources/learn-about-abuse/types-of-domestic-violence

Part 3

Resources and
Therapist Guides

Therapeutic Resources

Therapeutic Resources

These resources are designed to serve as helpful tools for clinicians when working with their clients. They have been formatted in a way that has proven effective for my clients and myself, but it is important to remember that each case requires careful consideration. Users are encouraged to adapt and utilize the templates provided as needed. Feel free to update and customize these guides to align with your own preferences and therapeutic style.

Drawing on my experience as a former public school educator, these resources are presented in a lesson plan format, accompanied by explanations of how I intended them to be used. However, I acknowledge that there may be alternative and more effective ways to utilize these tools. I encourage each clinician to discover their own best practices for incorporating the information provided.

Before presenting these resources to your clients, it is essential to familiarize yourself with each one. Select specific assignments that will benefit your clients based on their unique therapeutic needs, ensuring a comprehensive approach as they embark on their ENM journey. Assign the relevant tools that align with your clients' needs, and make sure to follow up within the designated timeframe to explore the impact of the activity on their mental, physical, and emotional well-being.

As you reflect on the effectiveness of these resources, consider the following:

• Was the assigned tool valuable for the client or couple?
• Did it have the intended impact or achieve the recommended outcome?
• Can the resources or tools be modified for future clients facing similar situations?

DOI: 10.4324/9781003464891-19

In addition, gather client feedback to ensure that they perceive the assignment as beneficial to their personal growth and development. This ongoing reflection and feedback process will help refine your approach and enhance the effectiveness of these resources in supporting your clients.

Couples Satisfaction Index (CSI): Therapist Guide

Couples Satisfaction Index (CSI)

Goals of This Activity

1 Assess the relationship satisfaction of couples.
2 Identify the presence of issues between individuals and the intensity of presenting problems.
3 Implement intervention strategies to increase relationship satisfaction.

Clinical Considerations

A 32-item scale designed to measure one's satisfaction in a relationship. The scale has a variety of items with different response scales and formats. The authors have also specified that the scale can safely be decreased to either a 16-item format or even a 4-item format, depending on a researcher's needs.

PERMISSION FOR USE: We developed the CSI scales to be freely available for research and clinical use. No further permission is required beyond this form and the authors will not generate study-specific permission letters.

SCORING: To score the CSI-32, you simply sum the responses across all the items. The point values of each response of each item are shown above. NOTE – When we present the scale to participants, we do not show them those point values. We just give them circles to fill in (on pen-and-paper versions) or radio buttons to click (in online surveys) in place of those point values.

INTERPRETATION: CSI-32 scores can range from 0 to 161. Higher scores indicate higher levels of relationship satisfaction. CSI-32 scores falling below 104.5 suggest notable relationship dissatisfaction.

CITATION: If you are using this scale, then you should cite the research article validating it as follows:

DOI: 10.4324/9781003464891-20

Reference

Funk, J. L., & Rogge, R. D. (2007). Testing the ruler with item response theory: increasing precision of measurement for relationship satisfaction with the Couples Satisfaction Index. Journal of Family Psychology, *21*, 572–583.

Couples Satisfaction Index (CSI)

Description of Measure

A 32-item scale designed to measure one's satisfaction in a relationship. The scale has a variety of items with different response scales and formats. Funk and Rogge have also specified that the scale should safely be reduced to a 16-item or even 4-item, depending on a researcher's needs.

Scale:
1. Please indicate the degree of happiness, all things considered, of your relationship.

Extremely Unhappy	Fairly Unhappy	A Little Unhappy	Happy	Very Happy	Extremely Happy	Perfect
0	1	2	3	4	5	6

Most people have disagreements in their relationships. Please indicate below the approximate extent of agreement or disagreement between you and your partner for each item on the following list.

	Always Agree	Almost Always Agree	Occasionally Disagree	Frequently Disagree	Almost Always Disagree	Always Disagree
2. Amount of time spent together	5	4	3	2	1	0
3. Making major decisions	5	4	3	2	1	0
4. Demonstrations of affection	5	4	3	2	1	0

DOI: 10.4324/9781003464891-21

	All the Time	Most of the Time	More Often than Not	Occasionally	Rarely	Never
5. In general, how often do you think that things between you and your partner are going well?	5	4	3	2	1	0
6. How often do you wish you hadn't gotten into this relationship?	0	1	2	3	4	5

	Not at All True	A Little True	Somewhat True	Mostly True	Almost Completely True	Completely True
7. I still feel a strong connection with my partner	0	1	2	3	4	5
8. If I had my life to live over, I would marry (or live with / date) the same person	0	1	2	3	4	5
9. Our relationship is strong	0	1	2	3	4	5
10. I sometimes wonder if there is someone else out there for me	5	4	3	2	1	0
11. My relationship with my partner makes me happy	0	1	2	3	4	5
12. I have a warm and comfortable relationship with my partner	0	1	2	3	4	5
13. I feel that I can confide in my partner about virtually anything	0	1	2	3	4	5
14. I have had second thoughts about this relationship recently	5	4	3	2	1	0
15. For me, my partner is the perfect romantic partner	0	1	2	3	4	5
16. I really feel like part of a team with my partner	0	1	2	3	4	5
17. I cannot imagine another person making me as happy as my partner does	0	1	2	3	4	5

	Not at All	A Little	Somewhat	Mostly	Almost Completely	Completely
18. How rewarding is your relationship with your partner?	0	1	2	3	4	5
19. How well does your partner meet your needs?	0	1	2	3	4	5
20. To what extent has your relationship met your original expectations?	0	1	2	3	4	5
21. In general, how satisfied are you with your relationship?	0	1	2	3	4	5

	Worse than All Others (Extremely Bad)					Better than All Others (Extremely Good)
22. How good is your relationship compared to most?	0		1	2	3	4	5

	Never	Less than Once a Month	Once or Twice a Month	Once or Twice a Week	Once a Day	More Often
23. Do you enjoy your partner's company?	0	1	2	3	4	5
24. How often do you and your partner have fun together?	0	1	2	3	4	5

Select the answer that best describes how you feel about your relationship for each of the following items. Base your responses on your first impressions and immediate feelings about the item.

25	INTERESTING	5	4	3	2	1	0	BORING
26	BAD	0	1	2	3	4	5	GOOD
27	FULL	5	4	3	2	1	0	EMPTY
28	LONELY	0	1	2	3	4	5	FRIENDLY
29	STURDY	5	4	3	2	1	0	FRAGILE
30	DISCOURAGING	0	1	2	3	4	5	HOPEFUL
31	ENJOYABLE	5	4	3	2	1	0	MISERABLE

Funk, J. L., & Rogge, R. D. (2007). Testing the ruler with item response theory: Increasing precision of measurement for relationship satisfaction with the Couples Satisfaction Index. *Journal of Family Psychology*, *21*, 572–583.

ENM Couple Questionnaire: Therapist Guide

Intake Ethical Non-monogamy Couple Questionnaire

Goals of This Activity

1 Lay the foundation for a successful therapeutic relationship
2 Keeps the therapist on track, ensuring they are gathering vital information to help create a thorough treatment plan
3 Streamlines the intake process, providing both the client and the counselor stay focused

Clinical Considerations

1 Client apprehensions: It is essential to acknowledge that couples seeking therapy for assistance with opening up about their relationship often experience feelings of nervousness, fear, and vulnerability. They may worry about being judged, shamed, or facing any other negative emotions that can arise when discussing intimate and personal aspects of their relationship.
2 The power of acceptance: When clients feel safe, supported, and accepted in therapy, they are more likely to open up and share their thoughts, emotions, and experiences. The therapist's non-judgmental and empathetic approach can create a pleasant surprise for clients as they realize they are met with understanding and validation.
3 Balancing comfort and focus: While client comfort is essential, it is crucial to maintain a balance between creating a safe space and staying focused on the therapeutic objectives. Tangents that uncover critical information can provide valuable insights. Still, they can also derail an intake session and make it difficult for the therapist to gather all the necessary information in the limited time available.
4 Individualize the approach: Every couple and individual have different experiences, preferences, and expectations. Adapting the approach to align with the therapist's style and the client's requirements ensures the delivery of personalized and effective therapy.

DOI: 10.4324/9781003464891-22

ENM Couple Questionnaire

1 What is the situation or problem, if any, that helped you decide to reach out and come to couples counseling?
2 How long have you been together?

   a Dating
   b Living together
   c Married

3 I would like each of you to tell me what initially attracted you to each other.
4 What was the beginning of your relationship like, and approximately how long did the new relationship energy last for each of you?
5 How are you both similar and how are you both different?
6 What do each of you do during times of conflict between you?
7 What strengths and weaknesses do you share as individuals and as a couple?
8 How would you describe your overall satisfaction with the current relationship dynamics?
9 Who brought up ethical non-monogamy, and what were the reactions to the suggestion?
10 What does ENM mean to each of you?
11 What does the term commitment mean to each of you?
12 What constitutes cheating to each of you?
13 What has been your experience so far in ENM?
14 What are your fears about ENM?

Activity for the Couple: Best Friend Fantasy

Have the couple close their eyes and imagine their partner being intimate with a close friend. Have the couple sit with that image for about 30 seconds.

DOI: 10.4324/9781003464891-23

When they open their eyes, have them face each other and tell each other what they saw and how it made them feel.

- The couple might say, "Oh, we are attracted to our best friends," or immediately react with, "Our best friends are off limits." That is not the point of this exercise. The point is to see how you feel about your partner sharing intimacy with someone who means something to you.
- Their therapist notes their reactions when retelling their imagined scenario to their partner.

  a. Did you identify feelings of jealousy?
  b. Did you observe distress or animosity toward each other?
  c. Was the couple comfortable fantasizing about this topic?
  d. How was their behavior when telling their partner?
  e. Did they seem embarrassed, or were they excited to tell each other?

Finding Your Why: Therapist Guide

Exploring Your Why

Goals of This Activity

1 Encourages the client to consider why they are exploring ENM individually and as a couple.
2 Develop an understanding of their goals for the ENM journey and what they want to learn about themselves.
3 Uncover possible coercion within the primary relationship.

Clinical Considerations

1 Activity expectations: Clarify that the activity is intended for each member of the relationship to complete independently, without the presence of their partner. This allows each individual to have the space and freedom to reflect on their thoughts, emotions, and experiences without feeling influenced or biased by their partner's input.
2 Privacy and confidentiality: Emphasize that the completed activity will be reviewed privately with the therapist and not shared with their partner unless the client and therapist agree that it benefits the relationship. Stress the importance of maintaining client privacy and confidentiality, as this is critical in building and maintaining trust between the therapist and the client.
3 Collaborative approach: Acknowledge that sharing the information depends on the therapist and the client's joint agreement that it would benefit the relationship. The therapist can work with each client to determine how to integrate the information into the couple's therapy sessions.
4 Individualize the approach: Encourage therapists to adjust the provided template to suit their practice best and meet the unique needs of their clients. Every couple and individual has different experiences, preferences,

DOI: 10.4324/9781003464891-24

and expectations. Adapting the approach to align with the therapist's style and the client's requirements ensures the delivery of personalized and effective therapy.

By setting clear expectations for the activity, maintaining confidentiality and privacy, adopting a collaborative approach, and customizing the approach to align with clients' unique needs, therapists can facilitate the effective delivery and integration of the activity in their sessions. This ultimately promotes clients' growth and development and improves their relationship dynamics.

Resource

Veaux, F., Rickert, E., & Hardy, J. W. (2014). *More than two: A practical guide to ethical polyamory.* Thorntree Press.

Finding Your Why

Directions: Answer the following questions to the best of your ability. This activity will be done independently and brought to your individual session to be reviewed with your therapist.

1 Have you ever experienced romantic love for more than one person at a time? If so, what was that like for you?
2 Do you feel as if only one person can be meant for you? For example, is your partner your "soulmate" or the only true love you can ever have?
3 How important is it for you to have multiple romantic relationships?
4 Are you open to multiple sexual relationships, romantic relationships, or both? If you would like more than one sexual relationship, what degree of closeness or intimacy would you be comfortable with, and what can you realistically offer an outside partner?
5 How important is transparency to you in your relationship? Do you want to know your consistent partner's other lovers? Do you want your compatible partner to know your other lovers?
6 In your own words, how do you define commitment? Do you feel it is possible to be committed to more than one partner at a time? What would that look like for you and your future relationships?
7 If you are currently in a relationship, does your desire for multiple relationships stem from dissatisfaction or unhappiness in your consistent relationship? Would you still desire multiple partners if all of your needs were being met in your consistent relationship?

DOI: 10.4324/9781003464891-25

Finding Your Fears: Therapist Guide

Finding Your Fears

Goals of This Activity

1 Uncover hidden fears about ENM for discussion.
2 It allows the therapist to normalize fears and uncertainties about ENM.
3 If no fears are identified, encourage the client to keep this guide handy so they can document fears if or when they arise.

Clinical Considerations

1 Introduce the activity: Explain to the couple that fears can sometimes be hard to identify and that this activity will help them identify their fears related to ethical non-monogamy relationships. Provide them with a copy of the "Finding Your Fears" handout.
2 Please review the list: Instruct each individual to review the overall list in the handout and identify common fears that spoke to them. They should mark or highlight the fear they relate to the most.
3 Encourage writing: Remind the couple that the list might not include their specific fears and encourage them to write out any additional fears that they may have in the blank spaces provided on the handout.
4 Start the discussion: Begin a discussion about the couple's fears. Normalize their feelings as much as possible and reassure them that their fears are valid. Use open-ended questions to explore their fears in more detail. Questions include, "Can you tell me more about why you feel that way?" or "Would you like to read your specific fear aloud to the group?"
5 Prepare for future fears: If the couple reports that they don't have any fears, encourage them to keep the handout close and write out any worries as they come up. Let them know that this activity can be revisited if necessary.

DOI: 10.4324/9781003464891-26

6   Complete in session: Let the couple know this activity can be completed during therapy. Plan for enough time to review the fears and facilitate the discussion.

By following these instructions, you can help the couple identify and explore their fears related to ethical non-monogamous relationships. This activity can help normalize their fears and provide a space to process and work through them together.

Finding Your Fears

Entering into ethical non-monogamy can evoke a range of emotions, including fear. Here's a list of 15 fears that someone might experience when embarking on this journey:

Type of Fear	Description of Fear	Yes	Unsure	No
Fear of Rejection	Worrying that your partner might leave you for someone else			
Fear of Jealousy	Anxiety about feeling jealous or unable to manage jealousy in a non-monogamous relationship			
Fear of Inadequacy	Feeling that you might not be enough for your partner or that you won't be able to fulfill their needs			
Fear of Comparison	Concerns about being compared to other partners and feeling inferior			
Fear of Abandonment	Worries that your partner will prioritize other relationships over yours			
Fear of Judgment	Fear of being judged by friends, family, or society for engaging in non-monogamy			
Fear of Communication Breakdown	Apprehension that open and honest communication might lead to conflict or relationship breakdown			
Fear of Missing Out	The fear of missing out on experiences or opportunities when your partner is with someone else			

(Continued)

DOI: 10.4324/9781003464891-27

Fear of Being Replaced	Feeling a sense of insecurity that your partner might find someone else who is better suited for them			
Fear of Losing Control	Concerns about losing control over the relationship dynamics and decisions			
Fear of STIs	Concerns about sexual health risks and the potential spread of sexually transmitted infections			
Fear of Time Management	Worrying about finding enough time to maintain multiple relationships and managing conflicting schedules			
Fear of Emotional Connection	Fearing that your partner might develop a deeper emotional connection with another person			
Fear of a Power Imbalance	Worries about feeling less valued or being disadvantaged in the relationship hierarchy			
Fear of Societal Norms	Concerns about how society might perceive and treat individuals in non-monogamous relationships			

Additional fears not listed above: _____

_____

_____

Sexual History Intake: Therapist Guide

Sexual History Interview

Goals of This Activity

1 Helps identify fractures in the primary relationship.
2 Explores possible sexual trauma and how it currently affects the primary relationship.
3 Provides insight into the sexual development of the client.

Clinical Considerations

When conducting the sexual history intake, it is best to have each partner participate in an individual session in case there are specific areas of concern the individual would like to discuss their sexual history. Traditionally, this is the second and third session when working with the couple. If information is presented regarding intense sexual trauma and you do not feel qualified to help the individual process the trauma, refer to a specialist for individual counseling.

As the clinician, you have the decision to make:

1 Do you stop the program with the couple and begin again when you feel the sexual trauma has been processed, or
2 Continue the program with the trauma partner in individual therapy. The sexual history intake is a discussion that will need to be had after the individual sexual history interviews have been concluded.

Here are some do's when conducting the sexual history intake:

• Maintain eye contact, even if you get embarrassed.
• Try to stay relaxed.
• Use familiar terminology or the client's language in the session.

DOI: 10.4324/9781003464891-28

- Ask detailed questions.
- Maintain an open mind and non-judgmental attitude.
- Be aware of your facial expressions, body language, and overall reactions when they detail their sexual preferences.

Here are some don'ts when conducting the sexual history intake:

- Don't assume the client's sexuality. Ask for clarification.
- Don't rush through the sexual history intake.
- Don't act as if you know everything. It is acceptable to ask clarifying questions.
- Don't assume you know what specific terms mean. Each individual has meaning in particular terms, and you are encouraged to ask the client, "What does that term mean to you?"

Reference

McCarthy, B. "Rekindling Desire." Modern Sex Therapy Institutes, 15 January 2021, online.

Sexual History Interview

Dr. Barry McCarthy, an esteemed professor of psychology at American University, as well as a certified sex therapist and couple therapist, has developed the Sexual History Interview, a comprehensive tool for practitioners to gain a deeper understanding of their client's sexual history. This valuable resource has been granted permission for adaptation and reproduction.

According to Dr. McCarthy's book, *Cognitive-Behavioral Therapy for Sexual Dysfunction*, the interview is recommended to be conducted individually with each client, separate from the couple's sessions. The initial session is advised to include the couple, followed by two subsequent sessions with each partner individually. By conducting these individual sessions, clients are more likely to express themselves freely, as they may feel apprehensive about being judged or rejected in the presence of their partner. Dr. McCarthy's approach emphasizes creating a safe and non-judgmental space for clients to share their sexual experiences openly.

Individual Session

Open the session by saying something similar to what is provided:

> I want to understand your psychological, relational, and sexual history before and during this relationship. I want to hear all your strengths as well as vulnerabilities. I appreciate your being as forthcoming and blunt as possible. Ultimately, I'll ask if there is anything sensitive or secret you do not want to share with your partner. I will not share it without your permission. However, I want to understand you and your experiences as much as possible so I can help resolve these problems.

DOI: 10.4324/9781003464891-29

Guidelines

Structure chronologically, move from less anxious to more anxiety-provoking questions, be non-judgmental about atypical behavior, ask open-ended questions, and probe for dysfunctional attitudes, behaviors, and emotions.

Initial Open-Ended Questions

1 "What did you value about growing up, and what caused you problems and regret?"

    a Formal education, including sex education

    b Religious background, including religious sex education

    c Parents as a marital and sexual model, including attitudes toward touching and privacy

Social and Sexual Experiences as a Child

1 Experiences with others (siblings or peers).

    a How have your siblings done sexually as adults?

    b As a child, were you comfortable with your body and gender?

    c Did you have a happy or troubled childhood?

Puberty and Adolescence

1 First orgasmic experience—age, situation, feelings

2 Masturbation—how learned, the technique used, first orgasmic experience, use of fantasies, and written or online material (has that changed or stayed the same?)

3 For females, menstruation is age at onset, preparation for, cognitive and emotional response of self and others.

4 Socially and sexually, what was high school like?

    a How did you feel about your body image?

    b Was dating a positive experience or a source of anxiety or guilt?

    c How old were you at first orgasm with a partner?

5 How old were you at first intercourse?

    a Was this a positive or negative experience?

    b How long did the relationship last, and how did it end?

6 Same-sex questions

    a Many men (women) have sexual thoughts, feelings, fantasies, and experiences with men (women). What were your experiences and feelings about being sexual with other men (women)?

7 Unwanted pregnancies or sexually transmitted infections

    a What were your experiences?

    b How did you feel about it at the time? In retrospect?

8 As you review your childhood and adolescence, what were your most important positive psychological, relational, and sexual learnings and experiences?

9 As you review your childhood and adolescence:

    a What was the most negative?

    b What was the most confusing?

    c What were the most guilt-inducing or traumatic psychological, relational, and sexual experiences?

Adult Sexuality

1 **(If attended college)** What was college like socially and sexually?

2 **(If work or service)** What were your young adult relationships and sexual experiences?

After Determining WHEN the Couple Met

1 As you review your dating and sexual history, what were the most positive and negative experiences?

2 What was happening in your life six months before meeting your spouse (partner)?

Present Relationship

1 How did you meet?

2 What was the initial attraction?

3 What were your first sexual experiences like?

4 When was sex best in this relationship?

    a What made it good for you?

    b How do you communicate sexually (verbally and non-verbally)?

    c When was desire/pleasure/eroticism/satisfaction best?

5 Are you attracted to your partner?

    a Do you have loving feelings?

    b When did sexual problems begin?

    c What caused this, and how has it played out?

    d Do you view sexual dysfunction as an individual or couple problem?

    e How much anger, guilt, resentment, and blaming are involved?

6   What are your strengths and vulnerabilities as a couple?

    a   What three changes would you request from your partner?

7   How is your general health, and are there health problems?

    a   What medications do you take, and what are the sexual side effects?

    b   Have you talked to your internist or specialist about sexual concerns?

8   Are financial issues a relational strength or vulnerability?

    a   What doesn't your partner understand about how you deal with work and financial issues?

9   **(If parents)** What are your strengths and vulnerabilities as a parent?

    a   Do you enjoy parenting?

10   Many people have thoughts, feelings, fantasies, and experiences regarding sex with others.

    a   What have your experiences been?

    b   Are you genuinely interested in trying ENM or exploring this to please your partner?

    c   Are you or would you be comfortable seeing your partner receiving pleasure from someone else?

    d   What are your fears about ENM?

    e   What have you not told your partner about your thoughts and feelings regarding ENM?

11   **(If there was an affair)** What did you feel during the extra-marital involvement, and how did it end?

"I" Messages – Therapist Guide

"I" Messages and Assertive Statements

Goals of This Activity

1 Provide a template for healthy communication with their partner.
2 Creates a framework for assertively expressing feelings, needs, and desires.
3 Allows each partner to label their feelings.

Clinical Considerations

Provide a copy of the "I" Messages and Assertive Statements handout: Begin by giving the couple a handout that explains the concept of "I" messages and how to construct assertive statements. This handout should provide examples and guidelines for effective communication.

1 Provide the feelings chart: Along with the handout, give the couple a feelings chart that lists a wide range of emotions. This chart can help them identify and express their feelings more accurately when constructing their statements.
2 Practice in the office: Encourage the couple to start practicing this form of communication in the therapist's office. They can begin by writing statements to their partner about things bothering them. This could include specific behaviors or actions that have caused harm or damage in the relationship.
3 Start small with everyday annoyances: If the couple finds it challenging to address more significant issues immediately, suggest starting with more minor daily annoyances. This could involve practicing communication around minor frustrations or irritations that occur regularly.
4 Understand the full usage of the statements: Emphasize the importance of fully understanding and integrating "I" Messages and Assertive

DOI: 10.4324/9781003464891-30

statements into their communication style. Explain that the goal is for them to become comfortable and skilled in using these statements so they are well-prepared to address future situations.

By following these directions, the couple can develop effective communication skills to openly express their concerns, needs, and emotions while promoting a healthier, more understanding relationship.

"I" Messages and Assertive Statements

The "I" Message (also known as an "assertiveness statement") can help you state your concerns, feelings, and needs in a manner that is easier for the listener to hear and understand.

- An "I-statement" focuses on your feelings and experiences.
- It does not focus on your perspective of what the other person has done or failed to do.

Suppose you can express your experience in a way that does not attack, criticize, or blame others. In that case, you are less likely to provoke defensiveness and hostility, which tends to escalate conflicts, or have the other person shut down or tune you out, which tends to stifle communication.

What an "I" Message Does

- Help reduce blaming, accusations, and defensiveness.
- Help you communicate your concerns, feelings, and needs **without** blaming others or sounding threatening. It helps you get your point across without causing the listener to shut down.
- Says, "This is how it looks from my side of things."

What an "I" Message Doesn't Do

- It is not about being polite. It's about being transparent.
- It is not concerned with how the other person might respond.
- It is not intended to force another person to "fix the problem."
- It clearly says, "This is how it looks from my perspective."

DOI: 10.4324/9781003464891-31

Pro-Tip

- If you expect the other person to respond as you want them to immediately, you probably have unrealistic expectations.
- An "I" Message is intended only to open *healthy conversation*. Using it alone will not resolve the conflict.
- If you expect an "I" Message to fix the conflict, you probably have unrealistic expectations.

Four Parts of an "I" Message

- "When you _____"
  state observation

- "I feel, or I think _____"
  state feeling

- "Because_____"
  state needs

- "I would prefer that_____"
  state preference

Here is Another Example of the "I" Message

How you feel	"I feel angry ... ."
What do you think about?	"how he spoke to me ... ."
Why do you feel this way?	"because it embarrassed me in front of my friends."
What you would like to see instead:	"I would prefer that we discuss these things in private."

Practice Your "I" Message

How you feel	"_____."
What do you have that feeling about?	"_____."
Why you feel this way	"_____."
What you would like to see instead:	"I would prefer _____."

Examples of How to Translate a Heated Remark into an "I" Message

"You never listen to anyone, and you're not really listening to me now."

- "I feel that my concerns are not being heard."

"I hate when you yell at the kids."

- "When you yell at the kids, I feel angry because I need the kids to be treated with respect. I would prefer you not raise your voice or curse in their presence."

"It's rude of you to be late all the time. You screw up everyone's schedule."

- "When you are scheduled to be at your desk at 8:30, but you do not come in until 9:00, I feel disrespected/frustrated, and being late means we can't start our meetings on time. I would prefer that you arrive at work at the agreed-upon time."

"The salaries in this department are inequitable and discriminatory."

- "I feel angry about the salary structure in this department. I am among the lowest-paid teachers here, which makes me feel underappreciated. I would like to understand more about how salaries are calculated, and I would like to talk to you about whether raising my salary is possible in the next budget cycle."

Feelings Wheel

We often use the exact words to describe our feelings to our partners; however, our comments often don't reflect our true feelings. Use the Feelings Wheel to identify your feelings when creating statements for your partner.

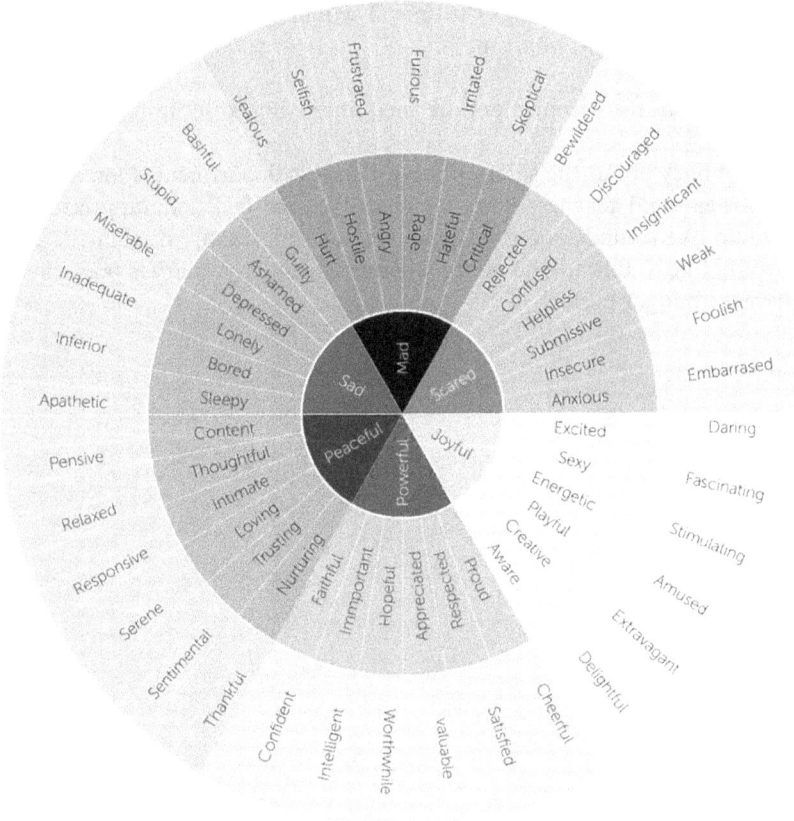

DOI: 10.4324/9781003464891-32

Behavior Change Request: Therapist Guide

Behavior Change Request

Goals of This Activity

1 Provide a framework for discussing behaviors one partner would like modified.
2 Increase awareness of hurtful behaviors and how they are affecting the primary relationships.
3 Indicate a plan of action for change.

Clinical Considerations

1 Explain to both partners that a BCR is a communication tool from Imago Relationship Therapy. Describe its purpose as a structured and non-confrontational approach to addressing behaviors that have caused harm or damage within the relationship.
2 The purpose of a BCR is to create a safe space for both partners to have a transparent conversation about specific actions or behaviors that one partner would like to see changed. Emphasize that the goal is to improve the relationship by establishing realistic expectations and working towards positive changes.
3 Provide a template or structure: Offer one that can guide the partners through the BCR process. This could include the following components:

- Encourage the partner initiating the BCR to begin by expressing appreciation for their partner and highlighting the positive aspects of the relationship.
- Ask the initiating partner to clearly and objectively articulate the behavior they want changed, providing specific examples if possible. Encourage them to use "I" statements to avoid blaming or accusing their partner.

DOI: 10.4324/9781003464891-33

- Invite the initiating partner to share how it affects them emotionally, physically, or mentally. This helps the other partner understand the significance of the requested change.
- Ask the initiating partner to propose alternative behaviors or changes they would prefer to see from their partner. Please encourage them to be realistic and specific in their suggestions.
- Facilitate a conversation between both partners, allowing the other partner to respond, ask questions, and express their thoughts and feelings about the request. Encourage active listening, empathy, and understanding.

Adapted from *Getting the Love You Want* by Harville Hendrix, Ph.D. (2008).

Behavior Change Request

Make an Appointment

Sender: "I would like to make an appointment to talk about a frustration I am experiencing and make a behavioral change request. Is now a good time?"

Receiver: Make time ASAP or indicate a time that works best for you.

Sender: Begin with sharing one positive: "First, I would like to express appreciation for ... ."

Receiver: Reflect: "You appreciate ... . Did I get that correct?"

Sharing Your Frustration

Sender: "I get frustrated when you ... ." State the frustration in one sentence. Example: "I get frustrated when you don't make time for us to reconnect after you have a playdate."

Receiver: Reflect on what you heard: "What I hear you saying is you get frustrated when I don't make time after a playdate to reconnect with you. Did I hear that correctly?"

Sender: Make corrections as needed, and when ready, share your frustration fully:

"When you (don't make time for us to reconnect after your playdates), I feel (insert feeling).

I imagine that (insert what you are imagining, ex: that I am not important to you), and I react by (insert how you tend to react, ex: withdraw, shutdown, etc.)."

Receiver: Reflect accurately: "So you are frustrated when I ... ."

Check for accuracy: "Did I get that correct?"

DOI: 10.4324/9781003464891-34

Connection to Previous Experience

Receiver: "Would you share with me what scares you about this behavior?"

Sender: Share your fear.

Receiver: "What hurts you so much about this behavior?"

Sender: Share your hurt.

Also, share with your partner a memory of a challenging time from your past that comes up when you experience this specific frustration:

"This behavior reminds me of a time in my past when ... (the main caregivers were not present or were there in negative ways) and then I would imagine that they ... (did not love me, did not want me, etc.)."

Summarize Feelings and Experience

Receiver: Provide an accurate reflection from the beginning:

"You get frustrated when I don't reconnect with you after a play date.

And when I do that, you feel ...

Which causes you to remember a previous experience when ...

And you experience those same feelings.

Did I get that right?"

The Behavior Change Request

Receiver: "What specific things could I do that would help meet your request?"

Sender: State three behavior change requests. Ensure they are specific, measurable, attainable, relevant, and time-limited. The Receiver will select one of the three options provided.

Receiver: Reflect on your choices to ensure you fully understand the request. Once you fully understand your options, choose the one you feel is best for you.

My Behavior Change Requests

Example: After a playdate, I agree to reconnect with you by:_____

_____
_____
_____

Notes: _____

_____
_____
_____

Mastering Difficult Conversations: Therapist Guide

Mastering Difficult Conversations

Goals of This Activity

1 Improve the quality of difficult conversations by eliminating barriers that hinder practical listening skills.
2 Provide a template for formulating topics of conversation and create a plan of action for receiving communication.

Clinical Considerations

1 Explain to the couple that the objective is to help them practice having difficult conversations. This activity aims to improve their communication skills and create a safe and open environment for discussing challenging topics.
2 Distribute the handout to the couple in the office. Ensure that each partner has a copy to refer to during the activity.
3 Instruct the couple to choose a topic they find difficult to discuss. Please encourage them to select a topic that is important to both partners and can benefit from improved communication.
4 Guide the couple through the handout, step by step, using their chosen difficult conversation topic. Please encourage them to follow the prompts and guidelines provided on the handout to structure their conversation.
5 Remind the couple to approach the conversation with patience, empathy, and active listening. Emphasize the importance of maintaining a safe and respectful environment during their discussion.
6 Emphasize that it is essential for the couple to continue practicing the art of difficult conversations outside of the therapy session. Instruct them to take a copy of the handout home to continue practicing these skills daily.

DOI: 10.4324/9781003464891-35

7 Advise the couple to set aside dedicated time to practice difficult conversations using the handout. Suggest that they schedule regular check-ins to discuss the progress of their communication skills and address any challenges or concerns that arise.

Mastering Difficult Conversations

As a society, we are not taught how to conduct difficult conversations effectively, and our first line of defense is to shut down. This behavior will end an ethical non-monogamous relationship before they even have their first date with another couple. Communication is one of the most critical elements of ENM relationships.

Step 1: Determine the Topic

Knowing what you will talk about BEFORE a difficult conversation will help you enter into the discussion focused on the issue at hand, ensuring unnecessary details do not sidetrack you.

The topic of conversation:

_____
_____
_____
_____
_____

Step 2: Be Solution-Focused

After determining the topic, list the possible solutions you would like to explore with your partner.

Possible solutions:

_____
_____
_____
_____
_____

DOI: 10.4324/9781003464891-36

Step 3: Out of Your Head and Down on Paper

Once you have your topic and list of possible solutions, you need to phrase it in a way your partner will understand. This is a great place to utilize the *"I" Messages & Assertive Statements* activity.

When you:_____

_____

I feel: _____

_____

Because:_____

_____

I would prefer: _____

_____

Step 4: Receiving Negative Feedback

Partner 1 might initiate a difficult conversation with Partner 2, but Partner 2 might have feedback they would like to share with Partner 1. This is not always easy, but it is necessary for relationship growth. You may not get the response you want, and/or, throughout the conversation, you might find that you were incorrect. That is common and reflects relationship growth.

Possible negative feedback:

_____
_____
_____
_____
_____

Step 5: Mental Preparation

You are armed with your "I" Message and ready to have a difficult conversation with your partner. Wrong! Factor in the nerves, the fear of rejection, and the judgment you have conjured in their head. You are your own worst enemy.

List your fears:

_____
_____
_____
_____
_____

Step 6: Take Care of Yourself and Yours

The heightened emotional state that difficult conversations can evoke in you can result in anxiety until the situation has been resolved. You must take care of yourself by participating in a self-care activity to relax and ensure you attend to the relationship's needs.

Self-care practices:

_____

_____

_____

_____

_____

Reflection Questions

1   What did we accomplish by having this conversation?

_____

_____

_____

2   What positives resulted from this conversation?

_____

_____

_____

3   What negatives resulted from this conversation?

_____

_____

_____

4   What is our plan of action moving forward regarding this topic?

_____

_____

_____

Attachment Styles: Therapist Guide

Dimensions of Attachment

Goals of This Activity

1 Educate the couple on how their attachment style affects their relationship dynamics.
2 Provide an understanding of each partner's attachment style.
3 Explore how each partner can move towards a secure attachment style.

Clinical Considerations

1 Explain to the couple that cultivating secure attachment is possible and necessary for successful non-monogamous relationships. Highlight that secure attachment involves effective communication, trust, agreement adherence, and honest dialogue about desired changes in the relationship.
2 Clarify that the purpose of the handout is to provide guidance and tools for the couple to work towards cultivating secure attachment in their relationships. Emphasize that it is intended to be used as a tool while they are in the office.
3 Provide each partner with a printed copy of the handout. Encourage them to refer to it and use it as a point of reference during discussions and exercises in the office.
4 Guide the couple through each section of the handout, explaining the significance and relevance of the information provided. Emphasize the importance of each element of secure attachment, such as effective communication, trust-building, agreement adherence, and open dialogue about desired changes.
5 Engage in a conversation with the couple about how they can apply and practice the principles of secure attachment in their relationships. Encourage them to share their insights, questions, and concerns related

DOI: 10.4324/9781003464891-37

to incorporating these principles into their non-monogamous dynamics.

6 Encourage the couple to take the time to reflect on their behaviors, emotions, and thought patterns concerning the concepts presented in the handout. Suggest that they explore their attachment styles and how they may impact their relationships.

Attachment Styles

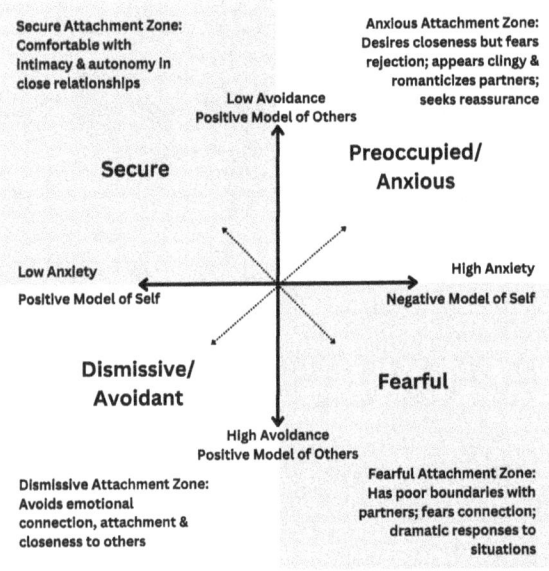

Figure 3.1b Dimensions of Attachment.

DOI: 10.4324/9781003464891-38

Directions: Using the information from the front of this page, create your attachment story detailing how you feel your attachment formed, providing evidence from past relationships or experiences from your current relationship.

Your attachment story:

_____
_____
_____
_____
_____
_____
_____
_____
_____
_____
_____
_____

While your attachment is a personal journey, how can your partner help you achieve secure attachment in your current relationship?

_____
_____
_____
_____
_____
_____
_____
_____
_____
_____
_____

Attachment and Trauma Integration Model: Therapist Guide

The Attachment and Trauma Integration Model

Goals of This Activity

1 Educate the clients about how trauma affects the dynamics in their primary relationship.
2 Encourage the client to explore how they might feel at each level as they come out to others about their ENM lifestyle.
3 Increase awareness of possible outcomes for revealing their ENM lifestyle.

Clinical Considerations

1 Begin by explaining to the client that the Attachment and Trauma Integration Model, as described by polyamorous psychotherapist Jessica Fern, provides insight into how emotional experiences impact significant relationships. Emphasize that trauma and attachment wounds are not solely individual or relational experiences but extend to the larger world we inhabit.
2 Highlight the importance of understanding the nested nature of attachment and trauma in the client's polyamorous relationships. Explain that this model encourages us to consider how various levels of attachment and trauma, from personal experiences to societal influences, can shape the dynamics and outcomes of our relationships.
3 Refer to Jessica Fern's book, Polysecure, and explain that she delves deeper into the concept of how trauma and attachment wounds are not limited to individual or relational experiences but stem from the broader world we live in. You may reference the specific page number in the book (e.g., pg. 76).
4 Urge the client to reflect on the potential impacts of different levels within the Nested Model of Attachment and Trauma. This could

DOI: 10.4324/9781003464891-39

include considering how personal traumas or attachment wounds, relational dynamics, and societal factors influence their polyamorous relationships. Ask them to evaluate and explore how these different levels interact and intersect within their experiences.

5 Encourage the client to share their thoughts, observations, and insights regarding the ramifications of level in the Nested Model. Create a safe and non-judgmental space for them to express their feelings and explore the complexities of their polyamorous relationships in relation to attachment and trauma.

Attachment and Trauma Integration Model

The Attachment & Trauma Integration Model

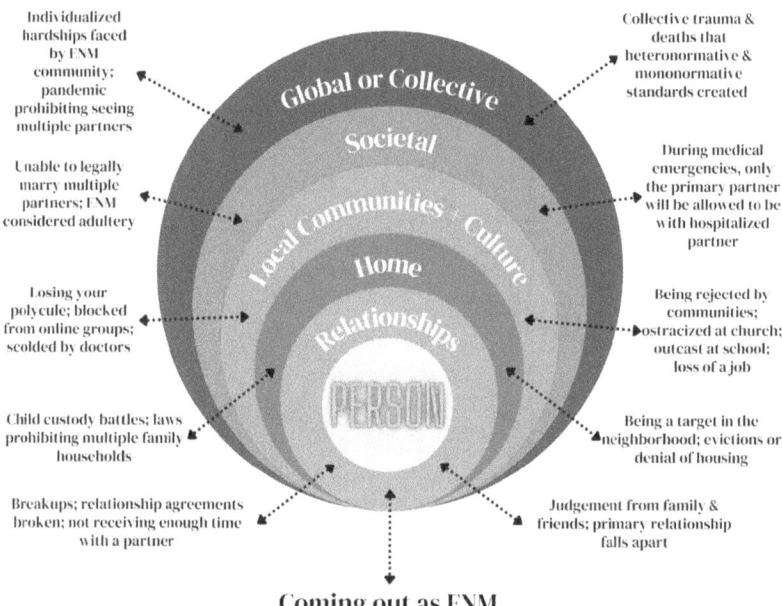

Individualized hardships faced by ENM community; pandemic prohibiting seeing multiple partners

Unable to legally marry multiple partners; ENM considered adultery

Losing your polycule; blocked from online groups; scolded by doctors

Child custody battles; laws prohibiting multiple family households

Breakups; relationship agreements broken; not receiving enough time with a partner

Collective trauma & deaths that heteronormative & mononormative standards created

During medical emergencies, only the primary partner will be allowed to be with hospitalized partner

Being rejected by communities; ostracized at church; outcast at school; loss of a job

Being a target in the neighborhood; evictions or denial of housing

Judgement from family & friends; primary relationship falls apart

Coming out as ENM

Coming out as ethically non-monogamous involves embracing your personal identity, understanding how multiple relationships align with your values, and addressing any internalized shame or negative beliefs associated with nonmonogamy.

Adapted from *Polysecure*, by Jessica Fern, 2020.

DOI: 10.4324/9781003464891-40

1   How do you see yourself being affected at the self-level?

_____

_____

_____

_____

_____

2   How do you see yourself being affected at the relationship level?

_____

_____

_____

_____

_____

3   How do you see yourself being affected at the home level?

_____

_____

_____

_____

_____

4   How do you see yourself being affected at the culture and community level?

_____

_____

_____

_____

_____

5   How do you see yourself being affected at the societal level?

_____

_____

_____

_____

_____

6   How do you see yourself being affected at the global level?

_____

_____

_____

_____

_____

Cognitive Restructuring: Therapist Guide

Cognitive Restructuring in ENM

Goals of This Activity

1 Express feelings associated with faulty thought patterns.
2 List faulty thought patterns.
3 Facilitate thought restructuring.
4 Address Demon Dialogues and identify their adverse effects on the primary relationship.

Clinical Considerations

1 Cognitive restructuring is a therapeutic technique for the client that involves identifying and replacing negative thought patterns with more positive and realistic ones. This technique can mainly promote vulnerability and emotional growth in relationships.
2 Provide the client with a quote from Shelley Sommerfeldt, PsyD, where she states that resisting vulnerability is a coping mechanism and a means of emotional protection (Sommerfeldt, 2019). Highlight that this suggests individuals may shut down to shield themselves from potential emotional harm.
3 Clarify that the goal is to help the client identify and replace negative thought patterns that impede vulnerability in their relationship. Emphasize that restructuring their thoughts can create a more open and authentic connection with their partner(s).
4 Instruct the client to take a moment to reflect on their thoughts and identify any negative patterns that arise when they resist being vulnerable. Please encourage them to write down these thoughts and explore their underlying beliefs and messages.
5 Prompt the client to challenge and reframe their negative thoughts by identifying alternative perspectives. Please encourage them to consider

DOI: 10.4324/9781003464891-41

evidence that contradicts their negative thoughts and generates more balanced or positive interpretations of their experiences.

6   Encourage the client to create affirmations or positive statements that challenge their negative thoughts and support vulnerability in their relationship. I suggest they repeat these affirmations regularly and integrate positive self-talk into their daily routine.

Cognitive Restructuring

Cognitive Restructuring in ENM

The American Psychological Association provided that cognitive behavioral therapy (CBT) "assumes that cognitive, emotional, and behavioral variables are functionally interrelated" and that those experiencing psychological issues can learn better ways of coping with them drastically improving the quality of their life and relationships.

1 · Identifying Faulty Thought Patterns

I am not enough for my partner so they want other partners.

Cognitive Restructuring

My partner wants us to grow as a couple and expand our intimacy by adding sexual partners to our relationship.

2 · Identifying Equivalent Feeling

~ Fear & Anxiety   ~ Sadness & Depression
~ Guilt & Shame   ~ Anger   ~Jealousy

Step 1: Select the strongest feeling first (guilt & shame), for this faulty thought and complete the remaining steps.

Step 2: If you identify secondary emotions (fear & anxiety) that need to be processed and complete the remaining steps.

3 · Flooded With Thoughts?

Please take a moment to identify any upsetting thoughts that may be present. Here are some guiding questions to help you with this process:

If XX were to happen, what significance or meaning would it hold for you?

If XX were to happen, what significance or meaning would it hold for you?

If XX were to happen, what significance or meaning would it hold for you?

4 · Processing the Faulty Thoughts

Step 1: Let's thoroughly analyze the accuracy of the identified faulty thoughts. In doing so, let's consider the evidence that supports this thought.
Step 2: Create a list of evidence that contradicts or does not support your faulty thought.

Guiding Questions

~ Is it possible to explore a different viewpoint regarding the current situation?

~ Is your concern primarily influenced by emotions rather than the objective facts?

5 · Make an Informed Decision

☐ NO, there is not enough evidence to support my faulty thoughts.

~ Formulate a precise thought that is backed by reliable evidence.

☐ YES, there is evidence to support my thought!

Step 1: Brainstorm and select the best option for your situation.
Step 2: Create a plan of action to best execute the identified option.
Step 3: Follow the plan and review for efficacy frequently

Figure 4.1b Cognitive Restructuring in ENM.

DOI: 10.4324/9781003464891-42

1 **Identify Distressing Situation:**

_____
_____
_____
_____

2 **Identify Equivalent Feeling:** (Select the strongest prevailing first for this situation)

    ☐ Fear & Anxiety   ☐ Sadness & Depression   ☐ Guilt & Shame
    ☐ Anger   ☐ Jealousy

3 **Flooded With Thoughts:**
   a What would it mean to me if _____ happened?

_____
_____
_____
_____
_____
_____

   b If _____ happened, what would happen then?

_____
_____
_____
_____
_____

   c What would be so bad about _____ happening?

_____
_____
_____
_____
_____
_____

4   **Processing the Thoughts:**
   Step 1: What evidence supports this thought?

   _____
   _____
   _____
   _____
   _____
   _____

   Step 2: List evidence that **DOES NOT** support the thought.

   _____
   _____
   _____
   _____
   _____
   _____

   Step 3: Is there another way of looking at the situation? Is my concern based more on feeling than on the facts?

   _____
   _____
   _____
   _____
   _____
   _____

5 **Make a decision:**

☐ No, there is no evidence to support my thought.

Create an accurate thought that is supported by your evidence:

Destructive Communication: Therapist Guide

Demon Dialogues in ENM

Goals of This Activity

1 Identify destructive cycles of dispute experienced by the couple.
2 Remove the roadblock that is hindering the connection between the partners.
3 Educate the client about the three patterns that stop couples from safely connecting.

Clinical Considerations

"Demon Dialogues" is a term coined by Dr. Sue Johnson and used to characterize the destructive cycles of conflict experienced within intimate relationships, resulting in feelings of disconnection from our partners.

This activity will educate the clients about the three patterns of behavior that frequently cause partners to withdraw from each other and provide a plan of action for moving forward.

DOI: 10.4324/9781003464891-43

Destructive Communication

Destructive Communication Patterns in ENM

The phrase "Demon Dialogue" was introduced by Dr. Sue Johnson, co-founder of Emotion-Focused Therapy, to describe the harmful patterns of conflict experienced in intimate relationships that lead to emotional disconnection from one's partner. In situations where multiple relationships are involved, these demon dialogues can become overwhelming and have a detrimental impact on all the relationships involved.

 Tit-For-Tat Arguments

- Back & forth verbal attacks
- Difference of opinions
- Reactive & defensive nature of a verbal exchange

Core Message

I am determined to assert my independence and prove that I am not under your control.

"To name is to begin to tame."
~Dr. Sue Johnson

 Engage & Disengage

- One partner irritates and finds fault
- The other partner protects themself from a verbal attack and withdraws.

Core Message

As one partner intensifies their protests and attacks, the other partner reacts by retreating and distancing themselves at an increasingly rapid pace.

 Negative Spiraling

- Stuck in "Tit-For-Tat" and/or "Engage & Disengage causing distance in the relationship
- Shutting down and avoiding issues
- Emotionally isolating from partner

Core Message

I am in pain and feeling frightened. I will choose to withdraw and allow us to gradually grow apart.

Adapted from *Hold Me Tight: Seven Conversations for a Lifetime of Love* by Sue Johnson, 2008.

Figure 4.2b Destructive Communication Patterns in ENM.

DOI: 10.4324/9781003464891-44

Navigating Risks and Stigma: Therapist Guide

Navigating Risks and Stigma

Goals of This Activity

1 Identify experiences where risks are present or could be experienced.
2 Explore how the client will navigate the risks associated with ENM.
3 Acknowledge the stigma associated with living an ENM lifestyle.

Clinical Considerations

1 Explain to the clients that all relationships involve emotional risks that must be considered. Emphasize that in ENM relationships, the potential for risks increases due to the complexity of multiple partners and their issues and baggage.
2 Explain that engaging in ENM can evoke common emotions, such as jealousy, resentment, and fear of abandonment. Highlight that these emotions are natural reactions and can be navigated and managed effectively with self-reflection and self-awareness.
3 Instruct the clients to take a deep look within themselves and explore their emotions and fears related to ENM. Please encourage them to reflect on any perceived or emotional risks they may encounter in their relationships. Remind them that understanding their emotions is crucial in navigating and managing risks.
4 Guide the clients to list perceived and real emotional risks associated with their ENM lifestyle. Instruct them to examine each risk and consider the context, possible triggers, and potential impact on their relationships and personal well-being.
5 Encourage the clients to brainstorm and develop coping strategies for each identified emotional risk. Discuss ways to address and manage these emotions effectively, such as open communication with partners,

DOI: 10.4324/9781003464891-45

practicing self-care, seeking support from a therapist or support group, and establishing clear personal boundaries.

6 Foster self-compassion and self-growth: Emphasize the importance of self-compassion throughout navigating emotional risks in ENM. Encourage the clients to approach themselves with kindness and understanding as they work through their emotions and fears. Highlight that this process can lead to personal growth and resilience.

Reference

Powell, D. L. (2018). *Building open relationships: Your hands-on guide to swinging, polyamory, and beyond!* Dr. Liz Powell.

Navigating Risks and Stigma

This activity will explore the risks associated with ENM and provide a plan of action if/when challenging situations arise.

Navigating Emotional Risks						
	Concerned, Yet Manageable					Frozen with Fear
	5	4	3	2	1	0
Vulnerability						
Resentment						
Fear of Abandonment						
Falling in Love						
Heartbreak						
Mismatched Interest Levels						
Other:						
Notes:						

DOI: 10.4324/9781003464891-46

Navigating Physical Risks						
	Concerned, Yet Manageable					**Frozen with Fear**
	5	**4**	**3**	**2**	**1**	**0**
STIs						
Unplanned Pregnancy Secondary Partner						
Unplanned Pregnancy Primary Partner						
Physical Injury						
Urinary Tract Infections						
Other:						
Notes:						

Navigating Social Risks						
	Concerned, Yet Manageable					**Frozen with Fear**
	5	**4**	**3**	**2**	**1**	**0**
Judgment from Family						
Loss of Employment						
Impact on Children						
Judgment from Friends						
Religious Concerns						
Position in Community						
Other:						
Notes:						

Answer these questions with yourself in mind, not your partners.

1 What protective measures can you put in place to help alleviate your fears?

2 What are the possible advantages of taking these risks?

3 Are the perceived risks worth the possible rewards?

4 What are the hard boundaries that you are not willing to cross, regardless of the possible rewards?

Vulnerability in ENM: Therapist Guide

Steps for Vulnerability in ENM

Goals of This Activity

1 Increase awareness of the importance of being vulnerable in romantic relationships.
2 Develop an awareness of where they might be stuck when trying to be vulnerable in their relationships.
3 Demonstrate active listening with their partners.

Clinical Considerations

1 Explain to the clients that being vulnerable in relationships is not a skill often taught in our society. Emphasize that many couples struggle with vulnerability and may not know how to begin or what vulnerability looks like in their relationship.
2 Explain that vulnerability is crucial in building trust and intimacy. Highlight that vulnerability allows for deeper connection and fosters a sense of emotional safety and security.
3 Instruct the clients to reflect on their relationship and identify potential barriers preventing them from being more vulnerable. These barriers could include past experiences, fear of rejection or judgment, a lack of trust, and communication issues.
4 Guide the clients to overcome identified barriers by providing examples of effective communication, such as using "I" statements, active listening, and expressing emotions nonjudgmentally. Encourage brain-storming strategies to build trust, such as regular check-ins, sharing personal stories, and establishing clear boundaries.
5 Provide clients with practical exercises to help them practice vulnera-bility in their relationships. These exercises could include sharing a

DOI: 10.4324/9781003464891-47

challenging personal experience, asking their partner for emotional support, or expressing gratitude and appreciation for their partner.

6   Emphasize that vulnerability is an ongoing process that requires self-reflection and self-awareness. Encourage the clients to reflect on their emotions regularly, reassess their communication skills, and adapt as necessary. Highlight that this process can lead to personal growth and development within the relationship.

Vulnerability in ENM

Steps for Vulnerability in ENM

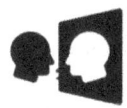

Mirror, Mirror on the Wall
Are you taking a look at your thought patterns & identifying the faulty thoughts?

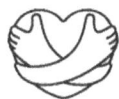

Self-Soothing Practices
What can you do when you are flooded with emotion to help you calm down & be fully present?
-- Conscious Breathing
-- Positive Self-Talk
-- Engaged Endorphins - listen to your favorite song

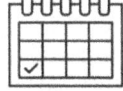

Pencil-in Check-ins
Schedule check-ins with your partner

Expand Comfort Zone
Pushing emotional boundaries by embracing emotional and/or hard conversations help couples create new homeostasis after every discussion.

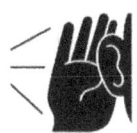

Practice Active Listening
Listen to understand, not listen to respond
Remember TOMCAT
T - Turn towards your partner
O - Open Posture
M - Maintain eye contact
C - Can't interrupt
A - Ask open-ended questions
T - Take time to reflect

DOI: 10.4324/9781003464891-48

Mixed Orientation Relationship: Therapist Guide

Mixed Orientation Relationship

Goals of This Activity

1 Establish a foundation for growth within the mixed-orientation relationship.
2 Identify emotional needs that have not been met since coming out.
3 Apply coping strategies to aid in the continued growth of the mixed-orientation relationship.
4 Explore what forgiveness looks like for each partner.
5 Increase awareness of hurtful actions toward each other.

Clinical Considerations

1 Explain to the clients that all relationships involve emotional risks that must be considered. Emphasize that in ENM relationships, the potential for risks increases due to the complexity of multiple partners and their issues and baggage.
2 Explain that engaging in ENM can evoke common emotions such as jealousy, resentment, and fear of abandonment. Highlight that these emotions are natural reactions and can be navigated and managed effectively with self-reflection and self-awareness.
3 Instruct the clients to take a deep look within themselves and explore their emotions and fears related to ENM. Encourage them to reflect on any perceived or actual emotional risks they may encounter in their relationships. Remind them that understanding their emotions is crucial in navigating and managing risks.
4 Guide the clients to list perceived and real emotional risks associated with their ENM lifestyle. Instruct them to examine each risk and consider the context, possible triggers, and potential impact on their relationships and personal well-being.

DOI: 10.4324/9781003464891-49

5   Encourage the clients to brainstorm and develop coping strategies for each identified emotional risk. Discuss ways to address and manage these emotions effectively, such as open communication with partners, practicing self-care, seeking support from a therapist or support group, and establishing clear personal boundaries.

6   Foster self-compassion and self-growth: Emphasize the importance of self-compassion throughout navigating emotional risks in ENM.

Resource

Taormino, T. (2008). *Opening up: A guide to polyamory*. Cleis.

Mixed Orientation Relationship

When one partner discloses their true sexuality to their partner after a significant period of presenting as heterosexual, many emotions arise, and questions swirl in the heterosexual's head. This activity will clarify, help establish boundaries, and allow you to design a relationship that works for your dynamic.

The Grieving Process

- Allow yourself space and time to grieve the relationship that you thought you had.
- This process is different for everyone, but generally, the stages are the same.

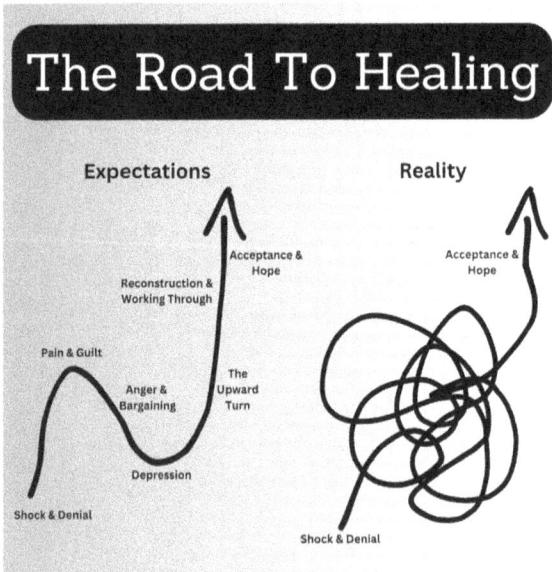

Figure 4.5b Mixed Orientation Relationship.

DOI: 10.4324/9781003464891-50

Strategies for a Successful Mixed-Orientation Relationship

- Tackle the situation from a friendship perspective, not a bitter, resentful mindset.
- Take time to reach acceptance instead of pushing for answers immediately
- Practice the Art of Difficult Conversations

  - Step 1: Determine the topic
  - Step 2: Be Solution-Focused
  - Step 3: Utilize 'I' Messages & Assertive Statements
  - Step 4: How will you process negative feedback?
  - Step 5: Practice Self-Care

- There will be stages of solid progress and stages of perceived setbacks.

  - Measure progress in small forward movements

- Create a support network or seek individual counseling
- Find an appreciation for the strength it took your partner to overcome their fear of coming out to you
- The heterosexual partner should create a list of boundaries needed for emotional and physical safety.

  - Boundaries will evolve and grow and are not set in stone

- Identify the LGBTQIA+ partner's emotional and sexual needs
- Be kind to each other and work toward acceptance

Forgiveness and Acceptance

Use this space to explore what stops you from forgiving your partner, if needed, and accepting their sexuality.

	YES/NO	Plan of Action
Fear of Being Vulnerable		
Religious or Moral Convictions		
Fear of Rejection from Family & Friends		
Inability to Control Emotions		
Other		

The Four Phases of Forgiveness

- The Uncovering Phase
  - How has your partner coming out to you impacted your life?
- The Decision Phase
  - Do you feel you can forgive your partner and move forward with the relationship, or do you think you need to separate?
- The Work Phase
  - Can you see things from your partner's perspective and work towards establishing positive feelings toward them again?
- The Deepening Phase
  - Explore the areas of personal growth and relationship growth.

Designing Your New Relationship

There is no right or wrong way to design your new relationship with your partner. Allow your imagination to run wild and forget what society says it has to look like.

The Four W's

Who Checklist (Who are you comfortable with at this time?)

Gender Preferences: __Women __Men __Transwomen/MTF __Transmen/FTM

Coupled Status: ___ Single ___ Married ___ NA

Sexual Orientation: __ LGBTQIA+ __bisexual __heterosexual __pansexual __NA

Age: ___ Older ___ Younger ___ Around Same Age ___ NA

D/s Orientation: ___ Dominant ___ submissive ___ NA

Degree of Familiarity: ___ Stranger ___NA

Other:_____

What Checklist (what are you comfortable with your partner or yourself doing?)

Relationship Dynamics: ___Romantic Involvement ___BDSM   ___Socializing
                       ___Friendship   ___Flirting   ___Dating
                       ___Sleepovers   ___Travel Partner
                       ___Emotional Connection ___Love   ___Commitment
                       Other: _____

Sexual Activity	Yes, To Give	Yes, To Receive	No	Yes w/ Conditions (List Boundaries Below)
Flirting				
Sensual Touch				
Chest/Nipple Play				
Handjob/ Digital Penetration				
Cunnilingus				
Fellation				
Analingus				
Vaginal Penetration with Fingers				
Vaginal Penetration with Toys				
Penis in Vagina (PIV)				
Anal Penetration with Fingers				
Anal Penetration with Toys				
Erotic Role Play				
Other:				
Other:				

When Checklist (when are you comfortable with you or your primary partner playing/being with secondary partners?)

Frequency of Contact	List Conditions Here If There Are Any
___ One time only	
___ Ongoing, Infrequent	(Specify)
___ Ongoing, Frequent	(Specify)
___ Other:	
Reserved dates & Special Occasions	

Where Checklist (Are there any places you feel the need to avoid?)

Place	List Conditions Here If There Are Any
___ Out of Town	
___ In Town	(Specify)
___ Public Setting	(Specify)
___ At Home	
Other:	

Designing Your ENM Relationship: Therapist Guide

Designing Your ENM Relationship

Goals of This Activity

1 Reimagine the dynamics of their primary relationship.
2 Verbalize an understanding of acceptance and appreciation toward their partner.
3 Increase awareness of available options for ENM.

Clinical Considerations

1 Explain to the clients that this part of therapy is where they reimagine their relationship dynamics and open it up to endless possibilities. This assignment can be done over several sessions or as homework to be discussed afterward.
2 Ensure that clients have a clear understanding of what ENM is and the different forms it can take. Discuss the importance of clear communication, boundaries, and consent in ENM relationships.
3 Instruct clients to brainstorm and discuss their partnership goals and desires for the relationship. This could include factors such as emotional intimacy, sexual exploration, shared experiences with other partners, or exploring different relationship dynamics.
4 Encourage clients to reflect on their values and boundaries in the context of ENM. This could include discussing what forms of ENM feel comfortable for each partner, what boundaries or rules need to be established for safety, and the kind of relationship hierarchy they envision.
5 Discuss the importance of effective communication in ENM relationships. Encourage clients to establish a communication plan that allows both partners to express their needs and feelings nonjudgmentally. This can include setting aside regular time to check in, discussing how issues

DOI: 10.4324/9781003464891-51

should be brought up non-confrontationally, or agreeing to examine the entire scope of each other's relationships with others.

6 Emphasize that designing an ENM relationship is an ongoing process that requires regular negotiation and self-reflection. Encourage clients to be open and honest with each other about their feelings and adjust their relationship design as their individual and collective needs change.

Designing Your ENM Relationship

Forging the Framework with The Four W's

Who Checklist (Who are you comfortable with at this time?)

Gender Preferences: __Women __Men __Transwomen/MTF __Transmen/FTM

Coupled Status: ___ Single ___ Married ___ NA

Sexual Orientation: __ LGBTQIA+ __bisexual __heterosexual __pansexual __NA

Age: ___ Older ___ Younger ___ Around Same Age ___ NA

D/s Orientation: ___ Dominant ___ submissive ___ NA

Degree of Familiarity: ___ Stranger ___NA

Other:_____

What Checklist (what are you comfortable with your partner or yourself doing?)

Relationship Dynamics: ___Romantic Involvement ___BDSM ___Socializing
___Friendship ___Flirting ___Dating
___Sleepovers ___Travel Partner
___Emotional Connection ___Love ___Commitment
Other: _____

Sexual Activity	Yes, To Give	Yes, To Receive	No	Yes w/ Conditions (List Boundaries Below)
Flirting				
Sensual Touch				
Chest/Nipple Play				

(Continued)

DOI: 10.4324/9781003464891-52

Handjob/ Digital Penetration				
Cunnilingus				
Fellation				
Analingus				
Vaginal Penetration with Fingers				
Vaginal Penetration with Toys				
Penis in Vagina (PIV)				
Anal Penetration with Fingers				
Anal Penetration with Toys				
Erotic Role Play				
Other:				
Other:				

When Checklist (when are you comfortable with you or your primary partner playing/being with secondary partners?)

Frequency of Contact	List Conditions Here If There Are Any
____ One time only	
____ Ongoing, Infrequent	(Specify)
____ Ongoing, Frequent	(Specify)
____ Other:	
Reserved dates & Special Occasions	

Where Checklist (Are there any places you feel the need to avoid?)

Place	List Conditions Here If There Are Any
___ Out of Town	
___ In Town	(Specify)
___ Public Setting	(Specify)
___ At Home	
Other:	

Which do you prefer?

Permission	Notification	Veto Agreements
☐	☐	☐
Primary partners are the gatekeepers for all secondary relationships, and permission from the primary partner must be attained before an activity.	Well-defined boundaries, negotiated agreements, and complex rules within the relationship allow the primary partners to notify their partners before or after an activity.	The power to say NO to potential secondary partners without question. The secondary partner does not have a say in the matter.

Use this space to make notes, jot down discussion topics to explore with your partners, or draw a picture of your feelings.

Finding Common Grounds: Therapist Guide

Finding Common Grounds

Goals of This Activity

1 Learn healthy communication skills that allow couples to fight fairly.
2 Begins the process of tough conversations without being flooded with emotion.
3 Increase sensitivity toward how negative words damage the relationship dynamic.

Clinical Considerations

1 Explain to the couples that the art of compromise is an essential skill for all couples, regardless of their sexual lifestyle. Emphasize that compromise is not about winning or losing but about finding a solution that meets the needs and desires of both partners.
2 John Gottman's research shows that compromise is key in resolving couple's arguments by considering both partners' views.
3 Clarify that the purpose of this activity is to help couples practice the art of compromise in situations where a partner is using a veto agreement and does not accept the demands put forth by the other partner.
4 Instruct the couples to find a calm and comfortable environment for open and honest conversation. Remind them to respect and listen to each other's perspectives without interrupting or becoming defensive.
5 Emphasize active listening and validation of each other's feelings and ideas to foster a productive dialogue for compromise.
6 Assign each partner a designated time to express their perspective, demands, or preferences regarding the issue. Please encourage them to be specific, clear, and respectful in communicating their needs and concerns.

DOI: 10.4324/9781003464891-53

7 Encourage partners to discuss and brainstorm alternatives, aiming for a compromise that meets both their needs.
8 Guide the couples to analyze the suggested compromises and identify each option's potential tradeoffs and benefits.

Finding Common Grounds

> Making sacrifices for the benefit of all:
> Please compromise with me, considering our love and respect for each other.

Questions that help guide the process of reaching a favorable agreement:

Essential Requirement	My firm boundary or critical condition regarding this matter is:
Areas Open for Negotiation	Areas where I am open to finding a middle ground on this issue are:

Questions that help guide the process of reaching a favorable agreement:

Please clarify why this aspect is essential and cannot be compromised or negotiated.	
What are the underlying emotions and principles that shape your perspective on this matter?	
What are the shared objectives or aspirations that can be collectively pursued?	
What strategies or actions can be implemented to achieve these objectives together?	

(Continued)

DOI: 10.4324/9781003464891-54

What measures can be taken to establish a temporary agreement or middle ground between the parties involved?	
What steps can be taken to fulfill your fundamental requirements, or assistance can be provided?	

An outcome that we both agree on considering our respective desires and needs, is:

Boundaries, Agreements, and Rules: Therapist Guide

Boundaries, Agreements and Rules, Oh My!

Goals of This Activity

1 Provide foundational knowledge for ENM.
2 Acknowledge the personal boundaries needed for each partner to feel safe.
3 Indicate agreements that will be established and the impact breaking an agreement will have on the primary couple.

Clinical Considerations

(*This resource should be paired with Designing your ENM Relationship)

Couples often use boundaries, agreements, and rules interchangeably; however, each term has a different meaning that must be explored with those in your office. While we will go into depth with each of these terms throughout this chapter, here is a brief explanation of each to help you understand better:

• A boundary concerns the self (me) and is established for the individual and their specific needs for obtaining emotional and physical safety within limits.
• An agreement is a negotiation for all involved parties that discovers a common ground with other individuals to support their needs and desires; arrangements are equivalent to consent.
• A rule, take it or leave it mentality is an irrevocable condition to solve problems and/or meet a need.

DOI: 10.4324/9781003464891-55

Boundary: All of my partners must wear protection with other partners.

Agreement: All of my partners agree to wear protection with their other partners.

Rule: If you don't wear a condom with other partners, then I will need a clear STI test before we have sex again.

Boundaries, Agreements, and Rules, Oh My!

- A boundary concerns the self **(me)** and is established for the individual and their specific needs for obtaining emotional and physical safety within limits.

  - Individuals create conditions based on their needs, wants, and refusals.

- An agreement is a negotiation for **all involved parties** that discovers a common ground with other individuals to support their needs and desires; arrangements are equivalent to consent.

  - Mutual Accords support ALL individuals' needs, wants, and refusals.
  - Re-negotiable at any time.

- A rule, take it or leave it mentality is an irrevocable condition to solve problems and/or meet a need.

  - Decisions the couple agrees to are based on their needs, wants, and refusals that may impact others.
  - Non-negotiable
  - Carries penalty for breaking a rule

Boundary: All of my partners must wear protection with other partners.

Agreement: All of my partners agree to wear protection with their other partners.

Rule: If you don't wear a condom with other partners, then I will need a clear STI test before we have sex again.

DOI: 10.4324/9781003464891-56

- Describe your boundaries:

- Describe your agreements:

- State your rules

The power of saying NO is vital for self-management. Saying NO to things you don't want to do or don't have time to do honors what is important to you and puts your NEEDS first!

Relationship Contract: Therapist Guide

Relationship Contract

Goals of This Activity

1 Ensures that everyone knows the boundaries, agreements, and rules of engagement.
2 Develop the ability to verbalize needs, wants, and desires.
3 Keep a living relationship contract available for all concerned parties.

Clinical Considerations

(*This resource should be paired with Designing your ENM Relationship)

1 Explain to the couple that this new document will serve as a contract and should be considered a living document that can be updated at any time. It is important to stress that modifications and adjustments can be made as needed.
2 Optionally, suggest that the couple incorporate specific times in the contract when they want to revisit and discuss any potential modifications. This can help ensure that their agreement remains up-to-date and relevant to their evolving needs and circumstances.
3 Encourage the couple to review the compiled work and make any necessary additions or adjustments to reflect their desires and requests accurately.
4 Once satisfied with the content, advise the couple to sign and date the document to formalize the contract.

DOI: 10.4324/9781003464891-57

Key Concepts

Permission – Each partner must ask permission BEFORE doing something with secondary partners.

Notification – Each partner shares what they did AFTER they have done something with secondary partners.

CAN Veto – Each partner has the right to stop their partner from seeing someone or from doing something with a secondary partner with no questions asked. This does not take the secondary partner's feelings into consideration.

CANNOT Veto – Each partner can discuss their concerns about the secondary partner with the other, but it is up to the individual to decide how they want to proceed. This decision takes the secondary partner's feelings into consideration.

Relationship Contract

Partner A: _____Commitment Level (1-10) _____

Partner B: _____Commitment Level (1-10) _____

1 Partner A: I am comfortable with my partner being in relationships
   with _____ as long as the secondary partner is
   _____(gender preference)_____

   _____. I am comfortable with the secondary partner being
   (coupled status)

   _____, and I prefer them to be _____.
   (sex orientation)   (age of 2nd partner)

2 Partner B: I am comfortable with my partner being in relationships
   with _____ as long as the secondary partner is
   (gender preference)

   _____. I am comfortable with thesecondary partner being
   (coupled status)

   _____, and I prefer them to be _____.
   (sex orientation)   (age of 2nd partner)

3 Partner A: I am comfortable with my partner having the
   following   relationship   dynamics   with   secondary   partners:

   _____.

   (list all relationship dynamics you are comfortable with currently)

4 Partner B: I am comfortable with my partner having the following   relationship   dynamics   with   secondary   partners:

   _____.

   (list all relationship dynamics you are comfortable with currently)

DOI: 10.4324/9781003464891-58

5   Partner A: I am comfortable with my partner participating in the following sexual activities, and if there are any conditions, those are listed as well:

_____

_____

6   Partner B: I am comfortable with my partner participating in the following sexual activities, and if there are any conditions, those are listed as well:

_____

_____

7   Partner A: I am comfortable with my partner seeing secondary partners: _____
        (frequency of contact)

8   Partner B: I am comfortable with my partner seeing secondary partners: _____
        (frequency of contact)

9   Partner A: I am comfortable with my partner seeing secondary partners: _____
        (where can they meet)

10 Partner B: I am comfortable with my partner seeing secondary partners: _____
        (where can they meet)

11 We reserve the right to the first choice on the following dates & special occasions:

_____

_____

12 We agree to: (circle one) **permission** or **notification** style relationship.

13 We agree to the following veto agreements: (circle one) **CAN veto** or **CANNOT veto**.

14 Partner A: List Boundaries

_____

_____

_____

_____

15 Partner B: List Boundaries

_____

_____

_____

_____

16   We agree to the following Agreements & Rules: (use additional paper if necessary)

_____

_____

_____

_____

_____   _____

Partner A   Date   Partner B   Date

*We agree to revisit this relationship contract on the following date: _____ or when: _____

Types of Jealousy: Therapist Guide

Types of Jealousy

Goals of This Activity

1 Explore past relationships, comparing and contrasting the types of jealousy experienced, if any.
2 Begin to reframe jealousy as an individual issue because the partner is not responsible.
3 Explore the root cause of their jealousy and reframe their mindset.

Clinical Considerations

1 Begin by acknowledging that jealousy is a complex emotion with various underlying layers, such as insecurity, fear of loss, fear of abandonment, inadequacy, and helplessness. Help the individual understand that experiencing jealousy is normal and beyond their control.
2 Emphasize that while the emotion is natural, the actions taken in response to jealousy can be controlled. Discuss how these actions often attempt to regain control over a situation and create a false sense of safety and security.
3 Explain that trying to control a partner's behavior to manage jealousy can harm the relationship. It undermines trust and intimacy, suggesting that the individual does not believe their partner's affection is genuine.
4 Offer an activity to explore and address jealousy. This activity can be done in the office during a session or assigned as homework to be discussed in the next session.
5 Guide the activity, allowing the individual to reflect on their own experiences with jealousy. Please encourage them to write down their thoughts, feelings, and reactions to situations that trigger jealousy.
6 Prompt them to explore the underlying emotions and beliefs associated

DOI: 10.4324/9781003464891-59

with their jealousy. Some potential questions to consider are: What specific insecurities or fears drive jealousy? What are the underlying assumptions they hold about themselves or their relationship?

7   Please encourage them to consider alternative perspectives and challenge their assumptions about the situations that trigger jealousy. Help them explore healthier ways to cope with jealousy, such as open communication, building trust, and focusing on self-improvement.

8   Instruct them to document their reflections and insights during the activity.

Types of Jealousy

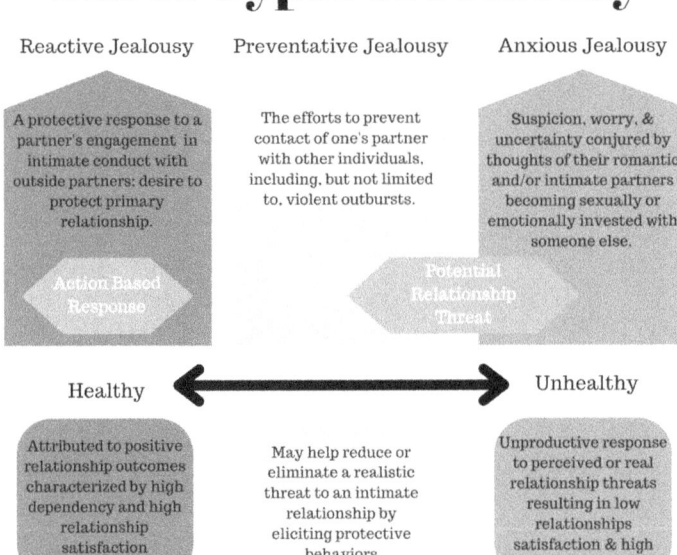

Three Types of Jealousy

Reactive Jealousy   Preventative Jealousy   Anxious Jealousy

A protective response to a partner's engagement in intimate conduct with outside partners; desire to protect primary relationship.

The efforts to prevent contact of one's partner with other individuals, including, but not limited to, violent outbursts.

Suspicion, worry, & uncertainty conjured by thoughts of their romantic and/or intimate partners becoming sexually or emotionally invested with someone else.

Action Based Response

Potential Relationship Threat

Healthy ⟵⟶ Unhealthy

Attributed to positive relationship outcomes characterized by high dependency and high relationship satisfaction

May help reduce or eliminate a realistic threat to an intimate relationship by eliciting protective behaviors

Unproductive response to perceived or real relationship threats resulting in low relationships satisfaction & high uncertainty

Adapted from *Personality, birth order and attachment styles as related to various types of jealousy* by B.P. Buunk, 1997

Figure 6.1b Types of Jealousy.

- How does your jealousy manifest?
- How has jealousy affected your current relationship?
- Provide examples of how you can reframe your jealousy into a positive outcome.

DOI: 10.4324/9781003464891-60

Navigating Jealousy: Therapist Guide

Navigating Jealousy

Goals of This Activity

1 Explore past relationships, comparing and contrasting the types of jealousy experienced, if any.
2 Begin to reframe jealousy as an individual issue because the partner is not responsible.
3 Explore the root cause of their jealousy and reframe their mindset.

Clinical Considerations

1 Begin by emphasizing the importance of exploring and understanding their personal experience of jealousy. Encourage clients to reflect on how jealousy manifests in their thoughts, emotions, and behaviors.
2 Guide clients towards discovering healthier and more manageable ways to deal with jealousy. Please encourage them to consider alternative perspectives and coping strategies that can help reduce the over-whelming aspects of jealousy.
3 Offer an activity that can be completed during a session or assigned as homework to discuss in the next session.
4 Provide specific guidance for the activity, allowing clients to delve into their jealousy patterns. Prompt them to identify particular triggers that provoke their jealousy and explore the underlying emotions and beliefs associated with these triggers.
5 Encourage clients to document their reflections, thoughts, and insights during the activity, either through writing or any other preferred method of self-expression.

DOI: 10.4324/9781003464891-61

Navigating Jealousy

Accept Your Feelings	List Your Feelings Here

~ Separate Triggers From Causation ~

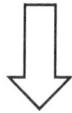

I feel insecure when you passionately kiss other partners because it has been a while since you have kissed me that way. You did not do anything wrong by kissing them, I am expressing my feelings in this moment.

~ Talk About Your Feelings ~

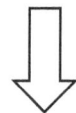

DOI: 10.4324/9781003464891-62

~ Try to Understand Your Feelings ~

Type of Fear	How Do You Want To Proceed?
Fear of being alone	
Fear of being abandoned	
Fear of being rejected	
Fear of losing your primary partner	
Fear of being left out	

~ Potential Sources of Jealousy ~

It is essential to note that jealousy can manifest differently for everyone, and these are just some potential forms that may arise in the context of ethical non-monogamy.

1. Fear of being replaced or feeling inadequate
2. Insecurity about the distribution of time and attention among partners
3. Jealousy triggered by seeing a partner engage in intimate acts with another person
4. Comparison and envy of the emotional connection shared with other partners
5. Fear of missing out on experiences shared between partners and their other relationships
6. Jealousy arising from perceived hierarchies or power imbalances within multiple relationships
7. Concerns about the level of commitment and emotional investment in comparison to other partners
8. Social jealousy, such as feeling left out or the fear of social judgment by others within the non-monogamous community
9. Fear of being emotionally replaced or the loss of intimacy with a partner
10. Jealousy triggered by knowledge of a partner's romantic or sexual encounters with others before discussing it together.

Use This Space to Explore Your Personal Fears

Brain in Love: Therapist Guide

The Brain in Love

Goals of this Activity

1 Understand new relationship energy (NRE) and how it can affect the primary relationship.
2 Encourage the partners to create a plan of action if one or both are experiencing NRE.
3 Become capable of handling negative emotions toward the partner experiencing NRE.

Clinical Considerations

New Relationship Energy (NRE) refers to the intense passion and excitement commonly experienced in the early stages of a new romantic relationship. Feelings of infatuation, euphoria, and a strong connection with a new partner characterize it. NRE can create a profound impact on one's emotional and physical well-being, often described as a "cocktail of neurotransmitters" that can induce addictive and overwhelming sensations.

During the NRE phase, individuals may experience increased feelings of happiness, giddiness, and a belief that everything is perfect. The exchange of affectionate messages or spending time with the new partner can heighten these emotions, even turning a bad day into an ideal one. This phase is often associated with a "you-are-my-missing-puzzle-piece" feeling, where the new relationship feels like a perfect match.

It is worth noting that NRE can coexist with other emotions, such as trauma and anxiety, as it brings intense changes in brain signals that can lead to both positive and challenging experiences. The duration of NRE can vary from a few weeks to a few years, depending on the individuals involved and the unique dynamics of the relationship.

DOI: 10.4324/9781003464891-63

Please remember that NRE is a complex topic, and individual experiences may vary. It is always important to communicate openly and honestly with all parties involved in a relationship to ensure that everyone's emotional needs are met.

Brain in Love

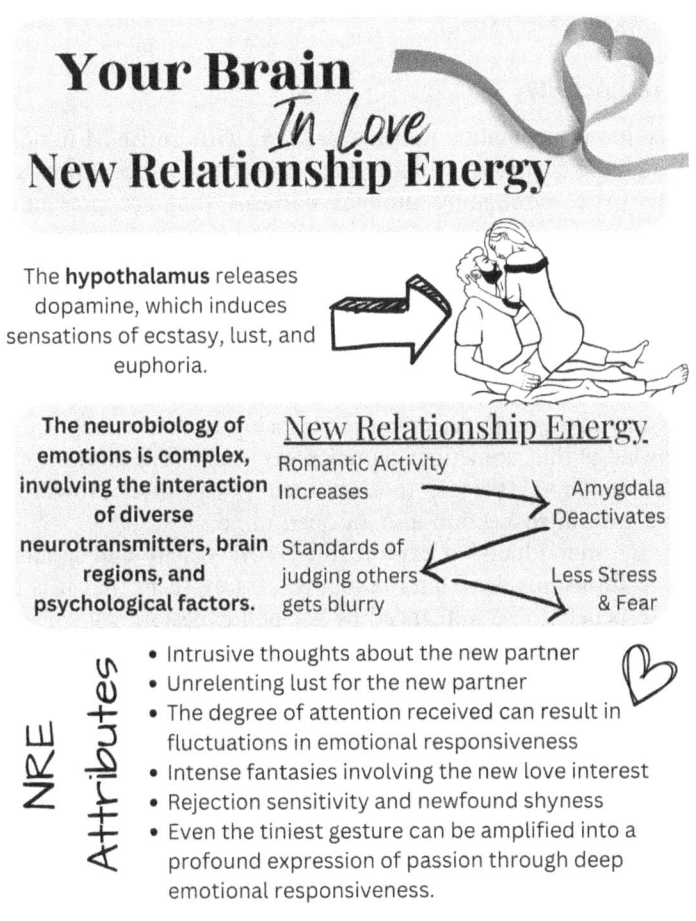

Figure 6.3b Your Brain in Love.

DOI: 10.4324/9781003464891-64

Mononormative No More!: Therapist Guide

Mononormative No More!

Goals of this Activity

1 Replace mono-normative thought patterns with an ENM mindset.
2 Challenge the clients to evaluate their core beliefs about monogamy.
3 Identify toxic monogamy thought patterns that are present in the relationship.

CLINICAL CONSIDERATIONS

1 Begin by acknowledging that transitioning into ethical non-monogamy can be challenging, mainly due to societal expectations that promote monogamy as the only accepted relationship structure.
2 Acknowledge that sometimes couples get stuck in a mono-normative mindset and may struggle to shift their perspective. However, it is possible with introspection and an open mind.
3 Encourage individuals to explore their core beliefs and assumptions about relationships, love, and sexuality. Assure them that it is normal for these beliefs to be influenced by societal expectations.
4 Help clients identify patterns or perspectives they may be clinging to that are no longer serving them. Explore how these beliefs may limit their ability to embrace ethical non-monogamy fully.
5 Guide clients to re-evaluate their beliefs and discover new ways of viewing love, relationships, and sexual partnerships that work for their new ideologies. Please encourage them to embrace the possibility of expanding and evolving their understanding of these concepts.

DOI: 10.4324/9781003464891-65

Mononormative No More!

Determine your core values. From the list below, choose and write down every core value that resonates with you. Do not overthink your selection. As you read through the list, simply write down the words that feel like a core value to you personally. If you think of a value, you possess that is not on the list, write it down.

ACHIEVEMENT	EXCELLENCE	NATURE
ADVANCEMENT	EXCITEMENT	OPEN & HONEST
ADVENTURE	EXPERTISE	ORDER
CHALLENGING ISSUES	FINANCIAL GAIN	PERSISTENCE
CHANGE & VARIETY	FREEDOM	PERSONAL
CLOSE RELATIONSHIPS	FRIENDSHIPS	PHYSICAL CHANGE
COMMUNITY	GROWTH	PRIVACY
COMPETENCE	HELPING SOCIETY	PROMOTION
COMPETITION	DEVELOPMENT	SELF-MOTIVATION
COOPERATION	HONEST	SELF-RESPECT
CREATIVITY	COMMUNICATION	SERENITY
CUSTOMER SERVICE	HONESTY	STATUS
DECISIVENESS	HUMOUR	SUPERVISING OTHERS
DEMOCRACY	INDEPENDENCE	TEAMWORK
ECOMONIC SECURITY	INFLUENCING	TIME FREEDOM
EFFECTIVENESS	OTHERS	TRUTH
ETHICAL PRACTICE	LOYALTY	WEALTH
	MEANINGFUL WORK	
	MONEY	

DOI: 10.4324/9781003464891-66

Narrow your selection above, by grouping like values together into 5 groups and writing them in the spaces below. Group together values that have a similar meaning to you, that you feel fit easily together.

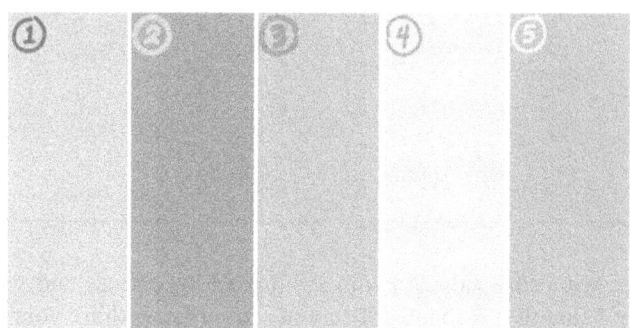

1 Compare the value you have placed in Section 1 to the value in Section 2. Which of these two core values is most important to you? Is one of them necessary for the other to exist? Draw an arrow from one section to the other, with the head of the arrow pointing toward the value that is most important to you.

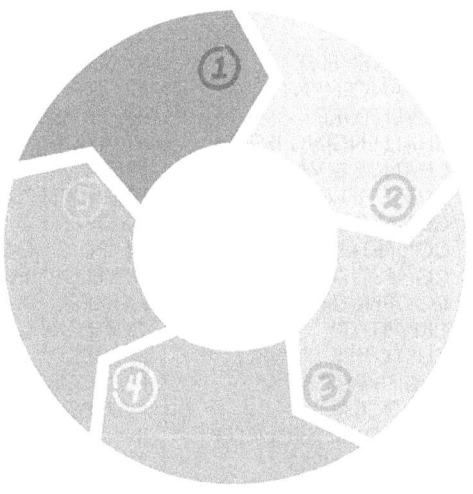

2 Continue by comparing the value in Section 1 to the values in Sections 3-5, drawing an arrow toward the one that is most important to you.

3 Working clockwise, compare the value in Section 2 to each of the values 3-5, then the value in Section 3 to the values in Sections 4 and 5, and so on. Continue until each value has been compared to the other 4 values, with the head of the arrow pointing to the most important value in each case.

4 Count the number of arrows that point to each value. The value with the most arrows is your top value, and the value with the second strongest value, and so on.

Choose one of the values included in the group, or a word that you feel best encompasses the meaning of the entire group name.

These are your top 5 Core Values

Examples

1 If wealth is not important to you unless you have wellness, you would draw your arrow pointing towards wellness.

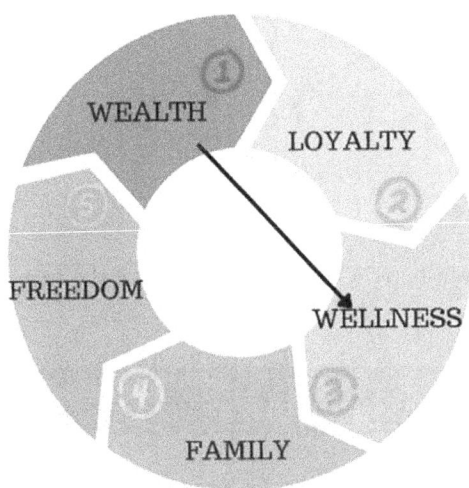

2.

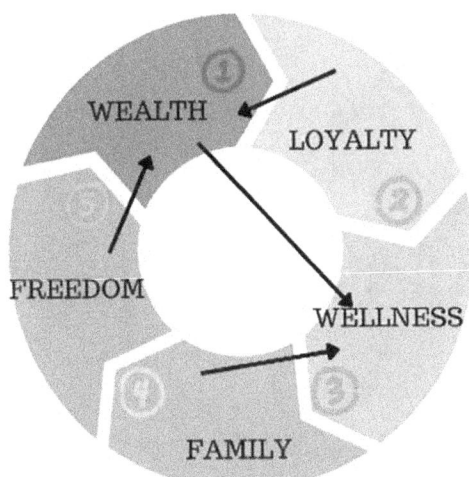

3.

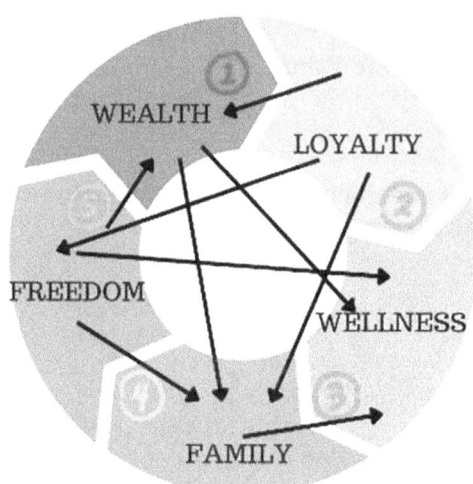

Write each of your Top 5 Core Values in one of the sections of the Values Wheel below.

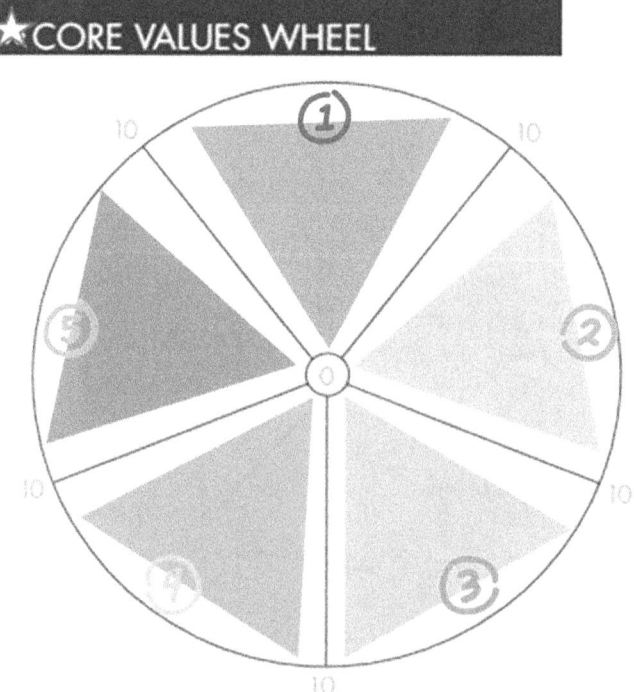

1   For each value, rate how well you are living that value by drawing a line between 1 and 10 in each section.

- If you feel you are living the value to its fullest, it will be a 10.
- If you feel you are only living the value some of the time, it might be a 5-6.
- If you are out of alignment with respect to the value, it could be less than 5.

Example:

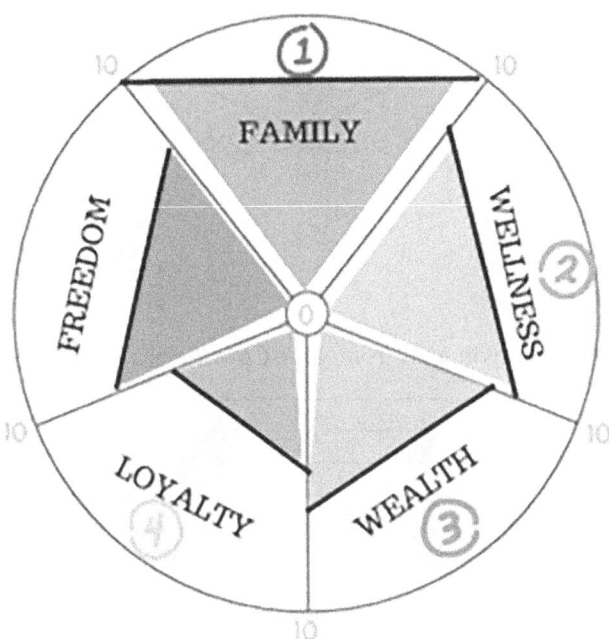

2   Once you have rated each value, you now have created a wheel.

- If uneven, like the example above, it indicates that you are not living each of your Top 5 Core Values equally. It will be more difficult to move forward in life if the wheel is unbalanced.
- A smoother, more even wheel will make it easier to move forward comfortably. If all values are at a 10 then your development will be quicker than if they are all at a 5.

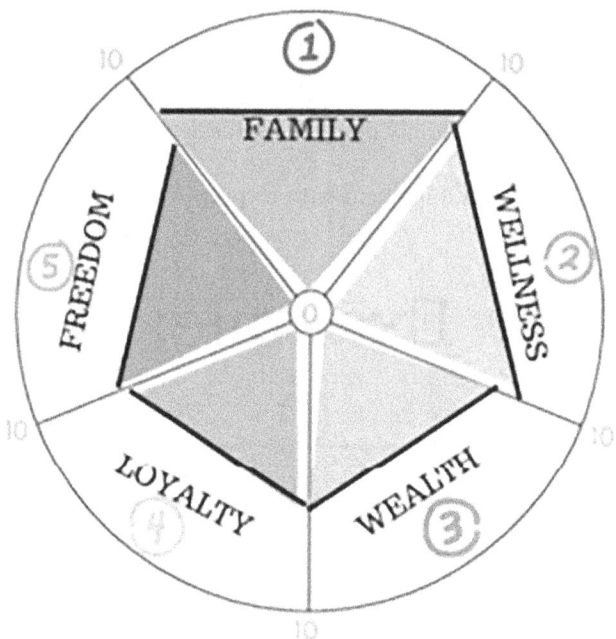

What insights can you gain from your Core Values Wheel?

_____
_____
_____
_____
_____
_____
_____

As a result of this activity, what might you start doing differently in your life to better address your identified core values?

_____
_____
_____
_____
_____
_____
_____

Mononormative No More!

Now that you have evaluated your Core Beliefs and Core Values, let us explore how toxic monogamy beliefs are contributing to the state of your relationship.

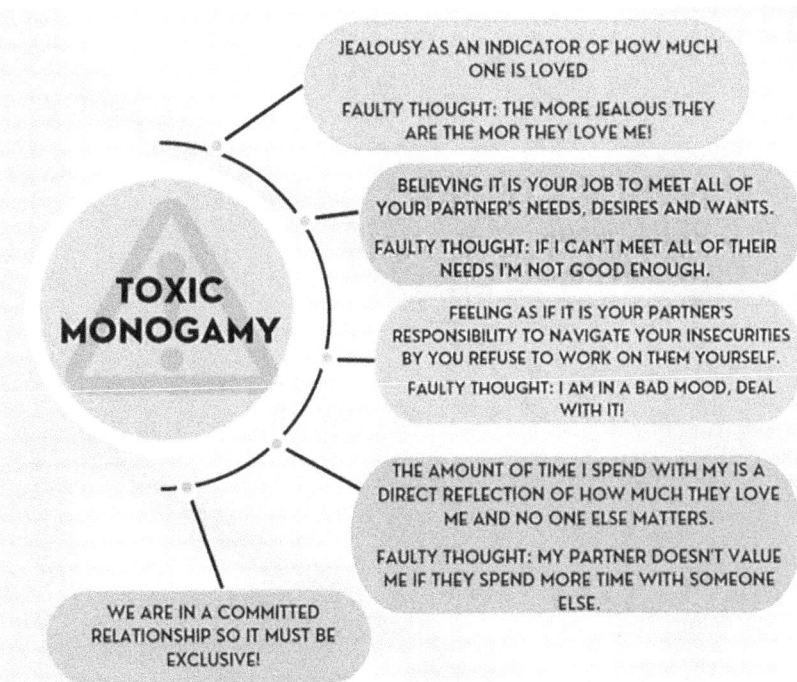

List other toxic monogamy core beliefs that you have struggled with since beginning ENM.

_____

_____

_____

_____

_____

_____

REFRAMING FAULTY THINKING

How can you reframe the statements above to reflect
healthy core beliefs?

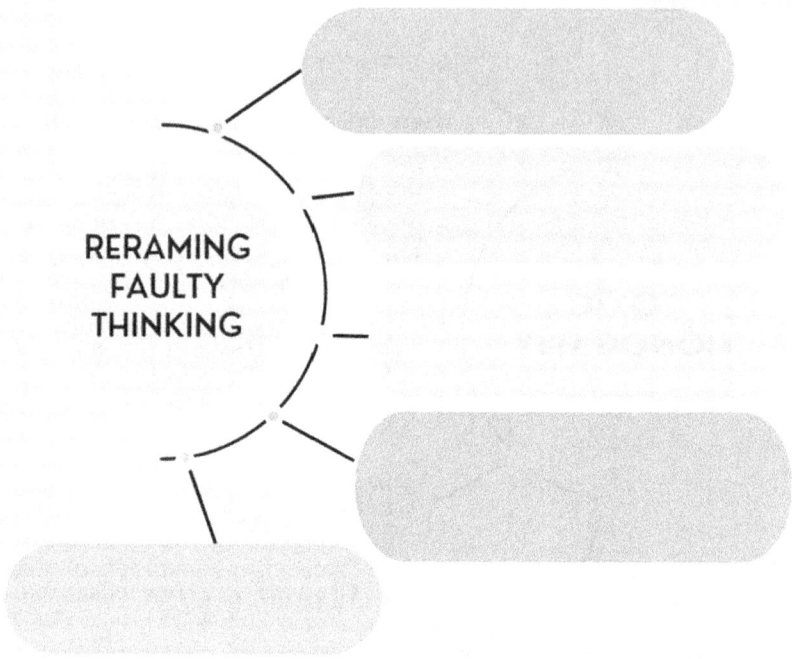

Reframe your listed struggles from the previous page below:

_____
_____
_____
_____
_____
_____
_____

Rejection Sensitivity Dysphoria: Therapist Guide

It's More Than Just Thin Skin

Rejection Sensitivity

Goals of this Activity

1 Form an understanding of Rejection Sensitivity Dysphoria.
2 Evaluate reactions to rejection, perceived or real.
3 Practice thought-stopping when needed.

Clinical Considerations

RSD can have a crucial impact on seeking and/or keeping relationships. Dating is complicated for those with RSD due to the hyper-focus placed on any feeling of rejection. The rapid mood changes can imitate the individual's perception of the trigger, ranging from an emotional breakdown with suicidal ideations to full-blown rage at the situation or person. Mood dysregulation can fluctuate quickly, resulting in multiple episodes daily (Dodson, 2022).

These individuals require constant reassurance from their partner(s) and will routinely second-guess their actions and behaviors. The fear of not being "good enough" contributes to them withholding their true feelings from their partner(s) at times of escalating conflict with exaggerated anger that feels harsher than the situation called for at the moment.

Reference

Dodson, W. (2022, July 11). New insights into rejection sensitive dysphoria. ADDitude. Retrieved September 26, 2022, from https://www.additudemag.com/rejection-sensitive-dysphoria-adhdemotional-dysregulation/

DOI: 10.4324/9781003464891-67

Rejection Sensitivity Dysphoria

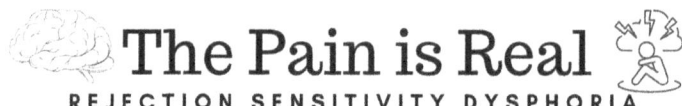

The Pain is Real
REJECTION SENSITIVITY DYSPHORIA
EXTREME EMOTIONAL SENSITIVITY TO CRITISISM OR REJECTION

CHARACTERISTICS OF RSD

- Emotional outbursts in response to perceived or actual criticism or rejection
  - Anger, rage, or burst into tears
- Disengagement during social situations
- Negative inner dialogue accompanied by thoughts of self-harm
- Habitual people-pleasers who avoid social settings where they might be criticized or fail at a task
- Constantly feeling attacked when in relationships leads them to be very defensive during times of confrontation
- Strive for perfectionism and will avoid starting projects or functions if there is a chance of failure
- Perseveration or the inability to move past a topic after the conversation has moved on
- Ruminations or obsessive thoughts that interfere with cognitive activity

I have to get out of here!

Who cares; that friendship wasn't worth it anyways!

RSD

Fine, I am leaving this group!

Everyone would be better off without me!

5 Ways to Thrive with RSD

1. **Thought Stop.** Evaluate your perspective of the situation BEFORE reacting. What do you think is happening compared to the reality of the situation?
2. **Ask Questions.** Don't assume that you know what others are thinking about, ask for clarification.
3. **Take A Moment.** Remove yourself from the situation before reacting. Does your reaction fit the situation?
4. **Be Open & Honest.** Talk to your partners about possible emotions BEFORE the clothes come off!
5. **Grace.** Give yourself the space to feel your emotions & forgive yourself if you overreact.

How has RSD affected your romantic relationships?

_____
_____
_____
_____
_____
_____
_____
_____
_____
_____
_____
_____

DOI: 10.4324/9781003464891-68

Rejection Sensitivity Dysphoria Quiz

REJECTION SENSITIVITY QUIZ

Do you have rejection sensitivity dysphoria?

1. Do you often feel like people are criticizing or rejecting you, even when there is no evidence to support this belief?
a) Never   d) Often
b) Rarely   e) Always
c) Sometimes

2. Have you ever avoided social situations because you are afraid of being rejected or criticized?
a) Never   d) Often
b) Rarely   e) Always
c) Sometimes

3. Do you often feel intense emotional pain in response to perceived criticism or rejection?
a) Never   d) Often
b) Rarely   e) Always
c) Sometimes

4. Have you ever lashed out or overreacted to perceived criticism or rejection, even when it was not intentional or directed at you?
a) Never   d) Often
b) Rarely   e) Always
c) Sometimes

5. Do you feel like your negative reactions to perceived rejection or criticism are difficult to control or manage?
a) Never   d) Often
b) Rarely   e) Always
c) Sometimes

6. Have you ever had difficulty maintaining relationships or friendships because of your intense response to perceived rejection or criticism?
a) Never   d) Often
b) Rarely   e) Always
c) Sometimes

7. Have you ever experienced physical symptoms (such as nausea, headaches, or muscle tension) in response to perceived rejection or criticism?
a) Never   d) Often
b) Rarely   e) Always
c) Sometimes

8. Do you feel like your fear of rejection or criticism impacts your daily life and functioning?
a) Never   d) Often
b) Rarely   e) Always
c) Sometimes

Scoring:
- Give yourself 1 point for every time you answered "Sometimes," 2 points for "Often," and 3 points for "Always."
- Add up your total score _____

Interpreting your results:
- 0-8 points: It is unlikely that you have rejection sensitivity dysphoria.
- 9-16 points: You may have some symptoms of rejection sensitivity dysphoria, but it is not severe.
- 17-24 points: You may have moderate to severe rejection sensitivity dysphoria. It is recommended that you seek professional help and support to address your symptoms.

This quiz in not a clinical diagnosis and should not be substituted for professional assessment or treatment.

DOI: 10.4324/9781003464891-69

Compersion: Therapist Guide

Compersion

Goals of this Activity

1 Provide an understanding of compersion and how it is achieved.
2 Accept that compersion may never be experienced.
3 Explore the benefits of compersion.

Clinical Considerations

While there is no unified definition of compersion, the majority agree that it is the opposite of jealousy and the happiness experienced when your partner is happy with or receiving pleasure from other partners. Research is limited at the time of this writing. Flicker and colleagues created a quantitative scale, The COMPERSe (Classifying Our Metamour/Partner Emotional Response Scale), explaining that it is "grounded in a qualitative understanding of consensually non-monogamous (CNM) individuals' lived experience of compersion" (Flicker et al., 2021, p. 1569).

Through their research, Flicker and colleagues found a three-factor scale for determining compersion:

• Happiness about Partner/Metamour Relationship (HPMR),
• Excitement for New Connections (ENC), and
• Sexual Arousal.

If clients are struggling with the concept of compersion or frustrated that they have not experienced it, yes, explore the components of compersion with them. Farrell (2022) strengthens the importance of open and honest communication when building compersion by suggesting that clinicians help reinforce healthy communication skills through mindfulness and acceptance.

DOI: 10.4324/9781003464891-70

Reference

Flicker, S. M., Sancier-Barbosa, F., Moors, A. C., & Browne, L. (2021). A closer look at relationship structures: Relationship satisfaction and attachment among people who practice hierarchical and non-hierarchical Polyamory. Archives of Sexual Behavior, 50(4), 1401–1417.

Compersion

DOI: 10.4324/9781003464891-71

COMPERSION

Compersion is our wholehearted participation in the happiness of others. It is the sympathetic joy we feel for somebody else, even when their positive experience does not involve or benefit us directly. Thus, compersion can be thought of as the opposite of jealousy and possessiveness.

(Dr. Marie Thouin, Love InSight)

What were your immediate thoughts after you read the quote above?

Describe a time when you felt jealousy.

Using the situation above, how where you able to navigate your jealous feelings?

What actions could have been taken in the above situation for you to have compersion?

New Relationship Energy: Therapist Guide

Handling New Relationship Energy

Goals of This Activity

1. Explore the possibilities of how NRE might affect an individual and create a plan of action to help combat damaging effects.
2. Create a roadmap to help the individual when experiencing NRE.
3. Provide a communication tool for the couple to utilize when NRE occurs.

Clinical Considerations

While NRE affects each person differently, some foundational principles can help sail their ship to calmer waters, including

- The person in the grips of NRE is not in their typical mindset; they are flooded with feel-good chemicals, so they should not make any significant decisions during this time.
- Communication is critical; if the NRE partner's actions and behaviors make their existing partner feel insecure, neglected, and/or unimportant, they must speak up.
- Ensure that the NRE client understands that their judgments and perceptions are biased, further impairing their judgment.
- Support the logical partner as they try to offer an objective view of the situation or express concern about the budding relationship; however, amid the NRE haze, their partner could accuse them of being jealous or unsupportive, and those feelings will need to be addressed as well.
- Encourage the NRE partner to use their newfound sexual energy and inspiration in all their relationships instead of focusing solely on the new relationship.

DOI: 10.4324/9781003464891-72

- Cautiously observe the client's patterns with NRE to ensure they are not jumping from one relationship to another when the NRE dissipates. Some individuals are addicted to the feelings they experience because of NRE and constantly seek new relationships to fill their needs. Frequently requiring NRE can be exceedingly hurtful for the consistent partners in their lives.

New Relationship Energy

Handling Relationship Energy!

Complete this activity and keep it accessible because you are going to need it. NRE hits everyone and this information will allow you to work through it with minimal damage to your other relationships. You are taking your own advice when you need it most.

The kind of person I want to be ... List 3 Qualities	How would you like to be described at your funeral? ☐ _____ ☐ _____ ☐ _____
In my most important relationships, I show those qualities by ... List 3 Actions	☐ _____ ☐ _____ ☐ _____
When NRE occurs, how does my partner need to approach me so I can hear them through the bliss?	When You I Feel Because I would Prefer
What actions or behaviors have I displayed in the past when I have experienced NRE? • Be honest with yourself. This will help you filter through harmful actions or behaviors when/if they occur.	

(Continued)

DOI: 10.4324/9781003464891-73

How can I ensure that I am not making emotional decisions when experiencing NRE? How can I stay grounded?	
How can I ensure that I am not making emotional decisions when experiencing NRE? How can I stay grounded?	

Mismatched Libidos: Therapist Guide

Navigating Mismatched Libido

Goals of this Activity

1. Develop an awareness of negative feelings associated with mismatched libidos.
2. Attain the required skills needed for effective communication and pleasurable sexual intimacy.
3. Eliminate any possible medical factors contributing to the low libido.

Clinical Considerations

A prevalent complaint that brings a couple, monogamous or ENM, to therapy is a difference in libido. One partner is upset that the other doesn't want sex as much as they once did, and now the high libido partner is conjuring up nonsensical ideas regarding infidelity, loss of attraction, and anything else that have read in the latest issue of their favorite magazine about why their partner no longer wants to have sex with them. It is unrealistic to believe that partners will be sexually in sync throughout their relationship. Liz Powell provided a great analogy in her book, Building Open Relationships, for describing mismatched libidos:

> If you had a relationship where one partner wanted to eat three times a day and the other wanted to eat one time a day, there's no good way for them to compromise and eat all of their meals together. Either one person is eating when they don't want to, or the other person is not eating when they want to. The person who wants to eat three times a day may feel resentful that their partner is starving them; the person who wants to eat once may feel like they don't even have time to get hungry before their partner is badgering them to eat again.
>
> (Powell, 2018, 276)

DOI: 10.4324/9781003464891-74

Mismatched Libidos

Normalizing Mismatched libidos

Mismatched libidos can be very frustrating; however, it does not mean the end of a relationship. But, it does mean more communication and compromise. It is very natural for sex drives to ebb and flows throughout the relationship, and a lifetime for that matter, but that does not mean something is wrong with an individual.

If you could have sex any way you wanted, don't be embarrassed, what would sex be like for you and your partner?

Are you experiencing any of the following:

Vulva Owners
• Vaginal dryness or general discomfort
• Pain during penetration
• Skin tags
• Shifts in menstrual cycles
• Abnormal breakouts on the face, chest, or back
• Hair loss
• Night sweats
• Darkening of the skin, notably around the groin, neck, and breasts

Penis Owners
• Tender breast
• Increase in breast tissue
• Decreased libido
• Inability to concentrate
• Decrease in bone mass
• Hair thinning or loss
• A decline in muscle mass
• Erectile disappointment

CHECK YOUR

1. How do you define sex?

2. How do you feel about scheduling sex?

Current Stressors in Your Life

1.

2.

3.

NOTES:

3. Do you need an orgasm to feel sexually fulfilled?

4. Would you feel comfortable participating in mutual masturbation? Why, or why not?

5. What does foreplay look like in your relationship? What would improve the quality of your foreplay?

DOI: 10.4324/9781003464891-75

Harm Reduction Sex Practices: Therapist Guide

Harm Reduction Sex Practices

Goals of this Activity

1. Explore and Identify risk-aware sex protocols that best fit their individual needs.
2. Negotiate and establish risk-aware sex protocols that best represent the couple's needs.
3. Acknowledge the risks associated with fluid bonding.

Clinical Consideration

We have already established that sex is risky with multiple partners. However, there are many ways of reducing the risk of transmitting an STI/STD by practicing safer sex. Everyone will create their own protocols for themselves. Then, the primary couple can explore those with each other and decide whether to add them to their combined risk-aware sex protocols. Theoretically, a couple's risk-aware sex protocols should match. However, sometimes they do not, and this is where they need to negotiate how they would like to proceed for them both to feel heard.

Fluid bonding with a partner or partners is a very personal and weighted decision that affects everyone within the relationship and their partners. Fluid bonding is having sex unbarriered with a partner or partners. When a client or couple is exploring fluid bonding with others, we have several discussions in our session together before the fluid bond with another. I want to ensure that they think about everything before deciding.

When clients want to fluid bond with another partner, they must clarify and set boundaries BEFORE they fluid bond. I have had many clients do the work on their end and go into a situation where they think that

DOI: 10.4324/9781003464891-76

everyone is on the same page, only to find out that the person they have fluid bonded with doesn't see the relationship dynamics the same way or didn't have a clear understanding, so boundaries are broken.

Resource

Dacker, E. M. (2022). The Relationship Talk Workbook. Maketimeforthetalk.com.

Harm Reduction Sex Practices

This activity is based on the research conducted by Dr. Evelin Dacker. This is a modified version of the workbook Dr. Dacker created, which can be found at maketimeforthetalk.com.

Talking About Sexual Health & STI Status

My last STI testing date was: _____/_____/_____

I test every:

- ☐ 3 months
- ☐ 6 months
- ☐ Yearly
- ☐ Before new sexual partners
- ☐ Other:

I was tested for the following and my results were:

(GC/Chlamydia Throat and Anal, Hep C, & HSV antibody testing are not done routinely, you have to ask specifically for those.)

	Positive	Negative	Not Tested
☐ GC/Chlamydia Genital	☐	☐	☐
☐ GC/Chlamydia Throat	☐	☐	☐
☐ GC/Chlamydia Anal	☐	☐	☐
☐ HIV	☐	☐	☐
☐ HPV with Pap Test	☐	☐	☐
☐ Hep B	☐	☐	☐
☐ Hep C	☐	☐	☐
☐ HSV 1 antibody	☐	☐	☐
☐ HSV 2 antibody	☐	☐	☐

DOI: 10.4324/9781003464891-77

I live with the following STIs:

☐   Genital Herpes: ☐ HSV 1   ☐ HSV 2
I have out-breaks about _____ times a year.
I ☐ Use or ☐ Do Not Use Antiviral Medication

☐   HIV
    o   On Antiretroviral Medication

☐   HPV
    o   I was diagnosed via pap test w/in last 2 years
    o   I had this in the past and now I am cleared

☐   Hep B
    ☐ Chronic ☐ Active ☐ Inactive

☐   Hep C

Risk Awareness:

☐   I currently have more than one sexual partner

☐   Since my last test, I haven't used a barrier with:
    ☐ Oral   ☐ Genital   ☐ Anal

☐   W/in the past 12 months, I had a partner with:
    ☐ Genital HSV
    ☐ Active HPV: Being treated or watched
    ☐ HIV: They ☐ Are or ☐ Are Not) medicated

☐   Other relevant risk factors to discuss:

Use this space to write your own sexual health statement:

Unveiling Turn-Ons for Connection & Intimacy Before intimacy, I prefer:

☐ Conversation

☐ Friendship

☐ Dates without sexual activity

☐ Romance

☐ Holding hands

☐ Sustained eye contact

☐ Tender touching

☐ Kissing

☐ Snuggling

My Lust Language is:

☐ Ambition

- Enjoys hearing their partner describe what they are doing to them

☐ Domination

- Sexting/dirty talk is about asserting control over the other person – a power exchange between lovers

☐ Sensation

- Turned on by descriptive texts/statements

☐ Transgression

- Sex is often associated with being bad, taboo, naughty or wrong, but that can be turned into pleasure

☐ I don't know

Answer the following questions:

1. What does consent look like to you?

2. Which specific areas do you find pleasurable when being touched?

3. What activities or actions do you find pleasurable and sexually satisfying to engage in with your partner?

4. What activities or actions do you find pleasurable and sexually gratifying for yourself?

5. What desires or activities would you like to explore with potential play partners?

6. Are there any activities or desires you enjoy but feel too shy to communicate or ask for now?

Navigating Aversions, Boundaries, and Triggers

☐ Alcohol Use
☐ Drug Use
☐ Public Display of Affection
☐ Proper Hygiene
☐ Talking loudly
☐ Not using a condom
☐ Exchanging Bodily Fluids
☐ Degrading remarks

☐ Impact play
☐ Anal play
☐ Humiliating remarks
☐ Deep throating
☐ Breath Restriction/Choking

Ejaculatory Fluids

On my body	__ Interested	__ No Thank you	__ Maybe
On/near my face	__ Interested	__ No Thank you	__ Maybe
Vaginally	__ Interested	__ No Thank you	__ Maybe
Anally	__ Interested	__ No Thank you	__ Maybe
Orally	__ Interested	__ No Thank you	__ Maybe

Answer the following questions:

1. Things that turn me off are:

2. Things that I would like to try but I am not too sure about just yet:

3. My hard nos are:

4. Some things that make me feel unsafe are:

5. The places I do not want to be touched are the following:

Trauma History
I have the following trauma triggers:

☐ Name calling   ☐ Touched or held without consent
☐ Yelling   ☐ Feeling trapped/confined
☐ Fighting   ☐ Violence/abuse
☐ Smells or tastes   ☐ Reminders of past traumatic events

Understanding Relationship Intentions and Communicating Expectations

1. What are your preferences regarding lights, sounds, and music? Are there any specific light levels, types of music, or soundscapes that you find enjoyable or soothing?

2. Do you enjoy pornography?   __ Interested __No Thank you __Maybe
3. Having sex frequently   __ Interested __No Thank you __Maybe
4. Using toys during sex   __ Interested __No Thank you __Maybe
5. Having sex occasionally   __ Interested __No Thank you __Maybe
6. Kinky sex   __ Interested __No Thank you __Maybe
7. Sensation Play   __ Interested __No Thank you __Maybe
8. Power Exchange (D/s)   __ Interested __No Thank you __Maybe
9. Anal sex   __ Interested __No Thank you __Maybe
10. Oral sex (inducing Anal)   __ Interested __No Thank you __Maybe

11. Sexual positions that I really enjoy:

12. Sexual positions that I would like to avoid:

Understanding Relationship Intentions and Communicating Expectations
I identify as:

☐ Heterosexual   ☐ Demisexual
☐ Bisexual   ☐ Pansexual
☐ Lesbian   ☐ Queer
☐ Gay   ☐ Sapiosexual
☐ Other: _____

Relationship Preference:
- ☐ Monogamous
- ☐ Ethical non-monogamous
- ☐ Open relationship
- ☐ Other: _____

- ☐ Poly: _____
- ☐ Don't ask, don't tell
- ☐ Relationship Anarchy

- ☐ Long term romantic relationship
- ☐ Domestic/Nesting partner
- ☐ Travel partner

- ☐ Casual sex
- ☐ Friend with Benefits
- ☐ Other: _____

Clarifying Expectations:
- After a sexual experience, I need:

- After a date, I would like:

- In terms of communicating, I prefer:

- ☐ Texting individually
- ☐ Group texting w/all partners included
- ☐ Chatting via messaging app

- ☐ Phone calls
- ☐ Video chats

- ☐ Other: _____

Prioritizing Safety Beyond Physical Protection
- I use barriers with: ___Oral ___Penetration ___Toys
- Preferred barriers include:
  - ☐ Condoms
  - ☐ Dental Dams

  - ☐ Gloves
  - ☐ Other: _____

From a neurological perspective, my perception of the world is shaped in this manner:
- ☐ Neurotypical
- ☐ Neurodivergent
- ☐ ADHD/ADD

- ☐ Autistic
- Other:_____

In terms of my physical safety, expect the following:
- ☐ Share my location with others
- ☐ Always keep cell phone near and on
- ☐ Check in with other partners before changing locations
- ☐ Other: _____

Based on the information above, write your 30 second elevator speech for future partners:

_____

_____

_____

_____

_____

_____

_____

_____

_____

Kinks and Fetishes: Therapist Guide

Accepting Kinks and Fetishes

Goals of this Activity

1. Recognize and understand how kinks and fetishes are present in individuals.
2. Gain an appreciation for their partner's kinks and fetishes.
3. Create a common language to help each partner communicate their needs and desires.

Clinical Considerations

Kinks and fetishes are personal and private windows into an individual's sexual soul. Opening up and sharing that world with someone can be terrifying. Therapeutically, shame presents one of the common issues when exploring kinks and fetishes. It can manifest through religious guilt, societal stigma, and shame experienced by previous partners and hinder one's ability to open up about their kinks and fetishes. If one of your clients entrusts their most sacred confession with you, that is an honor and should not be taken lightly. Verbalizing their kink or fetish to you, their therapist, might be the first time they have ever spoken these kinky desires out loud, and now, with your assistance, they want to share this information with their partner.

*Disclaimer: Holding space for the clients by providing sex-positive therapy does not mean you have to agree with their kinks or fetishes. You are providing the gift of acceptance without pathologizing them. If their kinks or fetishes do not hurt anyone or themselves and are not illegal, then simply accepting them as they are can increase the connection with clients and decrease their shame.

DOI: 10.4324/9781003464891-78

Kinks and Fetishes

DOI: 10.4324/9781003464891-79

Kinks & Fetishes

A kink is an activity or behavior that turns you on and can be included during sexy time with your partners. A kink is subjective and personal to the individual. For example, your mom might think sex toys are kinky but your best friend thinks sex toys are vanilla.

A fetish is an attraction linked to an inanimate object, activity, or part of the body other than sexual organs. The individual with the fetish cannot get aroused without fantasizing or actually engaging with the object or behavior in some form.

Think about it this way:

- You are laying in bed one night and you hear the upstairs neighbor having sex and get turned on; that is a kink.

- If you NEED to hear or watch others having sex to get sexually aroused then that is a fetish.

Talking to new partners about your Kinks & Fetishes

- All safe and consensual sex is healthy and acceptable. Try not to feel shame or guilt because of your kinks.

- Educate yourself about kinks. Kinks are more common than one might think.

- Talk about your kinks with your partner, help normalize your desires by using inviting terminology.

- Watch porn that showcases your kink and see how your partner reacts to that. Use the porn as a conversation starter for future exploration.

- Think of compromises that could be made ensuring everyone is comfortable and enjoying the experience.

Accepting & Understanding your partner's Kinks & Fetishes

- NORMAL sex is a myth, everyone likes different things and that is perfectly acceptable.

- Explore what about your partner's kink is making you feel uncomfortable.

- Begin sexualizing their kink or fetish in a way that might turn you on as well.

- If you are unable to provide your partner the exact kink or fetish they are requesting, is there an alternative?

- Accept your sexual differences and explore your own possible

- What message does society send regarding your, or your partner's kink/fetish?

- What about your kink/fetish is hard to share with your partner? Or Accept?

Kinks & Fetishes

How do you feel after disclosing your kink/fetish to your partner, or learning about your partner's kink/fetish?

- Shame
- Embarrassment
- Confused
- Self-Conscious
- Disturbed
- Reluctant
- Unsure
- Resistant
- Anxiety
- Guilt

- Accepting
- Curious
- Present
- Appreciative
- Trusting
- Loving
- Adventurous
- Proud
- Free
- Worthy

- Depressed
- Disappointed
- Heartbroken
- Resentful
- Bitter
- Incapable
- Nervous
- Worried
- Questioning
- Shocked

- Hopeful
- Optimistic
- Thankful
- Calm
- Vulnerable
- Daring
- Eager
- Inspired
- Interested
- Stimulated

Why might you feel this way?

Where did you learn to connect your identified feelings with kink/fetshes?

Is this belief one that you are willing to hold on to? How does this belief serve you? If the belief is not serving you, how can you adjust your belief to better serve you?

Sexual Preference Questionnaire: Therapist Guide

Sexual Preference Questionnaire

Goals of this Activity

1. Identify new sexual desires and interests.
2. Communicate sexual desires and interests to their partner.
3. Become accepting of their partner's sexual desires and interests.

Clinical Considerations

Each partner is given a copy of the sexual preference questionnaire and asked to highlight what they are interested in trying with their partner. After each partner has completed the questionnaire, they trade with their partner to see their highlighted requests. After both partners have reviewed their partners' lists, have them discuss their thoughts and feelings about their partners' desires compared to their own.

After this activity, provide them with the Sex Menu chart and have them complete that while in the office.

DOI: 10.4324/9781003464891-80

Sexual Preference Questionnaire

You are embarking on the exciting journey of exploring your sexual desires! Follow the rules carefully:

Be honest and complete this without your partner's influence.
Don't be embarrassed! Your sexual desires, sexuality, and kinks are perfect!
Highlight what you want to try on this questionnaire.
Have FUN!!!

Level 1:
Vanilla w/Sprinkles, Toys, Anal Play, Group and Public Fun

- Have longer teasing and foreplay sessions with your partner.
- Give your partner a sensual massage
- Take pictures of the partner
- Have pictures taken by the partner
- Take photos of us having sex
- Strip or give a lap dance to the partner
- Film ourselves having sex
- Use mirrors while having sex
- Be woken up with penetrative or oral sex by a partner
- Watch partner masturbate
- Be watched by my partner while I masturbate
- Watch porn together
- Show partner how I like something from the porn scene
- Be shown what your partner likes from porn
- Be more vocal towards your partner during sex
- Have your partner be more vocal
- Have partner talk dirty to me
- Call or be called obscene words (bitch, slut, whore, etc.)
- Increase sexy texts throughout the day
- Mutual exploration of erogenous zones

DOI: 10.4324/9781003464891-81

- Roleplay in costumes
- Wear stockings and high heels for your partner during sex
- Listen to romantic music while having sex
- Listen to aggressive music while having sex
- Mutually masturbate
- Be rougher in sex towards partner
- Have your partner be rougher towards you
- 69 with partner
- Swallow partner's cum
- Cum over your partner's breasts/neck
- Cum over your partner's face
- Have partner cum on my face
- Have a partner sit on my face and be orally pleasured
- Use dildos during sex
- Use vibrators during sex
- Wear a cock ring during sex
- Anally finger partner
- Be anally fingered by partner
- Rim partner's anus
- Have a partner rim you
- Have sex in front of an outward-facing window
- Let others watch you have sex
- Include another partner in sex, male or female
- Include another couple in sex
- Participate in large orgy
- Include more than two men in sex
- Include more than two women in sex
- Watch your partner have sex with another person
- Have a partner watch you have sex with another person
- Visit an adult novelty store and pick out new toys together
- Use intimacy wax candles during sex
- Learn each other's Erotic Blueprint for enhanced sexual pleasure
- Increase foreplay
- Have sex anywhere other than the bedroom

Level 2:
Advanced, includes BDSM

- Slap your partner's face during sex
- Have my face slapped during sex
- Use restraints during sex on a partner
- Be restrained by your partner during sex
- Pull the partner's hair

- Have your hair pulled
- Use a riding crop on partner
- Have your partner use a riding crop on you
- Be spanked by partner's hand
- Spank your partner with your hand
- Have your partner strike you with a cane
- Strike your partner with a cane
- Bite or be bitten by partner
- Be bitten by partner
- Wear a dog collar with a leash
- Be submissive to partner
- Be dominant toward partner
- Wear hoods or half hoods for partner
- Have your partner wear hoods/half hoods for you
- Sit on your partner's face to receive oral sex
- Be a submissive brat toward your partner
- Have your partner be a submissive servant
- Be a submissive servant toward your partner
- Wear a chastity belt for partner
- Have your partner wear a chastity belt for you
- Act as furniture to be used by partner
- Roleplay a forced sex scene
- Have your partner be a submissive brat for you
- Be suspended while having sex with partner
- Have your partner be suspended while having sex
- Double-penetrate your partner with another penis
- Triple penetrate your partner or be triple penetrated by your partner
- Wear or have your partner wear a play collar in private
- Wear or have your partner wear a former collar in public

Level 3:
Various Advanced Topic

- Make porn together
- Peg partners with a strap-on
- Be pegged by a partner with a strap-on
- Be forced by your partner to taste yourself
- Force partners to taste themselves
- Be forced to go down on another person
- Force my partner to go down on another person
- Watch my partner engage in same-sex sex acts
- Engage in same-sex sex acts
- Be forced to perform sex acts on another person by a partner

- Force my partner to perform sex acts on another person
- Eat food off my partner's body
- Straddle your partner while masturbating
- Have a partner straddle you while masturbating
- Roleplay a teacher/student scene
- Roleplay a cheating scene
- Mutual masturbation until orgasm
- Cum on your partner's belly
- Partner cum on my belly
- Give my partner oral sex while on my knees
- Create my kinky scene with my partner
- Learn Shabari
- Have sex in public
- Use nipple clamps on the partner
- Have my partner use nipple clamps on me
- Use a butt plug
- Have my partner use a butt plug
- Give my partner a prostate massage
- Have my partner give me a prostate massage
- Use anal beads
- I want my partner to edge me
- I want to edge my partner
- Try breath play – safely
- Use a ball gag on self or partner
- I want my partner to fist me or be fisted by me
- I want my partner to give me a golden shower
- I want to give my partner a golden shower

Sex Menu: Therapist Guide

Sex Menu

Goals of This Activity

1. Remove the pressure of thinking of new things to try during sex.
2. It provides a way to express specific requests they might not have had the courage to do in the past.
3. Evoke the client's sexual imagination.

Clinical Considerations

This activity can be used as a stand-alone activity or paired with the Sexual Preference Questionnaire. Encourage each partner to write five requests or ideas in the Things I Need and Things I Want to Try sections and as many items as they feel necessary in the No box. Have each partner give their menu to the other and request that they have at least three things off each list completed before the next session.

DOI: 10.4324/9781003464891-82

Sex Menu

Date for completion: _____

Sex Menu

Things I NEED More Of From My Partner:	Things I Want To Try With My Partner:
☐ _____	☐ _____
☐ _____	☐ _____
☐ _____	☐ _____
☐ _____	☐ _____
☐ _____	☐ _____
☐ _____	☐ _____
☐ _____	☐ _____
☐ _____	☐ _____
☐ _____	☐ _____
☐ _____	☐ _____
☐ _____	☐ _____
☐ _____	☐ _____

DOI: 10.4324/9781003464891-83

No Thank You!
These are the things that I am not interested in happening.

Intimate Partner Violence: Therapist Guide

Intimate Partner Violence in ENM

Goals of This Activity

1 Educate and inform clients about Intimate Partner Violence.
2 Provide a safe space to identify if these things are present in their relationship.
3 Open the conversation on how to leave a dangerous relationship.
4 Create a plan of action for correcting identified behaviors.

Clinical Considerations

If a therapist suspects that their client may be experiencing intimate partner violence (IPV), it is crucial to handle the situation with care and prioritize the client's safety. Here are five steps a therapist should take in such a situation:

1 Validate and create a safe space: Creating an environment where the client feels safe, supported, and validated is essential. Assure them that their experiences are taken seriously and that they are not to blame for the violence.
2 Assess the client's safety: Conduct a thorough assessment of the client's immediate safety by exploring the severity and frequency of the violence. Ask about any recent incidents and assess the client's risk level, taking note of any threats or escalating behaviors.
3 Develop a safety plan: Collaborate with the client to create a safety plan tailored to their needs and situation. This plan should identify practical steps the client can take to increase their safety, such as emergency contacts, safe places to go, and resources to access.
4 Provide resources and referrals: Offer information about local resources and support services specializing in domestic violence, such as shelters,

DOI: 10.4324/9781003464891-84

hotlines, counseling services, legal aid, or support groups. Share contact information and walk the client through the available options.

5 Consult and report if necessary: Consult with experienced professionals in the field of domestic violence to ensure a comprehensive understanding of the situation.

Therapists must approach IPV situations with sensitivity, respect, and knowledge. Each case is unique, and therapists should be prepared to adapt their approach based on the client's needs and specific circumstances.

Intimate Partner Violence

DOI: 10.4324/9781003464891-85

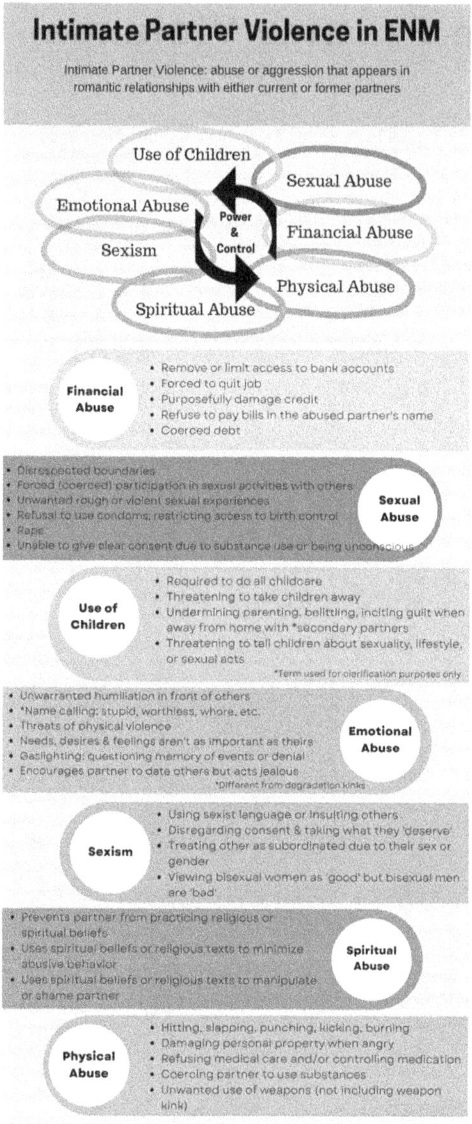

Figure 9.1b Intimate Partner Violence in ENM.

Notes:

_____

_____

_____

_____

_____

_____

_____

ENM Glossary

At the time of this book being written, these are common terms for those in ENM relationships; however, terminology changes daily and it is hard to keep up with the trending terms. This glossary is a broad explanation of the most common terms for the ENM lifestyle.

420   Refers to the usage of marijuana.

AC/DC   A person who enjoys sexual activity with both the same sex and the opposite sex (see BI, BISEXUAL).

ADULT   Colloquialism for pornographic.

AFF   Pertains to the website Adult Friend Finder.

ALL CULTURES   A person and/or couple who revels in all sexual activities and fetishes (see CULTURE).

AMERICAN CULTURE   The missionary position (man on top).

ANAL SEX   Intercourse of the anus (see GREEK, GREEK CULTURE).

ANALINGUS   Oral contact or stimulation of the anus by licking, sucking, and/or kissing.

ANIMAL TRAINING/ANIMALS   Sexual activity with animals (see B-EASTIALITY).

ARTS   Colloquialism for fetishes (see CULTURE).

B & D or B/D   Bondage and discipline. The use numerous methods used to restrain someone while delivering discipline, typically carried out by a "master" to their "slave" (see BONDAGE, DISCIPLINE, BDSM).

BBC   Acronym for Big Black Cock.

BBW   Acronym for Big Beautiful Woman; refers to women that are larger than medical standards and societal norms yet are satisfied and comfortable with their weight/size.

BDSM   A mixture of three terms: BD (Bondage & Discipline), DS (Dominance & Submission), and SM (Sadism & Masochism). Power-driven sexual activities on a large scale.

BEASTIALITY   (see ANIMAL TRAINING).

BI   Bisexual, also called Versatile (see AC/DC).

BI-COMFORTABLE   A female or male who is only open to bi-sexual acts while swinging. They do not identify as bi-sexual or homosexual in their everyday lives (see also HETERO-FLEXIBLE and SOCIALLY BI).

BI-CURIOUS   A male or female with at least some interest in participating in same-sex activities.

BIZARRE   Uncommon desires related to sex.

BONDAGE   A sexual fetish in which restraints such as chains, cloth, ropes, chains, or leather straps are used to tie, bind, or hold down a consensual partner during sexual activity. The binder is known as the "dominant," and the restrained one is known as the "submissive."

BUKKAKE   A Japanese sexual term that refers to a male or multiple males showering a participant with semen.

BYOB   An acronym meaning Bring Your Own Beer. This signifies that visitors must bring their own alcoholic beverages to an event that does not or cannot sell alcohol. Mixers (i.e., sodas, juices, ice) are typically provided (see also MIXERS PROVIDED).

CAN ENTERTAIN/CAN HOST   Indicates that a swinger is willing to provide a place where they and others can participate in swinging (typically their home).

CAN TRAVEL/WILL TRAVEL   Indicates that a swinger is willing to travel to participate in swinging.

CANING   A fetish involves spanking a participant with a light cane (typically bamboo or light wood).

CHEATING   Participating in sexual activity with another person(s) without the consent and/or knowledge of the other partner(s).

CLEAN   Being hygienic with no sexually transmitted diseases.

CLOSED DOOR   (see CLOSED SWINGING).

CLOSED SWINGING   Couples interact sexually in separate rooms but in the same house to allow privacy.

CLOSET SWINGER   A person who swings privately (see DISCREET).

COUGAR   Refers to a woman of an older age who boldly pursues younger men.

COUPLE   In swinging, this is typically a man and a woman. They may be spouses, living together, in a committed relationship, or a single couple dating to swing.

CPL   (see COUPLE).

CUCKOLD   Originally referred to as the husband of a cheating wife. Contemporarily, it is defined as a husband whose wife plays without his involvement yet tells him about her experiences. It can also refer to a husband who watches his wife play (whether the watching is forced or consensual). Sometimes, this term is used to describe a wife. There are many ways to define this. It is best to ask for clarification.

CULTURE   Colloquialism for Arts or Fetish.

CUNNILINGUS   Oral stimulation of the clitoris and vagina using the lips, tongue, and teeth in some instances (see FRENCH CULTURE).

D/D FREE   Refers to a person or couple being Drug/Disease Free. This person(s) does not use drugs and is free of STDs.

DILDO   A synthetic penis (typically comprised of plastic, rubber, or glass). It is used for sexual stimulation of the vagina and/or the anus.

HALL PASS   1. Consent is provided to one spouse by the other to autonomously locate and engage in sexual play with a separate party. 2. Consent to play outside the home without the other married partner being present or involved.

DIRECTOR   1. The main person who runs a swing club (typically the owner). 2. An individual employed by the director. Their duties consist of the operations of the club (also known as the Manager).

DISCIPLINE   A sexual fetish with one dominating partner. The submissive partner often receives physical punishment of some sort. This can range from being physically restrained, spankings, or being beaten. (All involved are willing participants.)

DISCREET OR DISCRETION   Preference of others not being made aware of participating in swinging-related activities.

DOCILE   The openness and willingness to receive bondage and/or discipline during sex (see SUBMISSIVE).

DOGGING   A British colloquialism for participating in or watching others participate in sexual activity in a semi-public place. Voyeurism and exhibitionism are closely related to dogging.

DOMESTIC TRAINING   Household chores of an intimate and shaming nature are carried out by the submissive.

DOUBLE PENETRATION   The penetration of two orifices simultaneously at the same time (typically the anus and vagina but can sometimes include the mouth).

DP   Double Penetration.

DOMINANT   The sexual partner who dominates/ is in control of a willing submissive partner.

ENGLISH CULTURE   Stimulation that is sexual in nature (typically received from being caned or spanked).

ENTERTAIN   (see CAN ENTERTAIN).

EUROPEAN STYLE CLUB   A club having the requirement that guests remove their clothing at some point in the day or night.

EXHIBITIONIST   A person who becomes sexually aroused or receives pleasure from his/her body being seen by others.

F   Female.

FELLATIO   The oral sexual stimulation of the penis.

FETISH   Non-sexual objects, actions, or non-genital anatomy used for sexual pleasure.

FFM or FMF   Two women and one man are involved in a threesome (see THREESOME). The acronym FFM sometimes refers to a threesome that is female-based, and the women involved are the focal points.

FLAGELLATION   Pain (such as spanking or caning) is used for sexual stimulation.

FLUID BONDED   Practice related to swapping genital fluids (also known as unprotected sex). Although the practice of fluid bonding is not limited to polyamorists, at the beginning of the relationship, it is crucial to focus on safer sex and overall sexual health when multiple partners are involved. Participants typically have agreements in place to protect the sexual health of those involved. Polyamorists have the propensity to require a great deal of self-accountability and blame for their sex partners.

FRENCH CULTURE   Sexual activity involving oral stimulation of the genitals (see FELLATIO, CUNNILINGUS).

FRIENDS FIRST   Developing some degree of friendship before engaging in sexual play (see INTERESTED IN FRIENDSHIP).

FULL SWAP   The sexual exchange of partners among two different couples.

FUN AND GAMES   Colloquialism for participating in sexual activity.

FURRIES   A subculture of individuals who enjoy dressing up as furry animals. This fetish is not always sexual and is sometimes used to have fun and/or temporarily escape reality.

GAY   A male or female who is homosexual.

GBM   Acronym for Gay Black Male.

GENEROUS   A term referring to exchanging money for sex.

GIRL-GIRL   Women engage in sexual acts while men watch.

GOLDEN SHOWER   Engaging in urine play (see WATERSPORTS).

GREEK CULTURE   Intercourse of the anus using the penis.

GROUP ROOM   A room assigned specifically for group sex. The floor of the room is typically adorned with mattresses.

GROUP SEX   Also referred to as swinging. Three or more people engage in sexual activity.

GWM   Acronym for Gay White Male.

HARDCORE   There is an assumption and expectation that sex will occur at the swing event.

HARD SWINGING   (see HARDCORE).

HEAD   Oral sexual stimulation of the genitals. (see FRENCH CULTURE, FELLATIO, CUNNILINGUS).

HEDONIST   An individual whose primary purpose is pleasure. This person can also be referred to as a swinger.

HETERO-FLEXIBLE   (see BI-COMFORTABLE).

HETEROSEXUAL   The sexual attraction to people of the opposite sex.

HOMOSEXUAL   The sexual attraction to people of the same sex (see GAY).

HORNY   Sexual tension. Someone who requires receiving pleasure from sex.

HUNG   Colloquialism for a male with a large penis.

HWP   Height-Weight Proportionate. This refers to an individual who is their ideal body weight for their height.

INTERESTED IN FRIENDSHIP   A person or couple looking for a sexual relationship involving emotions (see FRIENDS FIRST).

IR   Acronym for Interracial.

IRL   Acronym for In Real Life. This acronym is often used when chatting online or in ads.

ISO   Acronym for In Search Of. This acronym is often used when chatting online or in ads.

LEATHER   A fetish; the wearing or touching of leather provides sexual arousal.

LESBIAN   A woman who is emotionally and sexually attracted to the same sex (see GAY, HOMOSEXUAL).

LTR   Acronym for Long-Term Relationship.

M   Male.

MARITAL AIDS   Sexual toys and devices used for the sexual stimulation and pleasure of oneself and others (typically used among married couples).

MASOCHISM   Sexual satisfaction is achieved by receiving pain and being humiliated by another individual(s).

MASTER/SLAVE   This sexual relationship involves bondage and discipline among a dominant (master) and submissive (slave). (see B & D, BONDAGE, DISCIPLINE, BDSM).

MATROOM/MATTRESS ROOM   (see GROUP ROOM).

MBC   Acronym for Married Black Couple.

MBiC   Acronym for Married Bisexual Couple.

MEET & GREET (M&G)   An event for swingers meeting other swingers.

MEET FOR PLEASURE   Participants will meet for swinging. There is no implication for social and/or emotional interaction among those involved before engaging in sexual activity.

MENAGE A TROIS   Sexual interaction involving three people (typically two people of one sex and one person of the opposite sex) (see THREESOME, TRIAD).

MFM or MMF   Two men and one woman involved in a threesome (see THREESOME). MFM is typically two straight males and a female, while MMF can refer to two bisexual males and one female participant.

MILF   Acronym for "Mom I'd Like to Fuck." A term used to describe an older, attractive woman.

MIXERS PROVIDED   Indicates that an event will supply mixers (sodas, ice, juice) for guests, but the guests will have to bring their own alcohol (see BYOB).

MORESOMES A swinging interaction involving more than three people (see GROUP SEX).

MWC Acronym for Married White Couple.

NASCA The North American Swing Club Association. An association of swing clubs and literature to promote swinging as a valuable lifestyle

NEWBIES People who are new to swinging.

NSA Acronym for No Strings Attached. There are no expectations beyond the sexual interaction.

OFF-PREMISE Swinging does not take place at the event. Swingers meet up and make separate arrangements.

ON-PREMISE A club or event that permits sexual play. Rooms are typically provided for this to take place.

OPEN DOOR (see OPEN SWINGING).

OPEN RELATIONSHIP Partners can have other partners in this type of relationship. The other partners do not have to be polyamorous or swingers. Married couples refer to this as an open marriage.

OPEN SWINGING Swinging takes place between one couple and another couple. This occurs within the same room.

ORGY Sexual interaction among several participants within one room; also referred to as group sex.

PARTY This involves three or more people swinging (male and female).

PARTY CLOTHES Garments that are specifically worn to swing parties. This typically includes lingerie, robes, wrap-around, etc. These clothes provide easier access to body parts for possible sexual play.

PARTY HOUSE A place regularly that hosts swing parties (no membership required).

PASSIVE A person who does not contribute to sexual activity. This individual is quiet and submissive in swinging but has the willingness to undergo corrective training (see DISCIPLINE).

PASSIVELY BI A male or female that allows touch from someone of the same sex but will not reciprocate it ("you can touch me, but I won't touch you.")

PHOTOGRAPHY The interest in taking, recording, and/or exchanging sexually explicit photos and/or videos.

PLAYDAR The belief or feeling that another couple may be swingers. This is similar to "Gaydar" but for swingers.

PLAY PARTNER A partner selected for sexual play.

POLYAMORY An intimate relationship that involves over two persons.

P/P Photograph and phone number. This is typically used when chatting online or in personal ads.

PRO Short for Professional, refers to paid sex workers.

RECREATIONAL SWINGER An individual who engages in swinging for recreational purposes. There is no desire for the formation of an emotional relationship or connection.

RESTRAINT This bondage during sexual activity is mild.

ROMAN Involves group sex, the party scene, orgies, etc. (see ROMAN CULTURE).

ROMAN CULTURE Orgies of a sexual nature.

RUBBER 1. Also known as a condom (used for contraception). 2. Becoming sexually stimulated by the smell, look, and feel of rubber materials is also a factor (typically linked to B&D).

SAFE The description of an individual who cannot impregnate or become impregnated due to natural, chemical, or surgical sterilization.

SAME ROOM Sexual play in the same room.

SAME ROOM SWAP The swapping of partners in the same room.

SBF Acronym for Single Black Female.

SBiF Acronym for Single Bisexual Female.

SBM Acronym for Single Black Male.

SEPARATE ROOM Refers to couples splitting up to go into different rooms to swap partners for sexual play.

SGL Single (see SINGLE). Typically used for online chatting and ads.

S&M or S/M Abbreviation for Sadism and Masochism (see SADISM, MASOCHISM, BDSM).

SCAT The sexual use or arousal from fecal matter.

SDC References the website: Swingers Date Club.

SIGNIFICANT COUPLE Term for partners in an intimate relationship where they are each others' primary couple. Couple A is couple B's significant couple; therefore, they have a mutual understanding of the style of play, partners playing independently, and are often fluid bonded.

SINGLE A person who is a swinger but not in a relationship or married.

SLS Refers to the website: SwingLifestyle.com (a site for swingers).

SOCIAL A gathering with a magazine or swing club sponsors. No swinging takes place at the event, but arrangements for swinging may occur post-gathering.

SOCIAL SWING CLUB Private swingers' club membership offering regular swinging activities on the premises. Educational and traveling activities may also be offered. A membership fee may be involved.

SOCIALLY BI (See BI-COMFORTABLE).

SODOMY Sexual intercourse (primarily oral or anal) with an opposite-sex or same-sex partner.

SOFT SWINGERS These couples engage sexually only with one another. There is no swapping or intercourse involved with other individuals/couples.

SOFT SWAP Involves two couples exchanging partners for specific sexual acts. The participating couples decide this. Intercourse only occurs among primary couples.

SOFT SWINGING Used as a description of sex in the same room, being watched or watched, or any sexual act (besides intercourse) with someone other than the primary partner. This is often the initial experience for many couples new to swinging (see HARD SWINGING, HARDCORE).

SPLOSHING Sexual arousal and pleasure are derived from being covered in copious amounts of food products and beverages.

SRS Acronym for Same Room Sex (see SOFT SWINGING).

STD Acronym for Sexually Transmitted Disease.

STI Acronym for Sexually Transmitted Infection (see STD).

STR or STR8 Short for the term Straight (see STRAIGHT).

STRAIGHT An individual who has no sexual interest in the same sex. It also refers to a drug-free person. Swingers also use this term to define non-swingers.

SUBMISSIVE Refers to a passive individual yearning to be dominated by another. (see PASSIVE).

SWAP PICS A person's interest in exchanging sexually explicit/nude photos of themselves and/or others.

SWAPPING The sexual act of two couples exchanging partners (see SOFT SWAP; FULL SWAP).

SWEDISH CULTURE The usage of hands predominantly during massages, intended for sexual stimulation.

SWF Acronym for Single White Female.

SWING MAGAZINE The method by which swingers connected before the Internet existed. This magazine was geared toward the community of swingers. Personal ads and articles were included.

SWINGING Consenting adults participating in alternative lifestyles. These individuals enjoy engaging in recreational and social sexual activities with other consenting people.

SWINGING LIFESTYLE A swinging lifestyle involving recreational activities, friend selection, business, and social components.

SWINGING MARRIAGE A marriage that incorporates/allows swinging.

SWM Acronym for Single White Male.

THREESOME Three individuals (two of the same sex and one of the opposite sex) are swinging (see MENAGE A TROIS).

TICKET Males utilize this person (typically a woman) to gain entrance into swing parties/events.

TOYS Aids or items used during sexual activity (see MARITAL AIDS).

TRANSGENDER Individuals who do not identify with birth-assigned gender. This is unrelated to the individual's sexual orientation.

TRANSSEXUAL   A person who has undergone or is undergoing hormonal or surgical conversion from one gender to another.

TRANSVESTITE   An individual who is sexually satisfied by adorning oneself in garments that are typically identifiable to the opposite sex.

TRAVEL   (see CAN TRAVEL).

TRIAD   Three individuals (two of the same sex and one of the opposite sex) in an ongoing intimate relationship. Different from a threesome.

TRIOLISM   The indication of the desire for sexual threesomes. This is different from a TRIAD and is typically used in sexual ads.

TUBAL LIGATION   A procedure (surgical) comprised of the Fallopian tubes being cut and tied to render a female infertile.

UNICORN   A single female, bisexual or straight, willing to engage in sex with a couple. Some people once deemed this as mythical.

UTOPIAN SWINGER   An individual who considers and practices swinging as a lifestyle of self-actualization.

VANILLA   This term usually refers to people who are non-swingers (i.e., "vanilla acquaintances").

VASECTOMY   A procedure (surgical) consisting of the cutting and tying of the vas deferens for the artificial sterilization of a male.

VERSATILE   Also known as Bisexual (see AC/DC).

VIBRATOR   A vibrating electronic device used for sexual stimulation of oneself or another.

VOLUPTUOUS   This term is typically used to describe the form or frame of a well-formed or full-figured woman.

VOYEUR   An individual who achieves enjoyment watching others engage in sexual activity.

VOYEURISM   Sexual satisfaction gained by watching others participate in sexual acts.

WATERSPORTS   Usually related to urine play (see GOLDEN SHOWER).

WAY-OUTS/WEIRDOS   Individuals interested in sexual activities that are viewed as odd, kinky, or widely unfamiliar.

Index

Note: *Italicized* page numbers refer to figures and those in **bold** refer to tables.